Blind Vision

Blind Vision

The Neuroscience of Visual Impairment

Zaira Cattaneo and Tomaso Vecchi

The MIT Press
Cambridge, Massachusetts
London, England

This book was set in Stone Sans and Stone Serif by Toppan Best-set Premedia Limited.

Library of Congress Cataloging-in-Publication Data

Cattaneo, Zaira, 1979–.
Blind vision : the neuroscience of visual impairment / Zaira Cattaneo and Tomaso Vecchi.
p. ; cm.
Includes bibliographical references and index.
ISBN 978-0-262-01503-5 (hardcover : alk. paper)
ISBN 978-0-262-54988-2 (paperback)
1. Blindness—Pathophysiology. 2. Vision disorders—Pathophysiology. 3. Cognitive neuroscience. I. Vecchi, Tomaso, 1966–. II. Title.
[DNLM: 1. Blindness—physiopathology. 2. Blindness—psychology. 3. Cognitive Science—methods. 4. Perception—physiology. 5. Visually Impaired Persons—psychology. WW 276 C368b 2011]
RE91.C38 2011
617.7'12—dc22

2010018807

Contents

Acknowledgments vii
Prologue ix

1 Introduction 1

2 Blindness and Sensory Compensation 11

3 The Relationship between Visual Perception, Imagery, and Cognitive Functions 49

4 Imagery and Working Memory Processes in the Blind 75

5 Spatial Cognition in the Blind 113

6 Low Vision 137

7 The Importance of Blindness-Onset 155

8 Cortical Plasticity and Blindness 173

Conclusions 203

References 207
Index 265

Acknowledgments

This book wouldn't have been possible without the precious help of our friends and colleagues at the University of Pavia and Milano-Bicocca as well as in Boston (MA), Rochester (NY), and Utrecht (NL), where the authors had the opportunity to work in a warm and stimulating atmosphere. We are grateful to our colleagues from the University of Padova and Pisa who, since 2002, have been part of a research network on cognition and blindness together with the University of Pavia. This work has been partially supported by our departments and by the Italian Ministries for Research and for Foreign Affairs, the Fondazione Cariplo, and the Fondazione Banca del Monte di Pavia. A special thanks goes to all the blind and visually impaired individuals who participated in our studies, and to the Italian Blindness Union for its important collaboration. And finally, thanks to our partners Mario and Luisa for their support and encouragement to take the brief "sabbaticals" that were necessary to plan, discuss, and write this book.

Prologue

We have become convinced—by writing this book—that "blindness" for normally sighted individuals is somehow an incommensurable concept. We lack the words to describe it. In fact, as sighted individuals, we are used to define a blind person as someone that "cannot" see. In other words, we just describe blind individuals' experience borrowing from our lexicon of sighted subjects. But this probably doesn't make much sense to a congenitally blind person. In fact, we can have an idea of the limits of our sensory capacity—for instance, we know that our dog can discriminate ultrasounds whereas we cannot—but not of a sensory channel that we have never had. Accordingly, we have tried to make an effort in this book to convey the idea that blindness is not "less." In fact, blindness is "*alter*."

This book concerns research on imagery, spatial cognition and compensatory mechanisms at the sensorial, cognitive and cortical levels in individuals affected by a complete or profound visual deficit. Our aim is to offer a comprehensive view of the most recent and critical experimental findings rather than to focus on models or theories. We like to think of the different topics addressed in this book as puzzle pieces: although putting ideas together may require some effort, our expectation is that at the end a clear picture will emerge.

1 Introduction

I don't think we did go blind, I think we are blind, Blind but seeing, Blind people who can see, but do not see.
—Jose Saramago, *Blindness*

1.1 Blind Vision, a Paradox?

Can a blind person see? It may seem strange to ask such question at all. "Blind vision" indeed sounds like an awkward if not impossible binomium. But this is because we are used to thinking about vision strictly in terms of "seeing with the eyes." In fact, "to see" does not only require functioning eyes and optic nerves (peripheral structures), but also functioning brain structures. Peripheral (ocular) blindness only affects part of the circuit subtending vision: although blind individuals lack the visual input, their "central hardware" is spared. In this perspective, it appears less paradoxical to question whether the brain of a blind person can see, at least when we conceive of "seeing" as the ability to generate internal mental representations that may contain visual details. We don't pretend that this position is original—Plato had already used the same word, *idein,* to designate the act of looking and that of having an idea—still, we like to stress the logical possibility of "vision" in the blind, as far as this is regarded as an *imagery* process. And with this further open possibility (still to be verified): that crossmodal recruitment phenomena or brain stimulation may also induce some visual *qualia* in the blind.

A typical exercise that is proposed to explain how imagery works is to close the eyes and think about something familiar, such as a close friend, the kitchen table, a landscape we have admired. It's often impressive how vividly we can visualize these things in our mind, either when we imagine them or when we dream. "Have you ever had a dream, Neo, that you were so sure it was real?" asks Morpheus in *The Matrix*: "What if you were unable to wake up from that dream, Neo? How would you know the difference between the dream world and the real world?" Indeed mental images share many characteristics with their original visual percept. Nonetheless, we can also easily create a mental image of something that we have never seen: for instance, when a friend describes her/his new sofa and we can clearly "visualize" it in our mind. Without a doubt, our imagery processes are mainly visually shaped, and this because we normally rely on visual input in perceiving the world.

This, nevertheless, does not imply that a blind person cannot experience vivid mental representations of a friend's new sofa or of his/her own kitchen table. Touch and hearing can provide sufficient information for a blind person to generate a reliable internal representation of the external world. In fact, we can extract the shape of an object by touching it as well as by seeing it, we can identify and localize a person that is speaking through hearing his/her voice as well as through vision, and olfactory information also offers important details about objects (and people) and about where they are in space. Indeed, there are regions of the brain that, even when there is no sensorial deficit, process information regardless of its original sensorial source and respond to a specific object when this is either seen or touched (Pietrini, Furey et al. 2004). In this regard, mental representations do not "strictly" need vision, but may be generated through information acquired in other sensory modalities or by accessing semantic information stored in long-term memory. Notably, visual characteristics are also part of the semantic knowledge of a blind person: in other words, the congenitally blind know perfectly well that a banana is usually yellow, although they have never experienced this "yellow," and although the "pregnancy" of colors as a semantic category may be different in the blind compared to the sighted (see Connolly, Gleitman, and Thompson-Schill 2007). Hence, there are no *a priori* reasons to argue that a blind person cannot generate internal mental representations of the surrounding environment using tactile, proprioceptive, auditory and olfactory information, and relying on conceptual semantic knowledge.

Of course, one may object that blind individuals' mental representations are not comparable to those of the sighted so that, for instance, while sighted persons can picture in their mind a square in the form of a simultaneous image, a blind person can only represent it in the form of a "motor" trace, reflecting the successive movements associated with the tactile exploration of a square object. We disagree with this view. In fact, as we will argument throughout this book, we think that shapes and space are represented in an analog format in the blind (e.g., a line appears as a line, and not as a tactile memory trace), though with some intrinsic differences that derive from their dominant sensorial experience.

This book is about the effects that blindness and, more generally, different types of visual deficit exert on the development and functioning of the human cognitive system. There are a number of critical questions that can be addressed through the investigation of the nature of mental representations in congenitally and late visually impaired individuals. First of all, data can shed light on the relationship between visual perception, imagery, and working memory, clarifying the extent to which mental imagery (and more generally, the development of the cognitive system) depends upon normally functioning vision. Studying intersensory mechanisms in the blind may also help disentangle the functional and neural relationships between vision and the other senses, and may clarify whether and how "supramodal" mechanisms are affected by the absence of one sensory modality: Is vision necessary for the development of supramodal representations of objects (and space) and for normal intersensory interactions? Furthermore, studying both the totally blind and severely (but not totally) visually impaired individuals helps to shed light on which specific aspects of visual experience (e.g., binocularity, visual acuity, visual field) are critical for a correct cognitive development and/or for specific cognitive mechanisms. As we will discuss in the book, many variables—apart from the type, severity and etiology of visual deficit—may influence cognitive development and performance, such as the onset-time of the sensorial deprivation (congenital, early or late), the duration of the visual deficit, and other factors such as personal expertise and motivation. Finally, studying the blind offers the opportunity of knowing more about an extraordinary capacity of the brain: *plasticity*. In fact, the way the brain develops is mediated by everyday experience, and although this holds true especially in the first years of life, in adulthood brain structures still remain susceptible to experience-dependent changes: accordingly, portions of the brain that are not used due to the absence of the relevant percept—such as the visual cortex in blind or the auditory cortex in deaf individuals—may be reorganized to support other perceptual or cognitive functions. Moreover, in the absence of vision, the other senses work as functional substitutes and thus are often improved (i.e., sensory compensation), allowing blind individuals to interface with the external world and to cope with their everyday activities.

Our brain, indeed, doesn't need our eyes to "see": how this happens in blind and sighted individuals is the topic of this book.

1.2 The Tyranny of the Visual

Our culture is undoubtedly shaped by the visual: TV, computer interfaces, print images, written text, visual arts, photography, architecture, design—all of these are basic means we rely upon to acquire relevant information about what happens around us (Arlen 2000). Of course, most of our cultural experience of media is a hybrid of text, images and sounds, but still the visual format certainly plays the greatest role. This has not always been the case though: in a famous essay on this topic, "The Gutenberg Galaxy: The Making of Typographic Man," Marshall McLuhan (1962) analyzed the effects of mass media, especially the printing press, on European culture and human consciousness and argued that the invention of movable type was the decisive moment in the change from a culture in which all the senses played an important role in conveying cultural meanings, to a "tyranny" of the visual. Nowadays, although the Gutenberg era has come to an end and given way to the *electronic era* (in McLuhan's words), the tyranny of the visual is still obvious. However, a certain visual "prepotency" is not just culturally derived but likely has deeper biological bases, as suggested by the fact that it has also been observed in other species such as rats, cows and pigeons (Shapiro, Jacobs, and LoLordo 1980; Kraemer and Roberts 1985; Uetake and Kudo 1994). In fact, the majority of biologically important information is received visually.

But why is vision so important in our life? The answer is quite pragmatic: because the visual is "easy." In other words, when processing the stimuli coming from different sensory channels, individuals rely on the modality that is the most precise or accurate for a given task they are engaged in or preparing for (Welch and Warren 1980; Ernst and Bulthoff 2004). Now, imagine the situation of having to cross the street: normally you look left and right to see whether a car is coming. Actually, you could also look straight ahead and just pay attention to the sound of cars coming from one side or the other, but you never trust your hearing so much; what you always do is to turn your head and—only after having *seen* no car approaching—cross the street. Indeed, with a single gaze we can simultaneously embrace an enormous amount of information, and our foveal acuity allows us to focus on very detailed characteristics of what we are perceiving. Moreover, vision allows us to calibrate and coordinate movements in space, such as locomotion and hand gestures (just try to walk straight ahead or put a fork in your mouth while keeping your eyes closed. . .). Hence, thanks to the fact that of all the senses it has the greatest spatial resolution, vision is usually the primary sensory modality in spatial cognition and object identification (Rock and Victor 1964; Pick, Warren, and Hay 1969; Posner, Nissen, and Klein 1976; Power 1981; Heller 1992; Thinus-Blanc and Gaunet 1997; Eimer 2004), and is likely to offer a sort of "default" reference frame for multisensory and sensorimotor integration (Putzar, Goerendt et al. 2007). Interestingly, visual dominance may also derive from an original "weakness" of the visual system: in particular, Posner et al. (Posner, Nissen, and Klein 1976) hypothesized that humans have a strong tendency to actively (i.e., endogenously) attend to visual events in order to compensate for the poor alerting properties of the visual system (in comparison with the auditory or tactile systems; see also Spence, Nicholls, and Driver 2001; Spence, Shore, and Klein 2001). Accordingly, both animals and humans have been found to "switch" their attention more toward the auditory modality under conditions of high arousal in order to react more rapidly to potential threats (Foree and LoLordo 1973; Shapiro, Jacobs, and LoLordo 1980).

One of the most paradigmatic examples of visual dominance, or *prepotency*, has been described by Colavita (1974) (for early reviews, see Posner, Nissen, and Ogden 1978; and Welch, DuttonHurt, and Warren 1986). In Colavita's study, participants were asked to press one button whenever they heard a tone, and another button whenever they saw a light. In the majority of trials, only one stimulus (a tone or a light) was presented unpredictably, and participants responded both rapidly and accurately. However, a few trials interspersed throughout the experiment were bimodal, consisting of the simultaneous presentation of a tone and a light. Strikingly, in these bimodal trials, participants almost never responded to the sound and a number of subjects reported not to have even heard the auditory stimulus in that condition. Interestingly, participants typically responded more rapidly to the auditory targets than to the visual ones when these were presented in separate blocks of experimental trials. Another typical example of visual dominance is the "ventriloquist effect" for which the ventriloquist voice is mislocated toward the doll (see Bertelson 1999). Similarly, kinesthetic perception may also be misplaced toward simultaneously presented visual cues that appear elsewhere (Pavani, Spence, and Driver 2000).

The evidence discussed above suggests that the absence of vision must profoundly impact the perceptual experience of a blind person, affecting the ways in which their other senses interact and shaping their cognitive development. The next chapters will discuss whether this is the case.

1.3 Overview of the Book's Contents

There were several possible ways in which to organize the contents of this book, and we changed the chapter order several times before deciding to present it as it now stands. In fact, after weighing the costs and benefits of various orders, we decided that the best way to start a book like this was to begin with the "origin." And the origin, in our view, is our senses.

If vision is lost in the blind, then audition, touch and olfaction are still functioning and they represent the channels through which a blind person gets to know about the world. It is commonly believed that—on average—blind individuals possess a special talent for music, that they can discern voices more accurately than sighted people, and that their sense of touch and their olfactory capacities are improved (as in *Scent of a Woman*, where Al Pacino plays a late blind man who is surprisingly knowledgeable about women's perfumes). Beyond such common folk-beliefs, there is indeed experimental evidence that—where vision is lost or has never been present—other senses, and in particular touch and hearing, may gain acuity. Chapter 2 will offer a review of studies that have investigated sensory compensation phenomena in blind individuals, also discussing the implication that sensory changes play at a higher cognitive level. Moreover, the effect of blindness on intersensory interactions is considered: in fact, it has been hypothesized that visual inputs act as the driving force for setting up a common external reference frame for multisensory integration and action control (Putzar, Goerendt et al. 2007; Röder, Kusmierek et al. 2007). In this perspective, the lack of vision affects not only the way each of the other senses develops, but also the way in which multisensory information is treated.

Chapter 3 represents an "exception" in the structure of the book in that it doesn't directly deal with blindness. Rather, this chapter offers an overview of what has to be meant when speaking of "mental imagery" and "working memory," and provides a theoretical framework (and a basic lexicon) for understanding how imagery processes are possible in the blind and why they are so important for cognition. It will be clarified that mental images—whether essential or epiphenomenal (see the "imagery debate")—are of critical importance in domains such as memory, reasoning and creative problem solving. Moreover, behavioral and neuroimaging findings will be discussed, showing that although imagery can be viewed as a "quasi-pictorial" form or representation, analogous to perceptual experience, mental images are the result of complex processes which are similar (but not identical) to perception and in which long-term memory also plays a critical role.

Chapter 4 explores the functional characteristics and properties of mental images in blind individuals. It will be stressed how congenital/early blindness does not prevent the capacity to generate mental representations in an "analog" format, although these conditions are associated to specific limitations, mainly due to the characteristics of blind individuals' dominant perceptual experience. In fact, haptic and auditory experiences are necessarily *sequential*: the actual surface that can be simultaneously touched by our hands is limited (and fine discrimination only pertains to the fingers' tips), and even if we can perceive many auditory inputs at the same time, in this situation our auditory discrimination is poor and we often need to rely on short-term memory to "reconstruct" what we have heard. Conversely, vision generally allows parallel processing of multiple distinct inputs as well as their integration into a unique, meaningful representation, maintaining a high discrimination power. This different way of acquiring information plays a critical role in determining the performance of blind and sighted individuals in tasks which tap in on mental representation capacities. The analysis of similarities and differences between sighted and blind individuals' performance also extends our understanding of functional "supramodal" mechanisms within the human brain, which are capable of processing information regardless of its sensorial format.

Many researchers agree that spatial features play a major role in the generation of mental representations, providing a general "schema" that can then be fitted with other sensorial details. In fact, spatial mental representations are extremely important in everyday life, allowing individuals to orient in their environment, localize objects in order to interact with them, and so on. Not surprisingly, due to its greater spatial resolution, vision is usually the dominant sensory modality in spatial cognition. Chapter 5 describes how blind individuals represent peripersonal/near and extrapersonal/far space. Findings will be reported showing how the blind tend to rely on an egocentric/body-centered reference frame when representing objects in space and to generate "route-like"/sequential mental representations in navigation, whereas sighted individuals are able to generate allocentric mental representations (in which objects' locations are represented regardless of the observer's position) and to create "survey-like" representations of the navigational space. The importance of proper mobility and orientation training and of external devices (e.g., the voice system, auditory spatial displays) to support spatial cognition in the visually impaired will also be considered.

Research with completely blind subjects offers an "all-or-nothing" perspective on the impact of visual deprivation on cognitive abilities. Conversely, investigating whether and how different degrees of visual impairment differentially interact with cognitive processes sheds light on the *specific* aspects of the visual experience (i.e., visual acuity, visual field) that are critical in shaping cognitive mechanisms. Chapter 6 considers the case of "low-vision" individuals who suffer from a severe but not total visual deficit due to different pathologies (amblyopia, glaucoma, macular degeneration, retinitis pygmentosa, etc.). Findings will be reported showing how even a partial loss of sight can induce compensatory sensory phenomena and cortical plasticity changes and can affect cognitive processes. The particular case of individuals affected by monocular blindness will also be considered so as to explore the specific role of binocularity in modulating higher-level processes.

Research into the effect of blindness on cognitive abilities is usually carried out with individuals suffering from a congenital (or early) pathology. This reduces the effect of individual differences and allows researchers to evaluate the effects of functional and cortical plasticity in a homogeneous sample. However, the case of late blindness deserves specific attention because—by forcing a change in pre-existing normal strategies—it sheds light on whether and how the brain can reorganize its networks to deal with the new sensory experience. Overall, in chapter 7 we will see how having benefited from years of normal prior visual experience can result in certain advantages for the late blind over congenitally blind individuals in different cognitive tasks; at the same time, however, compensatory mechanisms are likely to be less robust in the case of a late onset than in congenital/early blindness. In fact, in evaluating the perceptual and cognitive skills of late blind individuals, the role of onset-age and duration of the visual deficit need to be considered. The case of late blindness deserves our attention especially in light of an increasing aging population in the developed world, for which rehabilitation and ad hoc training programs should be made available.

Finally, chapter 8 offers a summary of the most relevant findings on intramodal and crossmodal cortical plasticity phenomena occurring in case of blindness. Data from neuroimaging studies (based on functional magnetic resonance: fMRI, and positron emission tomography: PET), event-related potentials (ERPs) and transcranial magnetic stimulation (TMS) will be discussed. Notably, besides intramodal and crossmodal reorganization, the brain of blind individuals maintains a similar organization to that of sighted subjects in many respects, as is shown by the organization of the ventral ("what") and the dorsal ("where") streams. This supports the view that many areas of the human brain are "supramodal," i.e., they can elaborate information regardless its original sensory format.

1.4 Out of the Gutenberg Galaxy: Estimates and Definition of Visual Impairment

As we have summarized above, this book is more about the implications that blindness and visual impairment have at the cognitive and cortical levels than about optometric and ophthalmologic aspects of these conditions. Nevertheless, in order to better interpret the studies that we will review, it is important to get an idea of what we refer to when using the terms "blindness" and "visual impairment."

Indeed, "blindness" and "visual impairment" are very broad categories and different scales are used across countries to classify the extent of a visual deficit, making it difficult to precisely estimate the number of visually impaired individuals. In 2002, the World Health Organization (WHO) estimated that the number of visually impaired people worldwide was around 161 million, including 37 million individuals affected by blindness (Resnikoff, Pascolini et al. 2004). More recent estimations suggest that some 259 million people worldwide are affected by visual impairment: 42 million individuals with blindness and 217 million with less severe visual impairments (Dandona and Dandona 2006). However, when also considering individuals who are affected by low vision from uncorrected refractive errors, the number is even larger: in the vicinity of 314 million (Resnikoff, Pascolini et al. 2008).

Classification criteria for blindness and other forms of visual impairment are mainly based on measures of visual acuity and visual field. Visual acuity measures the sharpness of an individual's sight and is expressed as a fraction: the numerator indicates the maximum distance (in meters or feet) at which a person can stand and discriminate between two given objects, whereas the denominator refers to the usual distance at which a person with no visual deficits could discriminate between the same objects. Visual field refers to the total area in which a standardized test target can be detected in the peripheral vision while the eye is focused on a central point. Humans' normal visual field extends to approximately 60 degrees nasally (toward the nose, or inward) in each eye, to 100 degrees temporally (away from the nose, or outward), and approximately 60 degrees above and 75 below the horizontal meridian. The range of visual abilities is not uniform across our field of view: for example, binocular vision only covers 140 degrees of the field of vision in humans; the remaining peripheral 40 degrees have no binocular vision (due to no overlapping in the images from either eye for those parts of the field of view). Moreover, there is a concentration of color-sensitive cone cells in the fovea, the central region of the retina, in contrast to a concentration of motion-sensitive rod cells in the periphery.

According to the tenth revision of the International Classification of Diseases (ICD), blindness is defined as a best-corrected visual acuity less than 3/60 (meters), or corresponding visual field loss to less than 10 degrees in the better eye with the best possible correction, whereas low-vision (visual impairment less severe than blindness) is defined as best-corrected visual acuity less than 6/18 but equal or better than 3/60, or corresponding visual field loss to less than 20 degrees in the better eye with the best possible correction (World Health Organization 2007, http://www.who.int/classifications/icd/en/). If low vision is often characterized by low visual acuity and by a reduced visual field, other common types of visual deficit may affect contrast sensitivity and color vision, or result from an imbalance between the two eyes. *Contrast sensitivity* refers to an individual's ability to see low-contrast targets over an extended range of target sizes and orientations. In other words, contrast sensitivity is the visual ability to see objects that may not be outlined clearly or that do not stand out from their background; the higher the contrast sensitivity, the lower the contrast level at which an object can be seen. Many individuals—for instance cataract patients or individuals affected by diabetic retinopathy—may have good visual acuity, but still notice a loss of their visual capability. In all these cases, contrast sensitivity testing can provide a "real world" measurement of a patient's functional vision. *Color blindness* refers to the inability to perceive differences between some of the colors that normally sighted individuals can distinguish. Color blindness can be either acquired—due to eye, nerve or brain damage or exposure to certain chemicals—or more commonly, is congenital; it can be total or partial, and can take different forms (e.g., monochromacy, dichromacy, anomalous trichromacy). Another particular form of visual impairment consists of an imbalance between the two eyes that—in extreme cases—can result in partial or complete blindness in one eye. The most common cause of monocular blindness is *amblyopia* (from the Greek, *amblyos* = blunt; *opia* = vision), which affects 2–4 percent of the population (Ciuffreda 1991), and might derive from several conditions that degrade or unbalance vision prior to adolescence, including strabismus, image degradation (due to different causes, such as astigmatism and anisometropia) or form deprivation (for instance, congenital cataract and ptosis, i.e., drooping of one eyelid) (Doshi and Rodriguez 2007). In amblyopia, the brain favors one eye over the other: the less-favored eye is not adequately stimulated and the visual brain cells do not mature normally. In fact, although ocular examination and initial retinal function appear normal in amblyopia, processing abnormalities have been reported in the retina and primary visual cortex (for recent reviews, see Li, Klein, and Levi 2008). The severity of amblyopia depends on the degree of imbalance between the two eyes (e.g., dense unilateral cataract results in severe loss), and the age at which the amblyogenic factor occurs (cf. McKee, Levi, and Movshon 2003; Li, Klein, and Levi 2008). Nowadays, amblyopia is often successfully treated by patching the unaffected eye in infants and children, but has long been widely considered to be untreatable in adults (e.g., Mintz-Hittner and Fernandez 2000).

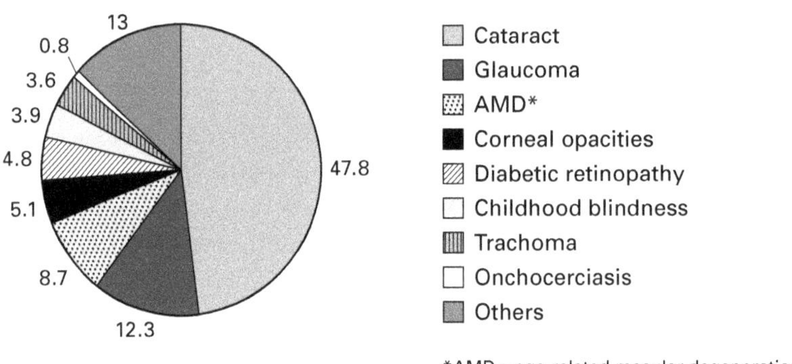

Figure 1.1

Global causes of blindness as a percentage of total blindness in 2002. Reprinted with permission from Resnikoff, Pascolini et al., "Global data on visual impairment in the year 2002," *Bulletin of the World Health Organization* 82 (11) (2004): 844–851.

The incidence of visual impairment in the population is not homogeneous throughout the world, following both socioeconomic factors and individual differences. Approximately 87 percent of visually impaired people live in developing countries, and females have a significantly higher risk of being visually impaired than males, in every region of the world and regardless of age. Overall, the most frequent causes of blindness are cataract (a clouding of the lens of the eye that impedes the passage of light), uncorrected refractive errors (near-sightedness, far-sightedness or astigmatism), glaucoma (a group of diseases that result in damage of the optic nerve), and age-related macular degeneration (which involves the loss of a person's central field of vision) (see figure 1.1). Other major causes include corneal opacities (eye diseases that scar the cornea), diabetic retinopathy (associated with diabetes), blinding trachoma, and eye conditions in children such as cataract, retinopathy of prematurity (an eye disorder of premature infants), and vitamin A deficiency.

2 Blindness and Sensory Compensation

Do you hear? The rain is falling
On the solitary
Greenness
With a crackling that persists
And varies in the air
According to the foliage
Sparser, less sparse.
Listen. The weeping is answered
By the song
Of the cicadas
Which are not frightened
By the weeping of the south wind
Or the ashen sky.
And the pine tree
Has one sound, and the myrtle
Another sound, and the juniper
Yet another, instruments
Different
Under numberless fingers.
—Gabriele d'Annunzio, *Rain in the Pine Wood*

2.1 Sensory Compensation

As humans, we can rely on different sensorial channels to experience the world: our several senses offer convergent but also *complementary* information about the external environment (Millar 1994). For instance, the position of an object in space can be perceived by touch, sight and audition (though using different spatial reference frames). It is commonly believed that when one sensory modality is lacking, the remaining senses improve to cope with this sensorial deficit. In fact, as pointed out by Röder and Rösler (2004), in investigating blind individuals' behavior in the remaining sensory modalities, three scenarios are theoretically possible: (1) if vision is necessary for the normal development and efficient use of the other sensory modalities, then blind individuals should also be impaired in the auditory and tactile domains; (2) if the different sensory modalities develop independently from each other, then no substantial differences in other sensory modalities should be observed between blind and sighted participants; and (3) if the remaining senses significantly improve to cope with the visual deficit leading to a "hypercompensation," then superior performances in the blind should be reported.

Indeed, many studies seem to suggest that auditory and tactile acuity might be enhanced in blind individuals, although experimental findings are not always consistent on the extent and significance of this "sensory compensation" (for recent reviews, see Röder and Rösler 2004; Théoret, Merabet, and Pascual-Leone 2004; Collignon, Voss et al. 2009). As we will often see in this book, contradictory findings may depend on the specific sample of participants tested (age at test, etiology of the visual deficit, degree of visual deficit, duration and onset-age of blindness, individual mobility abilities, specific abilities such as Braille reading, musical abilities, etc.) and on the specific task used (cf. Thinus-Blanc and Gaunet 1997). Moreover, sensory compensation phenomena observed at the behavioral level may depend on both cortical plasticity phenomena and/or changes in processing strategies: as noted by Röder and Rösler (2004), disentangling the behavioral consequences of these two variables is almost impossible since, on one hand, the use of different processing strategies likely causes a shift in the extent to which a particular sense is used, thus inducing a use-dependent cerebral reorganization; and, on the other hand, cortical reorganization may itself influence behavioral strategies.

In the following paragraphs we will review some of the latest and/or most critical findings on blindness-related compensatory phenomena occurring in non-visual sensory domains at different stages of information processing, specifically considering peripheral (sensory) and attentional mechanisms. Nonetheless, we will begin by offering a synthetic view on how the auditory and the tactile systems work in normal conditions in order to better understand possible functional changes occurring in these modalities as a consequence of blindness. Cortical plasticity phenomena accompanying these behavioral changes will be covered in chapter 8.

2.2 Hearing

Hearing is one of our most important senses. In everyday life, we unconsciously sort out meaningful sounds from background noise, we localize the source of sounds and we are able to (automatically) react to unexpected sounds. When a sound is produced, molecules of air are forced to move back and forth by a vibratory source at different frequencies, generating waves of compressions and refractions (Roeser, Valente, and

Hosford-Dunn 2000). The *frequency* of a sound refers to the number of oscillations or cycles produced by a vibrator in a given time: the frequency of audible sounds is measured in Hertz (Hz, i.e., cycles per second), and the human audible normal range is comprised between 20 and 20,000 Hz (although we are most sensitive to frequencies in a range comprised between 500 and 4,000 Hz). The *intensity* of a sound determines its *loudness* and reflects how tightly packed the molecules of air become during the compression phase of a sound wave; in other words, intensity refers to the amount of energy passing through a unit area normal to the direction of the radiated sound per unit of time and it is a vector quantity, having a magnitude and a direction. The greater the amount of displacement, the more intense the sound. Intensity is measured in decibels (dB), where a dB is a *relative* unit of measurement defined as the logarithmic ratio between two magnitudes of pressure or power. If the loudness of a sound is the psychological counterpart of its physical intensity, the *pitch* is the perceptual equivalent of frequency. Frequency and pitch are related in that as the frequency of a sound increases, an individual perceives a tone of a higher and higher pitch; nonetheless, the function describing the relation between frequency and pitch is not linear. The term *absolute pitch* refers to the capacity some individuals have to identify the pitch of a musical tone without an external reference pitch. Complex sounds are mixtures of pure tones and can be either harmonically related, thus having a pitch, or randomly related, resulting in noise. A sound *spectrum* is a representation of a sound in terms of the amount of vibration at each individual frequency. It is usually represented as a graph of intensity as a function of frequency. All natural auditory signals are spectrally and temporally complex, that is, they contain multiple frequencies and their frequencies composition, or spectrum, varies over time.

An important aspect of how the auditory system processes acoustic information is related to the ability to discriminate changes and/or differences in intensity and frequency. Individual threshold for intensity changes can be evaluated by measuring the smallest intensity difference required for a listener to judge which of two sounds is more intense or the minimum intensity increment that can be detected when added to a continuous sound. Similarly, different methods exist to measure frequency discrimination (decide which of two sounds is higher or lower in frequency, detect a small and transient change in the frequency of a continuous tone, etc.).

Another critical aspect of the auditory experience is *sound localization*. The source of a sound can be located in the three spatial dimensions as a function of the auditory system's ability to process the sound emanating from a source. These dimensions are azimuth, elevation and range. The azimuth refers to the direction of the sound source from the listener on the horizontal plane; it is expressed as angular degrees on a circle whereby 0 degrees is directly in front of the listener, and 180 degrees is directly behind him. Elevation refers to the vertical or up/down dimension and range refers to the distance or near/far dimension. We are able to determine the location of a sound by computing differences in the shape, timing and intensity of the waveforms that reach each ear. The path of a sound is influenced by the distance to the ears and by obstacles like the head (the so-called *head shadow* effect): in fact, because of the head, a sound emitted by a source on the side of a listener reaches one ear before the other (interaural time difference) and is less intense (interaural intensity—or level—difference). The human auditory system is very sensitive to even small interaural time and intensity differences. Beyond these *binaural cues* for sound localization, humans also rely on broadband, *monaural cues* provided by the filtering characteristics of the pinna, part of the external ear. Monaural cues are extremely important in the determination of the elevation and in the resolution of front/back confusions arising from ambiguous interaural time and intensity differences. Specifically, the pinna functions by funneling sound waves from the outside environment into the ear canal. The intricate shape of the pinna affects the frequency response of incoming sounds differently, depending on where the sound source is located. Hence, when a sound is in front of the listener, the spectral representation arriving at the tympanic membrane will be different from that of a sound arriving from behind the listener, even if the interaural cues are the same. Finally, other non-auditory factors including vision (e.g., the *ventriloquism effect* discussed in chapter 1), memory and listener expectations also play a role in sound localization.

The term *echo* refers to the perception of two distinct sounds resulting from the difference in arrival times of sound waves traveling over different paths but coming from a single source. Usually individuals are faced with several waveforms from which they have to infer the location of the sound source. If the direct sound will come from the source, several reflected waveforms—highly correlated with the direct sound source—will come from many other disparate locations, depending on the specific environment (positions of the room's walls in respect to the listener and the sound source, etc.). Depending on the delay with which reflected sounds reach the listener's ear relative to the direct source, the reflected sounds can either be integrated into the direct waveform (for short delays), increasing the sound level of the signal, or interfere with the original direct sound (longer delays), degrading the quality of the original signal. If the reflected sounds arrive quite late relative to the direct sounds, they may be perceived as an echo. According to the so-called *precedence effect*, the waveform that reaches the listener first will be used to identify the sound source, even if later-arriving waveforms may have a higher intensity. Individual *echo threshold* is defined as the time delay below which delayed sounds are not perceived as coming from different locations relative to the original sound.

Humans are also good at discriminating the *temporal order* of sounds, particularly if the sound, when presented in a particular order, is meaningful (e.g., speech) (Roeser, Valente, and Hosford-Dunn 2000). In these situations, humans can discriminate order changes for sounds lasting 7 milliseconds (ms) or shorter (cf. Divenyi and Hirsh 1974).

However, if the sounds are unrelated, longer intervals are needed—from 10 to 20 ms—to reach a comparable level of discrimination accuracy (Hirsch 1959; Warren and Platt 1974).

2.3 Enhanced Auditory Capacities in the Blind?

Intensity and Frequency Sensitivity

Early research comparing congenitally blind and normally sighted individuals didn't show significant differences in elementary auditory sensitivity, such as frequency, loudness perception and hearing threshold (Benedetti and Loeb 1972; Yates, Johnson, and Starz 1972; Starlinger and Niemeyer 1981; Bross and Borenstein 1982). According to Weaver and Stevens (2006), an auditory perceptual enhancement in early blind individuals is likely to be reported in more complex auditory perceptual tasks (for instance, when backward masking is manipulated). In line with this view, blind subjects outperformed sighted controls in discriminating the intensity of a tone presented to one ear in the presence of masking sounds in the other ear (Niemeyer and Starlinger 1981). More recently, Gougoux and colleagues (Gougoux, Lepore et al. 2004) required early blind participants to listen to pairs of pure tones of different frequencies and to decide whether the pitch was rising (second sound with higher pitch) or falling. Early blind individuals performed better than sighted controls in this task, even when the speed of change was ten times faster than that perceived by controls (Gougoux, Lepore et al. 2004). Similarly, Rokem and Ahissar (2009) found an overall lower threshold in a group of early blind subjects in psychoacoustic frequency discrimination tasks of different complexity, in which one tone had to be compared to a reference tone of 1 kilohertz (KHz), and in conditions in which two tones had to be compared with no fixed reference tone available (pitch discrimination).

Importantly, one may argue that enhanced auditory capacities in the blind depend on their usually greater musical experience, rather than to differences related to vision loss per se. This aspect has been considered by Wan and colleagues (Wan, Wood et al. 2010a), who compared auditory perception skills in blind and sighted individuals while controlling for musical training and pitch-naming abilities (absolute pitch). Congenitally blind, early blind, late blind and sighted subjects were tested on three tasks tapping different aspects of auditory processing: pitch discrimination (i.e., decide which of a pair of tones was higher), pitch-timbre categorization (i.e., make judgments on both pitch and timbre) and pitch working memory (i.e., listen to a series of tones and determine whether the first and the last tones were the same). Wan and colleagues (Wan, Wood et al. 2010a) found that blind subjects having a functional vision until late childhood (>= 14 years) performed similarly to the sighted matched subjects in all the tasks. Conversely, both congenitally blind and early blind subjects performed better than their matched group in the pitch discrimination and in the pitch-timbre categorization tasks, whereas no differences between blind and sighted individuals were observed in the working-memory task. These findings seem to suggest that enhancement of auditory acuity related to pitch stimuli in the blind is restricted to basic perceptual skills rather than extending to higher-level processes such as working memory, and that such enhancement does not depend on prior musical experience but is due to vision loss.

Temporal Resolution

Early blindness is likely to be associated with a higher auditory temporal resolution capacity: as in case of elementary sound perception though, the nature of the task seems to play a critical role. Hence, in very basic tasks, differences between sighted and early blind individuals may not be significant: for instance, Weaver and Stevens (2006) found no significant differences between early blind and sighted controls in detecting silent gaps (ranging from 1 to 7 ms) randomly intermixed within constant-duration intervals of sound noise.

On the other side, several studies suggest that blind individuals may be superior in temporal discrimination of meaningful sounds like speech. In fact, there is evidence that blind individuals may be able to understand ultra-fast synthetic speech at a rate of up to about 25 syllables per second, whereas the usual maximum performance level of normal-sighted listeners is around 8–10 syllables per second (see Hertrich, Dietrich et al. 2009). In one of the earlier reports on the topic, Niemeyer and Starlinger (1981) showed better speech discrimination ability in their sample of early blind individuals. In a subsequent study involving a large sample of early blind individuals, Muchnik and colleagues (Muchnik, Efrati et al. 1991) reported that blind individuals performed better than matched sighted controls in sound localization, temporal auditory resolution and discriminating speech material in noise (but notice that Muchnick et al.'s results might not be conclusive given the abnormally higher threshold of their control subjects compared to previous studies; see Stevens and Weaver 2005; Weaver and Stevens 2006). Hertrich and colleagues (Hertrich, Dietrich et al. 2009) in a single-case study have recently analyzed the enhanced speech perception capabilities of a blind listener suggesting that superior auditory skills in the blind may engage distinct regions of the central-visual system; in particular, the left fusiform gyrus and the right primary visual cortex (see chapter 8 for a more extensive discussion on the neural correlates associated with enhanced auditory capacities in the blind population).

In a series of experiments, Röder, Rösler, and Neville (2000) have examined verbal processing enhancement in the blind, reporting more rapid responses in early blind subjects on a semantic judgment task. Nonetheless, the effect is not likely to be placed at a semantic level of the auditory input processing. Since early blind participants were found to respond more rapidly to both words and pseudo-words, their advantage relative to the sighted controls is likely to reflect a more rapid perceptual processing of the stimuli, rather than a semantic level effect (Röder, Demuth et al. 2002). In fact, rapid auditory processing enhancements have also been found in other auditory non semantic studies: for instance, Rokem and Ahissar (2009) measured perceptual threshold in a group of congenitally blind individuals for identifying pseudo-words (the task required to correctly repeat pseudo-words previously heard) either in a quiet background or embedded in a background of speech noise; in both cases congenitally blind individuals showed lower threshold compared to matched sighted controls (see also Liotti, Ryder, and Woldorff 1998). Accordingly, Hugdahl and colleagues (Hugdahl, Ek et al. 2004) reported that blind individuals outperformed sighted controls in correctly reporting a series of syllables presented via headphones in a dichotic listening procedure.

Support to the hypothesis of an enhancement of auditory processing in early blind individuals also comes from electrophysiological evidence. Event-related potentials (ERPs) are voltage fluctuations, derived from the ongoing electroencephalogram (EEG), that are time-locked to specific sensory, motor, attentional or cognitive events. Thanks to their great temporal resolution, ERPs are a particularly useful technique in investigating the processing of auditory information. Focusing attention on a sound source in the environment is indexed by a negative ERP beginning 80–100 ms after the onset of the stimulus (the N1 component: see Röder, Teder-Salejarvi et al. 1999), which is normally greater for sounds in attended than in unattended locations. Early studies using ERPs have found shorter latencies for auditory brain ERPs in blind individuals compared with sighted individuals (Niemeyer and Starlinger 1981; Röder, Rösler et al. 1996). In an ERPs oddball study, congenitally blind subjects were found to have shorter refractory periods of the N1/P2 waveform in response to non-target stimuli that followed another non-target stimulus after various stimulus onset asynchronies (Röder, Rösler, and Neville 1999; Neville and Bavelier 2002): since refractory periods are likely to reflect the time needed to complete sensory processing by the underlying neural population, after which that population can respond to new stimulation, these data further support the view of enhanced temporal auditory processes in the blind (Röder, Rösler, and Neville 1999).

There is also evidence for enhanced *echo processing* and a better use of echo cues for navigation purposes in early blind individuals (e.g., Kellogg 1962; Rice, Feinstein, and Schusterman 1965; Strelow and Brabyn 1982). Importantly, it has been demonstrated that enhanced echo processing does not depend on blind individuals paying more attention to echo cues, as we will later discuss (cf. Dufour, Déspres, and Candas 2005). In fact, more rapid auditory processing may account for many of the perceptual and cognitive enhancements reported in early blindness (Neville and Bavelier 2000).

Sound Localization

Sound localization is the result of a complex perceptual process: in fact, the integration of multiple acoustic cues (e.g., interaural time difference and/or interaural intensity differences) is required to extract the horizontal coordinate of the sound with respect to the head (i.e., sound-source azimuth), whereas the analysis of the complex spectral shape cues provided by the pinna makes it possible to determine the sound position in the vertical plane (elevation) and disambiguate frontal from rear sound sources (cf. Blauert 1997; Roeser, Valente, and Hosford-Dunn 2000). The question of whether and how a total visual deprivation affects sound localization capacities has been largely debated, and two main models have been proposed: the "deficit model" states that auditory space needs visual calibration to properly develop (Axelrod 1959; Zwiers, Van Opstal, and Cruysberg 2001a,b; Lewald 2002a,b); the "compensation model" argues that although vision affects the normal development of spatial hearing abilities, compensation phenomena may occur through multimodal mechanisms (Jones 1975; Ashmead, Wall et al. 1998a; Ashmead, Wall et al. 1998b; Lessard, Paré et al. 1998; Röder, Teder-Salejarvi et al. 1999).

Animal evidence supports both views. On one side, findings with owls, ferrets, guinea pigs, cats and other mammalian species (Knudsen and Knudsen 1985; King, Hutchings et al. 1988; Withington-Wray, Binns, and Keating 1990; Heffner and Heffner 1992; Knudsen and Brainard 1995; Wallace and Stein 2000) suggest that visual feedback plays a critical role in the development of auditory spatial mapping. For instance, blind-reared owls have been found to localize sounds less precisely than normal owls, and—at the neural level—to possess a degraded representation of auditory space in their midbrain optic tectum (cf. Knudsen and Knudsen 1985; Knudsen and Brainard 1995). Also, in guinea pigs, ferrets and cats, the early loss of vision prevents the normal development of auditory spatial maps in the superior colliculus (Withington 1992; King and Carlile 1993). On the other side, early visual deprivation has been found to be accompanied by compensatory plasticity phenomena in the remaining sensory domains: for instance, in cats, early blindness improved certain aspects of sound localization (Rauschecker and Kniepert 1994) and resulted in a sharpened spatial tuning of auditory cortical neurons (Rauschecker 1999). Improved spatial hearing has also been reported in blind-reared ferrets (King and Parsons 1999).

Human studies on whether blindness is accompanied by enhanced auditory spatial localization capacities are also controversial. Sighted newborns are able to orient to sounds even in darkness and before the emergence of any visual orientating capacities (cf. Morrongiello 1994; Röder, Teder-Salejarvi et al. 1999), suggesting that spatial auditory maps can also be generated on the basis of non-visual feedbacks only. Accordingly, Ashmead et al. (Ashmead, Wall et al. 1998b) found that blind children can discriminate changes in sound elevation and sound distance as well as or even better than sighted controls, again suggesting that auditory spatial calibration might rely on changes in sound localization cues arising from self-motion, such as turning the head or walking. In general, whether or not the blind show enhanced auditory spatial skills depends on the specific task used, in terms of how stimuli are presented (e.g., monaural vs. binaural presentation), where they are presented (central vs. peripheral space), and on the overall complexity of the task.

In one of the most critical studies on spatial auditory capacities in the blind, Lessard et al. (Lessard, Paré et al. 1998) required blindfolded normally-sighted and early blind participants (some of whom had residual peripheral vision) to point with their hand to the apparent source of a sound, delivered from one of an array of sixteen loudspeakers. All participants showed a high level of performance in the task, suggesting that a three-dimensional map of space can be generated even in the total absence of visual input (note that the totally blind performed significantly better than the blind with residual vision, see chapter 6 for a larger discussion). In a further experimental condition, sound localization had to be performed monaurally (one ear was blocked with a soft foam earplug and a hearing protector muff): overall, individuals performed worse in this condition compared to the binaural condition, showing a localization bias toward the unobstructed ear. Nonetheless, while the control and residual vision groups demonstrated positional biases by localizing in favor of the unobstructed ear, half of the totally blind subjects localized the sound on the appropriate side, even when it was presented on the side of the obstructed ear. According to Lessard and colleagues (Lessard, Paré et al. 1998), these findings suggest that in monaural conditions, (at least some) blind individuals may have used spatial cues—such as the spectral content of the sound—more efficiently than sighted individuals (a compensation not available to individuals with residual vision). Although quite critical, these findings (Lessard, Paré et al. 1998) are not conclusive: first, it cannot be excluded that blind individuals have made small head movements to localize sounds in the monaural conditions; second, since a constant sound intensity (40 dB) was used throughout the experiment, changes in sound pressure at the ear over trials may have been used by the blind as a cue for location (see Morgan 1999; Zwiers, Van Opstal, and Cruysberg 2001b). Nevertheless, later studies confirmed that enhanced localization performance associated to blindness indeed depends on an improved use of subtle auditory cues, such as the spectral content of the sound. In fact, in a study in which the spectral content of the auditory stimuli and the ability of participants to process it was manipulated—respectively by sound-frequency filtering and by obstructing the pinna—increased localization errors were reported in blind subjects who previously performed well in the monaural task (Doucet, Guillemot et al. 2005).

Notably, better spatial localization in blind individuals seems to be particularly evident in peripheral space. Voss et al. (Voss, Lassonde et al. 2004) required early blind, late blind and sighted control individuals to discriminate the relative positions of two sounds presented in auditory space, either centrally in front of the listener, or in the periphery with stimuli presented 90 degrees from the mid-sagittal plane. Importantly, no difference between the three groups of participants was reported for stimuli presented centrally (probably due to a ceiling effect); however, when stimuli were presented in the periphery, both early and late blind individuals outperformed the sighted. Similar results were obtained in a previous study by Röder and others (Röder, Teder-Salejarvi et al. 1999), requiring participants to identify infrequent deviant sounds emanating from the most peripheral or most central speaker out of an eight-speaker array placed on the horizontal azimuth. Subjects had to ignore sounds coming from all other speakers. Blind and sighted subjects performed equally well at detecting deviant stimuli coming from the central auditory space; however, when asked to detect deviant sounds coming from the most peripheral speaker, blind outperformed sighted subjects, thus demonstrating superior auditory capabilities in far-lateral space. In the same study (Röder, Teder-Salejarvi et al. 1999), ERPs were also recorded that were consistent with the behavioral results: in fact, blind participants showed a steeper N1 gradient compared to the sighted controls for the peripheral but not for the central sounds, indicating a sharper attentional tuning mechanism operating at early spatial attention stages (first 100 ms) in blind individuals. Critically, as noted by Röder and Rösler in their review (Röder and Rösler 2004), these findings parallel those with deaf individuals, who show better visual detection in the peripheral visual field compared to the normally hearing subjects (e.g., Bavelier, Tomann et al. 2000).

It might be argued that differences in compensation for central and peripheral space are only *indirect*, rather reflecting an increase in the level of task difficulty, given that the task is more complex in the periphery than in the central visual field. However, available evidence suggests that when the task complexity increases for sounds to be localized in the central space, the blind do not outperform the sighted. For instance, Zwiers and colleagues (Zwiers, Van Opstal, and Cruysberg 2001b) designed a spatial auditory experiment containing complex hearing conditions in which background noise was added to the target while the stimuli were presented in frontal vertical space (within 50° from the midline). Blind subjects performed similarly to sighted controls when no background noise was present; however, when background noise was added, thus increasing the difficulty of the task and providing a more natural setting, blind subjects showed more difficulties than sighted controls in extracting the elevation-related spectral cues, and performed more poorly. In fact, in peripheral space, visual information becomes degraded and inputs from other sensory systems (tactile and motor feedback or both) may be required for a good spatial localization of the sounds, thus explaining why, in these circumstances, the blind may show superior abilities. However, visual feedback may be critical for accurate localization of sounds in frontal space (especially in complex contexts), given that reliance on vision is predominant in the central field.

Interestingly, visual calibration may play a more important role in *vertical* than in horizontal sound localization (Zwiers, Van Opstal, and Cruysberg 2001b; Lewald 2002b). For instance, Lewald (2002b) found that blind subjects made significantly larger absolute errors compared to the sighted in pointing with their head to sounds coming from different locations in the vertical plane. In fact, in the vertical dimension the primary cues for sound localization are distortions in the spectrum of the incoming sound which are produced by sound diffraction and reflection at the pinna: changes of these spectral cues cannot always be easily and directly related to sound elevation, so that vertical audiomotor cues may be less effective than for horizontal localization.

Overall, the studies reviewed above suggest that vision is not a mandatory prerequisite for the calibration of space and it is likely that this calibration in the blind comes from experiencing changes in sound-localization cues arising from self-motion, such as turning the head or the body, or walking in the environment toward the sound sources (Ashmead, Hill, and Talor 1989; Ashmead, Wall et al. 1998a). Nonetheless, lack of calibration by the visual system may be detrimental in certain situations.

Auditory Egocenter

In order to estimate the relative direction of one object with respect to another, we need to have a reference point. In the visual modality, this reference point is usually indicated with the term "Cyclopean eye" (cf. Hering 1879/1942; Le Conte 1881), and it is located at the center of the interocular axis. The "egocenter" has been found to exist in the kinesthetic and auditory modalities as well. In the kinesthetic modality, the egocenter is generally located at "the individual's front body surface or its near inside" (Shimono, Higashiyama, and Tam 2001). The auditory egocenter has been found to be located proximally to the visual egocenter when the sound source is located in the "frontomedial" field (within +/– 30° from the head's medial plane) and near the midpoint of the interaural axis or the center of horizontal head rotation for sound sources located outside the frontal field (beyond +/– 60° of the head's median plane) (Neelon, Brungart, and Simpson 2004). In a study by Sukemiya and colleagues (Sukemiya, Nakamizo, and Ono 2008), it has been found that the location of the auditory egocenter in congenitally blind individuals is different from that of late blind and normally sighted individuals. In particular, the auditory egocenter of the congenitally blind participants was found to be close to the midpoint of the interaural axis or the center of head rotation. Conversely, in normally sighted and late blind subjects the auditory egocenter was close to the midpoint of the interocular axis of visual egocenter (see figures 2.1 and 2.2).

In another study by Zwiers et al. (Zwiers, Van Opstal, and Cruysberg 2001a) early blind and sighted controls were required to point either with the left arm or with their nose in the direction of a sound of various duration and spectral contents presented within the two-dimensional frontal hemifields. Head-pointing and arm-pointing methods led to similar responses in both groups, indicating that the transformation needed to map the head-centered acoustic input into the appropriate coordinates of either motor systems was equally developed in both blind and sighted subjects.

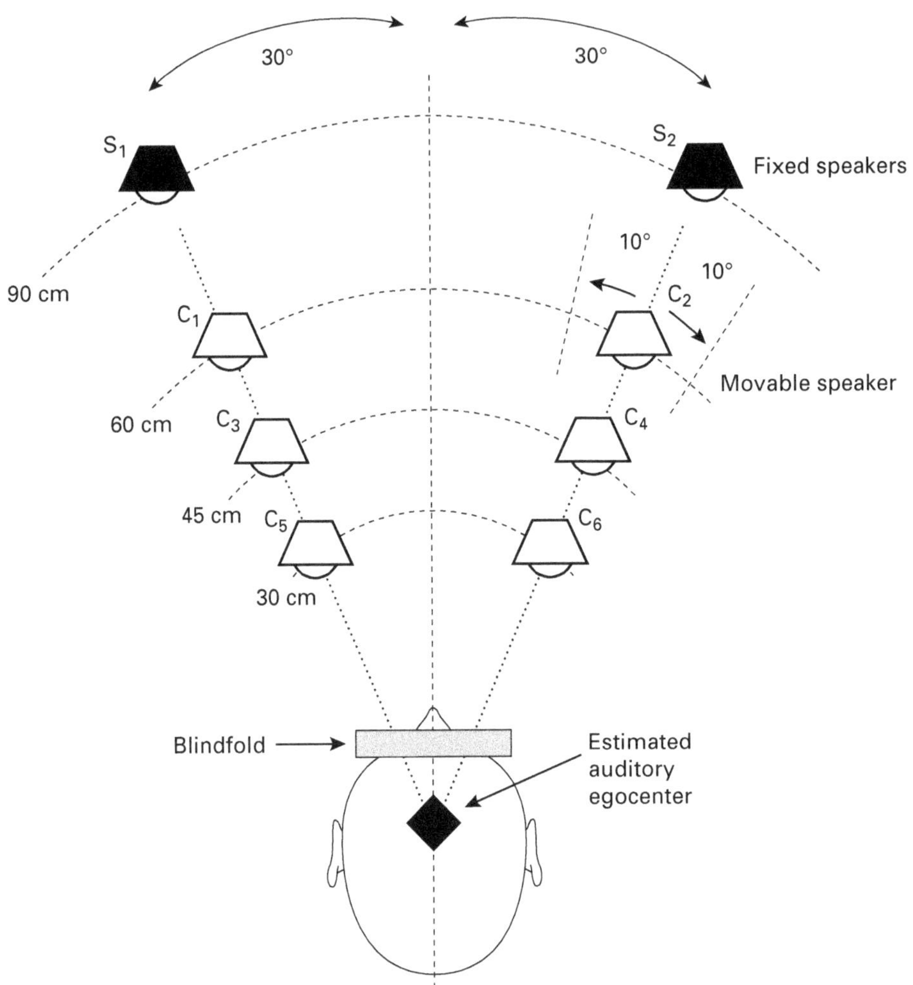

Figure 2.1
Schematic representation of the method used by Sukemiya, Nakamizo, and Ono to estimate the auditory egocenter in a group of congenitally blind, late blind and blindfolded sighted participants. S1 and S2 (solid speakers) were the two stationary loudspeakers, which were located at 30 degrees to the right and to the left of the median plane of the subject's head in a circular arc with a 90 centimeter radius centered on the midpoint of the interocular axis, and used as the standard stimuli. C's (blank speakers) indicate the locations of the movable speakers, and where the comparison sound was presented. The observer judged whether the apparent direction of the sound from one of C1, C3 and C5 (C2, C4 and C6) was right or left of that from S1 (S2). A line was fitted to the mean directions of C's at three distances. The egocenter was defined as the intersection of the two fitted lines.
Reprinted from Sukemiya, Nakamizo, and Ono, "Location of the auditory egocentre in the blind and normally sighted," *Perception* 37(10) (2008): 1587–1595. (Reprinted by permission of Pion Ltd.)

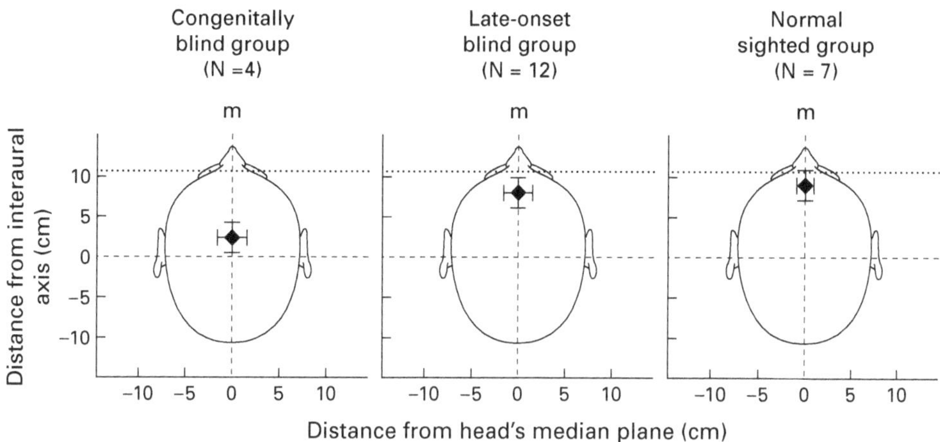

Figure 2.2

This figure reports the estimated locations of the auditory egocenter for the congenitally blind, the late blind and the normally sighted groups in Sukemiya et al.'s study (Sukemiya, Nakamizo, and Ono 2008). The solid black diamonds represent the mean locations of the auditory egocenters. The short horizontal and vertical lines represent the standard deviations for each group. The means (standard deviations) in centimeters calculated from the *x* and *y* coordinate values of the auditory egocenters are reported, for the congenitally blind, late blind and normally sighted groups.

Reprinted from Sukemiya, Nakamizo, and Ono, "Location of the auditory egocentre in the blind and normally sighted," *Perception* 37(10) (2008): 1587–1595. (Reprinted by permission of Pion Ltd.)

However, when pointing with the arm, the origin of pointing was much closer to the cyclopean eye than to their shoulder joint in sighted participants; conversely, for the blind, the pointing origin resulted to be at their shoulder joint. According to this study (Zwiers, Van Opstal, and Cruysberg 2001a), findings suggest that the functional shift in the frame of reference from the arm is mediated by an intact visual system, and thus acquired by learning, rather than being a pre-programmed movements strategy.

Lewald (2002a) investigated blind and sighted individuals' ability to relate body position to auditory spatial information. In fact, when sighted subjects are required to point toward a light spot presented in a dark environment, they usually undershoot stimulus eccentricity by a few degrees, an error probably due to a perceptual shift of spatial coordinates as a function of head position (Lewald, Dörrscheidt, and Ehrenstein 2000): the eyes usually move in the direction of the head rotation when fixating a stimulus to the side, but this deviation in orbital eye position is not completely taken into account when estimating the relationship between trunk, head and target position, thus inducing small errors (Lewald, Dörrscheidt, and Ehrenstein 2000). This error also occurs in sighted individuals when pointing to sounds in a dark environment: the error in this case is "indirect," reflecting visual calibration of auditory inputs. Therefore, this error should not be reported in the blind, who by definition lack calibration by retino-visuomotor inputs. Interestingly, Lewald (2002a) reported opposite systematic errors in blind and sighted individuals when localizing or lateralizing sounds with eccentric head position, although the overall accuracy was almost identical (the opposite systematic error showed by the blind may depend on a residual misadaptation of the transformation of the originally head-centered auditory information into a body-centered frame of reference).

Overall, these findings suggest that the blind differ from the sighted in the perceptual mechanisms that relate the coordinates of auditory space to those of the head and the body.

2.4 Enhanced Auditory Spatial Attention in Blindness?

It is well known that orienting attention both in space (Posner 2004) and in time improves the efficiency of visual, auditory and tactile processing (Ahissar and Hochstein 1993; Correa, Lupianez et al. 2006; Lange and Röder 2006). Therefore, higher performances in many auditory tasks may reflect either more efficient basic perceptual functioning, but also result from improved spatial attention devoted to auditory inputs. In this section, we report studies on auditory attention in blind subjects.

Röder and colleagues (Röder, Krämer, and Lange 2007) have suggested that blind individuals may direct attention more to temporal aspects than to spatial aspects of auditory input. Specifically, the authors hypothesized that given the generally improved temporal skills (both temporal auditory acuity and temporal tactile acuity) of congenitally blind subjects, they may give temporal cues a higher priority than spatial cues for stimulus selection, while the opposite should be observed in sighted individuals. In their task, participants were presented with either short (600 ms) or long (1200 ms) empty intervals which were demarcated by two sounds: the auditory onset marker (S1) appeared centrally, whereas the auditory offset marker (S2) could be presented either on the left or right hemifield. Participants were instructed to attend to the offset marker of one interval (short or long) and one location (left or right). Four possible combinations were thus possible: the offset target could be presented (1) at both attended location and point in time, (2) at both unattended location and point in time, (3) at attended location but unattended point in time, and (4) at unattended location but attended point in time. ERPs were recorded throughout the experiment. According to this hypothesis (Röder, Krämer, and Lange 2007), temporal attention effects precede spatial attention effects in blind individuals.

In line with this expectation, both spatial and temporal attention affected the N1 component in sighted participants, whereas in blind subjects only temporal attention did—supporting the higher priority of reliance on temporal aspects for stimulus selection in the blind.

Other studies have suggested that blind individuals may be better in selectively allocating attention to pre-attended portions of the external space. For instance, Hugdahl, Ek et al. (2004) reported enhanced ability in blind subjects to report correct syllables presented via headphones in a dichotic listening procedure. In non-forced attentional conditions, both blind and sighted individuals tended to report more correct syllables when coming from the right ear, reflecting the dominant role of the left temporal cortex in speech perception (Kimura 1967). However, blind individuals were better in modulating this effect through focusing attention in the forced-left-ear conditions.

As we have already mentioned in this chapter, superior capacities of blind individuals compared to sighted individuals may become significant only in complex situations. In the attentional domain, a complex situation subsists for instance when the task requires a subject to devote attentional resources to many different aspects at the same time (divided attention). In this regard, Kujala and colleagues found faster reaction times in blind compared to sighted individuals during divided-attention tasks, requiring the division of attention to simultaneously process auditory and tactile spatial information (Kujala, Alho et al. 1995; Kujala, Lehtokoski et al. 1997). However, other studies—beyond the previously discussed study by Hugdahl et al. (Hugdahl, Ek et al. 2004)—indicate that blind subjects can be more efficient than sighted subjects also in *selective* attention tasks involving spatial discrimination (Röder, Rösler et al. 1996; Röder, Teder-Salejarvi et al. 1999; Hötting, Rösler, and Röder 2004).

Quite surprisingly, eye movements (as an index of spatial attention) have been recorded during auditory localization in congenitally blind humans (Déspres, Candas, and Dufour 2005a). In fact, in normally sighted individuals eye movements are known to play a critical role in spatial processing of auditory information (Jones and Kabanoff 1975; Rorden and Driver 1999), with planned eye movements acting to elicit sensory processing toward the target of the planned action (Rizzolatti, Riggio et al. 1987). There is evidence that blind subjects can control voluntary eye movements (Hall, Gordon et al. 2000; Hall and Ciuffreda 2002), although ocular saccades precision is likely to decrease with increasing blindness duration (Hall, Gordon et al. 2000), suggesting that prior visual experience is necessary to achieve optimal control of eye movements. Déspres et al. (Déspres, Candas, and Dufour 2005a) found that blind subjects could voluntarily direct their gaze in the horizontal plane, and that this ocular saccade control affects the precision of auditory spatial localization to a similar extent in blind and sighted individuals.

2.5 Changes in Auditory and Verbal Memory and Language Processes

Superior auditory capacities may also affect higher-level processes, such as memory for auditory and verbal information and language processes. Déspres, Candas and Dufour (2005b) investigated self-positioning abilities in different individuals affected by different types of visual deficit (see also chapter 6). Subjects were led blindfolded in a dark anechoic and sound-attenuated room, where they sat at random locations and listened to eight sounds played in a random order from each of eight loudspeakers (two per wall and at subjects' ear-level). Once out of the room, participants were required to reproduce their position in the room. Early blind individuals performed significantly better than late blind and sighted controls in this task. According to Déspres et al. (Déspres, Candas, and Dufour 2005b) a better auditory memory in the blind is likely to have determined this pattern of results. Amedi et al. (Amedi, Raz et al. 2003) found superior verbal memory capacities in the blind, and this was related to activation in the occipital cortex in the blind but not in the sighted subjects (see chapter 8 for a deeper discussion of this study). In a verbal memory task requiring that the subject memorize lists of words (and their serial order), Raz et al. (Raz, Striem et al. 2007) found that blind participants recalled more words than the sighted (indicating better item-memory), and were most notably superior in recalling longer word sequences according to their original order. The superior serial memory of the blind and their higher serial-learning abilities likely depend on blind individuals' experience: in fact, the blind typically adopt serial strategies in order to compensate for the lack of immediate visual information. The results by Raz et al. (Raz, Striem et al. 2007) thus suggest the refinement of a specific cognitive ability to compensate for blindness. Other evidence has indicated superior short-term memory (e.g., digit and word span: Hull and Mason 1995; Röder and Neville 2003) and better long-term memory capacities (e.g., for voices: Bull, Rathborn, and Clifford 1983; Röder, Rösler, and Neville 2001; Röder and Neville 2003) in blind individuals (but see Cobb, Lawrence, and Nelson 1979).

Earlier in this chapter we reported how blind individuals have been found to possess enhanced speech-perception skills (e.g., Muchnik, Efrati et al. 1991; Röder, Rösler, and Neville 2000; Röder, Demuth et al. 2002). Röder and colleagues (Röder, Demuth et al. 2002) have carried out a study to clarify which subsystems (syntactic or semantic) of speech comprehension play a role in determining this rapid understanding of speech in the blind. Röder et al. (Röder, Demuth et al. 2002) used a lexical decision task in which adjectives were presented as primes and nouns or pseudo-words as targets. Some of the target-related words were semantically and syntactically correct; some only semantically, some only syntactically; and some neither semantically nor syntactically. Similar semantic and morphosyntactic priming effects were reported in both groups; nevertheless, overall lexical decision times for the blind subjects were shorter, especially for pseudo-words. According to Röder et al. (Röder, Demuth et al. 2002), these findings contradict both the hypothesis that blind people's semantic concepts are impoverished and the hypothesis previously put forward by Röder et al. (Röder, Rösler, and Neville 2000) that the blind make more use of syntactic context. Rather, the general reaction-time advantage reported in blind individuals in all conditions (even when pseudo-words were used) suggests that perceptual processing aspects, rather than specific language functions, are enhanced in the blind.

2.6 Perceptual, Attentional, and Cognitive Factors in Enhanced Auditory Capacities

A critical aspect to be considered when reviewing studies that report superior auditory abilities in blind individuals is the possible confounding between sensory, attentional and cognitive mechanisms (Collignon, Renier et al. 2006). In other words, the reported superiority of early blind subjects in many auditory spatial attention tasks may depend on the subjects' higher perceptual sensitivity; but vice versa, blind subjects' perceptual advantages may indeed reflect top-down modulation by attentional and cognitive mechanisms (Stevens and Weaver 2005). The same logic holds for tasks involving higher cognitive functions such as language and memory.

In one of the few studies that have specifically addressed this issue, Dufour, Déspres and Candas (2005) measured the extent to which blind and sighted subjects relied on echo-cues processing in an auditory localization task in which subjects' attention was either directed on echo-cues or on other features of the stimuli. Specifically, early blind, late blind and sighted participants had to judge the position of a wooden board on the basis of sounds that were reflected by the board; in a further condition, a task was used that *was not* directly focused on echo-cues, instead requiring that subjects localize a direct sound source. Nonetheless, the role of non-informative echo-cues was manipulated by having subjects positioned either at an equal distance from the lateral walls of the testing room, or closer to one of the two walls, the distance from the two walls being relevant in terms of echo-cues. In this second task, both late and early blind showed a greater localization bias in the direction of the closer wall, indicated enhanced sensitivity to reflected sounds. These results suggest that blind subjects have a lower echo threshold and fuse direct and reflected sounds with shorter delays, when compared to normally sighted individuals. Therefore, echo-cues processing is likely to be really enhanced in case of blindness and does not depend on a higher level of familiarity or on more attentional resources.

Collignon and colleagues (Collignon, Renier et al. 2006) designed an experiment in which they compared the performance of blind and sighted individuals in sensory sensitivity tasks, simple reaction times and selective and divided-attention tasks using individually adjusted auditory and tactile stimuli. By controlling for individuals' sensory sensitivity, the authors could assess attentional performance independently of sensory influence. No differences were reported between the two groups in either sensory sensitivity or in a simple reaction times task. However, a significant advantage of blind individuals emerged in the attentional tasks requiring that they detect either right-sided sounds or left-sided tactile pulses (selective attention condition), or the combination of a right-sided sound and a left-sided pulse (divided attention condition). These findings suggest that a more efficient modulatory role of attention in blind subjects may help them when stimuli have to be selected according to modality and spatial features (see also Collignon and De Volder, 2009). Accordingly, Liotti et al. (Liotti, Ryder, and Woldorff 1998) found that even when the task was adjusted to each participant's sound threshold, early blind subjects were faster at detecting changes in sound intensity in a dichotic listening paradigm. Given that sensory discrimination differences were controlled for, faster responses depended on attention-based mechanisms.

Rokem and Ahissar (2009) have specifically investigated the role of improved auditory processing in determining superior auditory memory in the blind. Specifically, the authors measured both cognitive and perceptual abilities in congenitally blind individuals and in a group of matched sighted controls. Short-term memory was assessed by means of a standard digit-span task and by a task requiring that subjects repeat sequences of pseudo-words (one to five items long). Blind subjects outperformed the sighted in both conditions; however, when the perceptual threshold of sighted and blind subjects was matched by adding noise, memory spans of the two groups overlapped. These data suggest that the blind subjects' improved memory abilities depend on improved stimulus processing at an early stage of encoding, rather than on superior abilities at subsequent memory-related processes. In fact, improved sensory encoding may allow the sequencing and "chunking" that support better memory performance, a hypothesis also put forward by Raz et al. (Raz, Striem et al. 2007), who suggested that memory advantages in the blind may depend on their ability to "chunk" together consecutively presented items. Hence, it is likely that the short-term memory advantage of blind individuals results from better stimulus encoding, rather than from superiority at subsequent processing stages.

Stevens and Weaver (2005) have suggested that blind individuals may benefit from a faster auditory perceptual consolidation. This phrase "perceptual consolidation" refers to the time needed for a complete representation of a stimulus to emerge, following an appropriate temporal integration of all its elements. Once generated, the perceptual representation and all its elements are accessible to further analysis and manipulation by other higher cognitive functions, such as reasoning or memory. A good tool to measure auditory perceptual consolidation is the auditory backward masking task (Kallman and Massaro 1979), which requires discriminating between two stimuli, with a backward mask presented at various delays after the second stimulus. The delay at which a mask no longer disrupts discrimination represents the time needed to generate a stable representation of the stimulus. In an auditory backward masking task in which complex auditory stimuli were used (Stevens and Weaver 2005), early blind subjects showed significantly greater accuracy at shorter mask onset delays than did sighted controls, even when adjusting for the spectral-temporal sensitivity difference between blind and sighted subjects. Critically, since perceptual consolidation can be regarded as the encoding phase of working memory that logically precedes the maintenance phase, improved perceptual consolidation mechanisms in the early blind might also be interpreted as an index of enhanced auditory working-memory capacity.

2.7 Touch

When we touch a surface or manipulate objects, we are engaged in a haptic experience. According to Loomis and Lederman (1986) the phrase "haptic perception" refers to the combined use of cutaneous and kinesthetic sense, and generally, it is an "active" experience under the individual's own control (see also Lederman and Klatzky 2009).

Cutaneous (or tactile) afferents are fast-conducting afferent neurons that transmit signals to the brain from a number of mechanoreceptors placed on the body's surface. Four main afferent types innervate the skin, and these differ in rate of adaptation and the size of their receptive fields, thus responding to cutaneous motion and deformation in different ways (see Johnson 2001; Johansson and Flanagan 2009 for reviews): fast-adapting type I (FA-I) receptors (Meissner corpuscles); slow-adapting type I (SA-I) receptors (Merkel cells); fast-adapting type II (FA-II) receptors (Pacini corpuscles); and slow-adapting type II (SA-II) receptors (Ruffini corpuscles). Meissner and Pacini corpuscles are rapidly adapting receptors that respond to transient, phasic or vibratory stimuli; these receptors respond to each initial application or removal of a stimulus but fail to respond during maintained stimulation. Merkel cells and Ruffini corpuscles are slowly adapting receptors which are active during the entire contact with the stimulus, thus responding to sustained indentation, and contributing to the perception of texture and local form, as well as static touch. Meissner corpuscles are particularly sensitive to low-frequency vibrations (roughly 5–50 Hz); they do not respond to static skin-deformation but can accurately detect dynamic skin-deformation. Meissner corpuscles are likely to be responsible also for the detection of slip between the skin and an object held in the hands, thus being extremely important in grip control (cf. Hager-Ross and Johansson 1996). Pacini corpuscles are very sensitive to high-frequency vibrations (roughly 4–400 Hz), but their spatial resolution is minimal: in fact, the receptive field of a Pacini corpuscle may be so large as to include the entire hand. Pacini corpuscles seem to be involved in coding the temporal attributes of the stimuli, such as the vibration of an object manipulated by the hand, and thus are important in responding to distant events acting on hand-held objects. In fact, it seems that when individuals become skilled in the use of a tool, they can perceive events at the working surface of the tools as though their fingers were present—and this thanks to Pacini corpuscles (cf. Brisben, Hsiao, and Johnson 1999). Afferents ending in the Merkel cells have a high spatial resolution thanks to the their small receptive fields (they can resolve spatial details of 0.5 mm, although their receptive-field diameter is around 2–3 mm) and are important in transmitting local spatial discontinuities (e.g., edge contours, Braille reading marks), being selectively sensitive to points, edges and curvatures. Ruffini corpuscles have a smaller spatial resolution due to their large and less localized receptive fields. Ruffini afferents are critical in providing the brain with motion signals from the whole hand: in fact, they signal skin-stretch accurately, and are thus important (together with proprioception receptors) in the perception of hand shape and finger position, both of which are critical for grip control.

The accuracy at which a tactile stimulus is detected depends on both the density of receptors and the size of their receptive fields. In fact, the greater the density and the smaller the receptive field, the higher the tactile acuity. Not surprisingly, cutaneous receptors are more densely present on the tips of the glabrous digits and in the perioral region. Accordingly, receptive fields are smaller on the finger tips, where each receptor serves an extremely small area of the skin. At the cortical level, densely innervated body parts are represented by a larger numbers of neurons occupying a disproportionately large part of the somatosensory system's body representation: in fact, the finger tips and lips provide the cortex with the most detailed information about a tactile stimulus.

Proprioceptive afferents are fast-conducting afferents that provide information about static limb and joint position or about the dynamic movement of the limb (kinhestesia) and thus are critical for balance, posture and limb movements. Proprioceptive receptors are located in muscles (muscle spindles, providing information about length of the muscle and speed of change of this length), tendons (the Golgi tendon organs, providing information about the tension of the muscle and hence the level of force employed and its variation over time) and joint capsules (joint-capsule mechanoceptors, probably important for angle, regulation and/or facilitation of muscle proprioception). Sensory information coded by cutaneous and proprioceptive receptors is conveyed to the brain mainly through the dorsal column medial-lemniscus pathway. This pathway underlies the capacity for fine form and texture discrimination, form recognition of three-dimensional objects, and motion detection, and is also involved in transmitting information about conscious awareness of body position in space.

Tactile spatial acuity is usually measured by way of two-point discrimination (but see Craig and Johnson 2000), texture discrimination, gap detection, grating resolution and letter recognition tasks. It has been estimated that the limit of tactile spatial resolution in young normally sighted individuals range from about 1.2 to 1.7 mm in the human fingerpad under conditions of static touch (see Legge, Madison et al. 2008 for a review). As we have already mentioned, the receptors defining this limit are the slowly adapting type I afferents or Merkell cells (see Johnson 2001). Tactile temporal sensitivity can be investigated in gap-detection paradigms, masking paradigms, tasks measuring the absolute sensitivity to vibration as a function of temporal frequency, and so on (see Loomis and Lederman 1986 for a review). In evaluating possible compensatory phenomena associated with blindness, it is important to consider whether the compensation occurs at the level of spatial acuity or temporal acuity, and whether possible superior haptic capacities in blind individuals depend on enhanced sensitivity occurring at the basic cutaneous/tactile level.

2.8 Enhanced Tactile Capacities in the Blind?

As in case of the auditory capacities, experimental findings are not always consistent regarding whether blind individuals develop superior tactile acuity compared to normally sighted individuals. Again, inter-subject variability and the type of task used in the different experiments (different involvement of cutaneous/proprioceptive receptors, etc.) are likely to be responsible for discrepancies in the literature. Unfortunately, standardized tests and batteries to assess perceptual and cognitive abilities in the haptic domain are limited and available in developmental settings only: Kainthola and Singh (1992) developed a test to assess tactile concentration and short-term memory in blind children of different ages; more recently, Ballesteros, Bardisa, and colleagues (2005) have developed a "haptic test battery" to test tactual abilities—ranging from tactual discrimination, systematic scanning and shape coding, short and long-term memory—in sighted and blind children of different ages (see figure 2.3).

In this section we review some of the most critical findings on the tactile discrimination capacity of blind individuals.

Tactile Pressure Sensitivity

Tactile *pressure* sensitivity as measured through Von Frey-like filaments (widely used in pain research) does not seem to differ between blind and sighted individuals (Axelrod 1959; Pascual-Leone and Torres 1993; Sterr, Green, and Elbert 2003; but see Sterr, Müller et al. 1998a).

Tactile Temporal Perception

Blind and sighted individuals were found to perform equally well in a vibrotactile frequency discrimination task, using frequencies of 100–150 Hz (thus based upon the Pacini afferents) (Alary, Duquette et al. 2009). In fact, although the threshold was lower in the blind group (16.5 Hz) compared to the sighted group (20 Hz), this difference was not statistically significant.

Röder, Rösler, and Spence (2004) have demonstrated that the congenitally blind are superior than both sighted and late blind individuals in temporal-order judgment

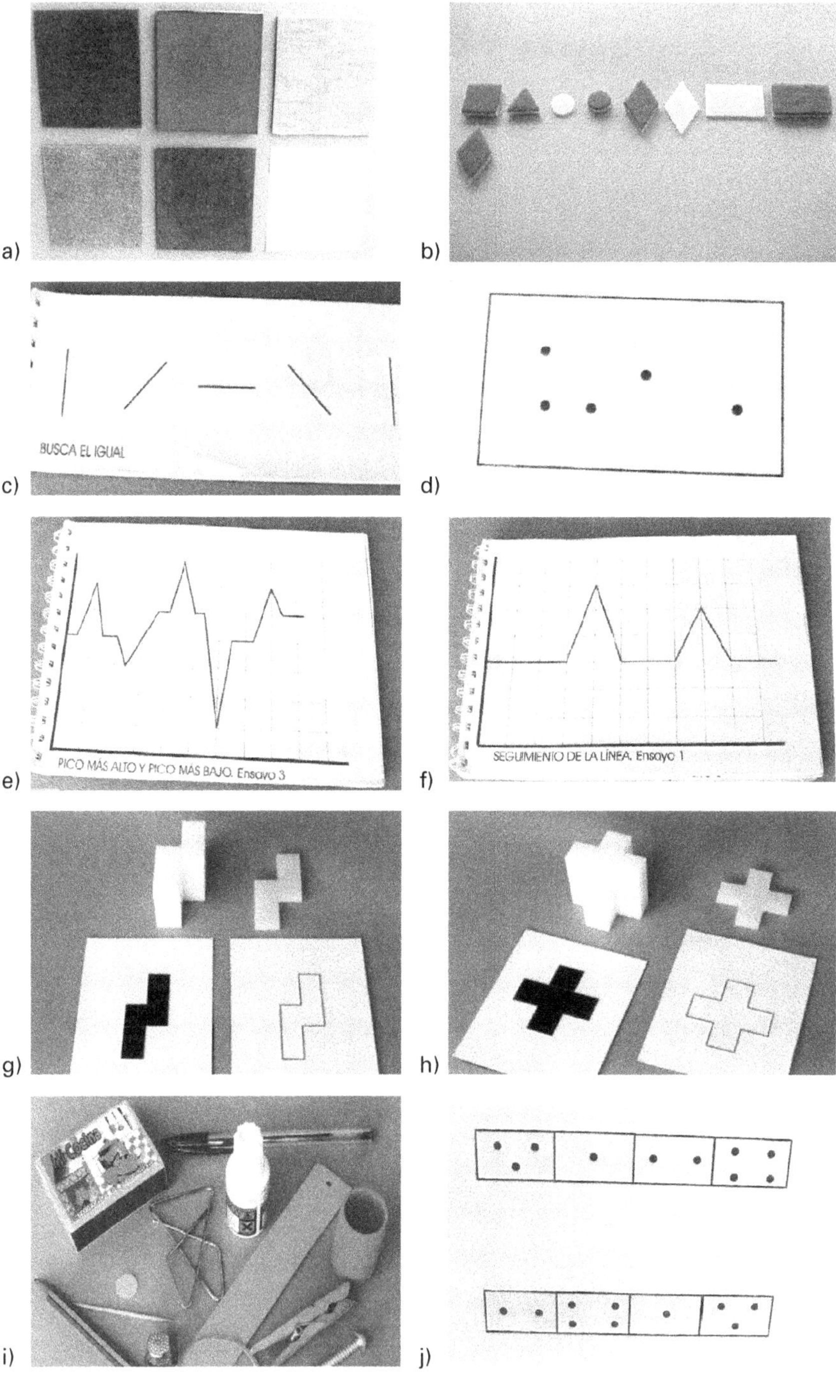
a)
b)
BUSCA EL IGUAL
c)
d)
PICO MÁS ALTO Y PICO MÁS BAJO. Ensayo 3
e)
SEGUIMIENTO DE LA LÍNEA. Ensayo 1
f)
g)
h)
i)
j)

tasks in which two tactile stimuli, one applied to either hand, were presented (with the hands being either crossed or uncrossed).

Tactile Spatial Discrimination

The texture-discrimination task, the gap-detection task, the grating-orientation task (GOT), the tasks of discriminating grating-ridge width and Braille-like dot patterns are among the most common tests used to measure *spatial* tactile acuity (see Sathian, Goodwin et al. 1989). In texture-discrimination tasks, subjects are usually required to move their fingers over a surface (or a surface is moved over the subject's static fingers) and to indicate possible changes in texture. This task likely depends on signals conveyed by SA-I afferents (Merkel receptors) (Connor and Johnson 1992), although rapidly adapting afferents may also play a role (Hollins and Risner 2000). The GOT requires that subjects discriminate the orientation of a grating applied to their fingertip, and is generally considered a rigorous test of passive tactile acuity (Johnson and Phillips 1981; Craig 1999). The orientation of a tactile grid is represented by the locations of activated SA-I afferents that correspond to the location of the edges in the grating (see Johnson and Phillips 1981; Gibson and Craig 2002). Grating-ridge width discrimination is usually tested with the subject's fingerpad sweeping across stationary gratings, a similar movement to what is used in Braille reading. Periodic gratings consist of alternating ridges and grooves, whose width can be specified to an accuracy of 0.01 mm (Sathian, Goodwin et al. 1989): perceived grating roughness increases with the increase in groove width and with the decrease of ridge width. Changes in groove and ridge width are detected by SA-I, fast-adapting receptors and Pacini corpuscles (Sathian, Goodwin et al. 1989). In gap detection (see Stevens and Choo 1996), an edge that is either solid or contains a gap is pressed against the skin; participants have to indicate whether the stimulus contains a gap or not. Gap width is then varied in order to find the individual's threshold, with gap-sensitivity again mainly depending on SA-I receptors. Braille-like dot-pattern tasks have also been used to measure tactile acuity: basically, the subject is required to tactilely recognize a number of dot patterns, usually with dot diameter and spacing being similar to Braille (although the size of the matrices in which the dots appear can be different from those used in Braille).

Figure 2.3

Examples of tests used by Ballesteros and colleagues in their haptic test battery: (a) texture discrimination; (b) dimensional structure; (c) spatial orientation; (d) dot scanning; (e–f) graphs and diagrams; (g–h) symmetry (three-dimensional objects, surfaces and raised-line shapes); (i) object naming; and (j) memory span (dots).

Reprinted from Ballesteros, Bardisa et al., "The haptic test battery: A new instrument to test tactual abilities in blind and visually impaired and sighted children," *British Journal of Visual Impairment* 23 (2005): 11–24. (© 2005. Reprinted by permission of SAGE)

Braille reading, like grating discrimination, is likely to rely in large part on SA-I receptors' activity (Phillips, Johansson, and Johnson 1990).

Alary et al. (Alary, Duquette et al. 2009) showed that (early and late) blind subjects performed better than sighted controls in a texture-discrimination task. Conversely, congenitally blind, late blind and sighted subjects did not differ in a task requiring discrimination of the texture of sandpaper (Heller 1989a). Notably, Heller (1989a) obtained similar results with or without movement on the part of the subject, according to other evidence suggesting that texture discrimination does not vary with active and passive touch (Chapman 1994). As suggested by Alary et al. (Alary, Duquette et al. 2009) discrepancies between their results and those reported by Heller may reflect differences in the physical properties of the textures used.

Van Boven et al. (Van Boven, Hamilton et al. 2000) compared 15 early blind Braille readers and 15 sighted subjects in a grating orientation task by manually applying the gratings to the index and middle fingers of both hands: overall, blind individuals showed superior tactile acuity on all four fingers. Goldreich and Kanics (2003) used a fully automated GOT task—thus controlling for unintended variability in stimulation parameters such as contact onset velocity, force, stability and duration that characterize manual application of the stimuli—to investigate tactile acuity capacities in a group of sighted and blind individuals. The blind group was heterogeneous, with participants differing for onset-age and degree of blindness (some participants could count on some residual light-perception), Braille-reading abilities, age at learning Braille, years reading Braille and daily Braille-reading hours. The authors found that tactile acuity was superior in the blind group, regardless of the degree of childhood vision, light-perception level or Braille-reading differences (see figure 2.4). In fact, the "average" blind subject showed a tactile acuity that was comparable to that of the average sighted subject 23 years younger. These findings suggest that blind individuals may have a superior capacity for decoding the spatial structure of the activated SA-I afferent array through central processing mechanisms (Goldreich and Kanics 2003).

In a following study, Goldreich and Kanics (2006) found that (early and late) blind outperformed sighted subjects in a grating-detection task requiring that they distinguish a thinly grooved surface from a smooth one. Since SA-I receptors respond well to edges, grooved surfaces elicit overall a greater SA-I population response-magnitude than do smooth surfaces (and hence, unlike a grating-orientation task, successful grating detection does not rely on the activated SA-I spatial structure cue) (see Johnson and Phillips 1981). The results of this study (Goldreich and Kanics 2006) show that blind individuals can make a better use than sighted subjects of the SA-I population response-magnitude cue present in the grating-detection task. As in their previous study (Goldreich and Kanics 2003), blind subjects' tactile acuity did not depend upon the onset-age of blindness or on Braille-reading experience (be that the age at which Braille was learned, years reading Braille or daily Braille reading time). Moreover, the

A

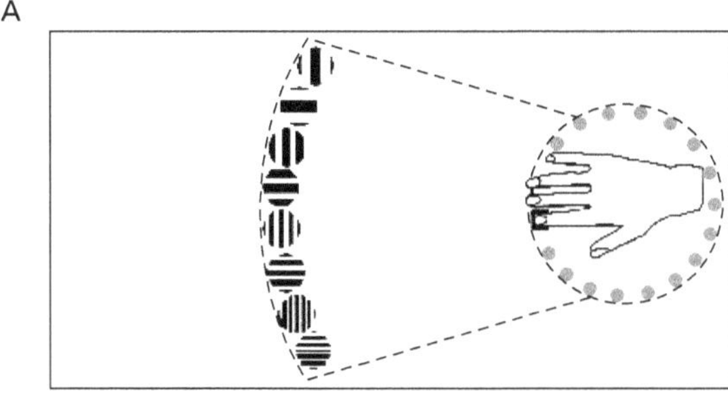

Upper Table (top view)

B

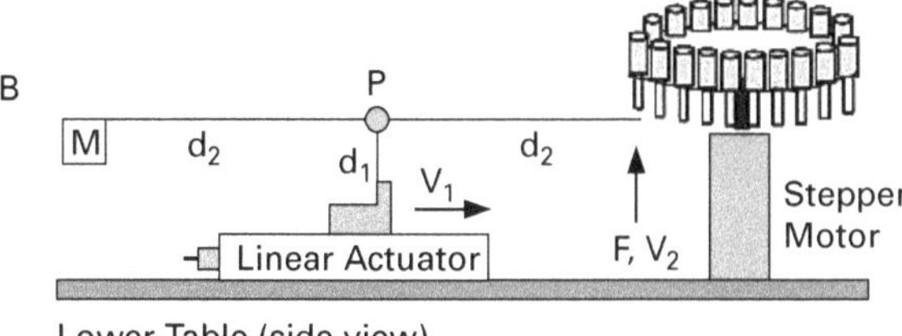

Lower Table (side view)

Figure 2.4

Schema of testing apparatus used by Goldreich and Kanics (2003). (A) *Top view*. The hand rested palm-down on an upper table, with the index finger positioned over a tunnel (not shown) through which the stimulus surfaces rose. Plastic barriers surrounding the fingertip prevented lateral and forward finger movements. Upward, downward and backward movements were detected by a force sensor on the fingernail (not shown) and were announced by an error tone. A rotatable disk (dashed circle) just below the table housed the stimulus surfaces (partial expanded view on left). (B) *Side view* of the lower table, concealed during testing. Rotation of the stepper motor positioned the appropriate stimulus surface under the finger, after which the linear actuator moved with velocity V1, freeing the rod supporting mass M to pivot around point P. The stimulus surface contacted the finger with force F = Mg and velocity V2 = (V1)(d2/d1). After a one-second contact period, the actuator retracted to return the rod and stimulus surface to their resting positions. M = 10 or 50 gm; V2 = 4 cm/sec. For clarity, only 19 of the 40 stimulus surfaces are shown.

Reprinted from Goldreich and Kanics, "Tactile acuity is enhanced in blindness," *Journal of Neuroscience* 23(8) (2003): 3439–3445. (See also Goldreich, Wong et al. 2009.) (Reprinted by permission of Society for Neuroscience) fact that the degree of childhood vision did not influence performance of blind individuals (Goldreich and Kanics 2003) argues against the importance of childhood visual deprivation in tactile acuity enhancement. Stevens, Foulke, and Patterson (1996) found superior ability of blind individuals in non-grating measures of passive tactile acuity, such as gap detection and line orientation. Röder and Neville (2003) reported better accuracy in blind participants compared to sighted in a two-points discrimination task.

On the basis of a review of the literature, Legge et al. (Legge, Madison et al. 2008) have reported that spatial tactile thresholds in young sighted individuals range from about 1.2 to 1.7 mm, whereas the threshold for blind subjects is roughly 0.2 mm lower, varying from 1 to 1.5 mm, thus representing about 15 percent better tactile acuity compared to sighted controls (see figure 2.5). Moreover, Legge et al. (Legge, Madison et al. 2008) demonstrated that enhanced tactile acuity in blind individuals is retained into old age (but only when measured with active touch: see Stevens, Foulke, and Patterson 1996; Goldreich and Kanics 2003; Goldreich and Kanics 2006), whereas tactile acuity has been found to decline with age in sighted individuals.

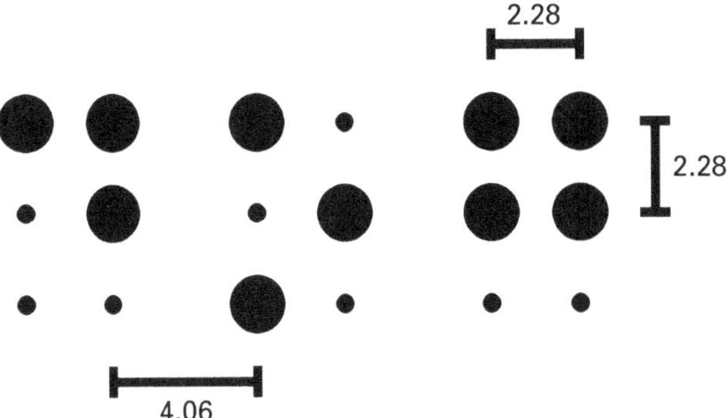

Figure 2.5
Three adjacent Braille cells are shown, illustrating the standard dimensions of the Braille cell and the rendering of the three-letter word "dog." There are six possible dot positions in each Braille cell; the larger black circles represent the dots in the character, and the smaller black circles represent the unused dot positions. For instance, the Braille character consisting of the top four dots of the right-hand cell represents the letter "g." According to Nolan and Kederis (1969), individual dots have a base diameter of 1.5 mm and a height above the surface of the page of 0.43 mm. Horizontally or vertically adjacent dots within a cell have a center-to-center separation of 2.28 mm.
Reprinted from Legge, Madison et al., "Retention of high tactile acuity throughout the life span in blindness," *Perception and Psychophysics* 70 (2008): 1471–1488. (Reprinted by permission of Psychonomic Society)

Importantly, according to Legge et al. (Legge, Madison et al. 2008), such a preservation of tactile acuity across the lifespan in blind individuals is likely to depend on the use of active touch in blind individuals' daily activities, rather than on Braille reading per se (see sections 2.9 and 2.10 for a discussion of the difference between active and passive touch and its importance in Braille reading). Interestingly, blind individuals may also manifest enhanced tactile spatial discrimination of the tongue, compared to sighted controls (Chebat, Rainville et al. 2007).

Nonetheless, other studies do not seem to support the view that blind individuals can count on an enhanced tactile spatial acuity. Pascual-Leone and Torres (1993) reported an expansion of topographic representation of the Braille reading finger within the primary somatosensory cortex in their blind group, but no differences were observed between blind and sighted individuals in the two-points discrimination threshold on the same reading finger, thus suggesting that an intramodal cortical expansion is not necessarily associated with a general improvement in tactile sensitivity. Alary et al. (Alary, Duquette et al. 2009) did not find differences between sighted and blind individuals in a grating-orientation discrimination task. Accordingly, Grant, Thiagarajah, and Sathian (2000) found no difference in tactile acuity between their early blind Braille readers, late blind readers and the control group of sighted subjects in a (manual) grating-orientation task and in discriminating gratings with variable ridge widths. Instead, Grant et al. (Grant, Thiagarajah, and Sathian 2000) found an advantage of early and late blind individuals in a hyperacuity tactile task using Braille-like dot patterns. However, in the last blocks of the experimental session, the two groups performed similarly, suggesting that sighted participants could achieve a good level of accuracy in a tactile acuity test thanks to practice. In light of these results, Grant and colleagues (Grant, Thiagarajah, and Sathian 2000) argued that blind individuals do not have a truly supernormal tactile sense but rather acquire greater proficiency with non-visual modalities thanks to high-level processes such as learning and attention. Furthermore, Grant et al. (Grant, Thiagarajah, and Sathian 2000) suggested that if Braille reading practice made it possible for the early blind to outperform the sighted in the initial sessions of the Braille-pattern dot-discrimination task, this initial advantage did not transfer to other tactile tasks, and thus that transfer of perceptual learning effects due to tactile experience has finite limits.

As we have already mentioned, methodological discrepancies between the different studies make comparisons difficult. Moreover, the threshold values reported by the different blind groups and sighted groups in similar tests is often different across studies. This is a critical point to stress, because if the threshold of either the blind group is particularly high or that of the sighted control group is particularly low, the comparison between the two groups might fail to reach significance (see Alary, Duquette et al. 2009). Finally, the importance of a specific ability for everyday activities represents a critical factor to be considered: for instance, if recognition of fine spatial structures could be relevant for blind individuals in facing their everyday activities (e.g., Braille reading), a high level of performance in the judgment of tactile stimulation intensity per se may not be crucial for them.

2.9 Is Braille Reading Important for Tactile Acuity?

The results discussed above raise questions about the importance of Braille reading practice in determining the level of performance in spatial tactile acuity tests. Braille characters consist of the combination of six dots, appearing in a 3 × 2 rectangular matrix called a Braille "cell" (see figure 2.5). Individual dots have a base diameter of 1.5 mm and a height above the surface of the page of 0.43 mm; the center-to-center dot spacing is 2.28 mm within the Braille cell (Nolan and Kederis 1969). The sixty-four possible arrangements of dots in the Braille cell (including the blank cell) represent the 64 characters of the Braille code. Of these 64 characters, 26 represent letters of the English alphabet. As we have mentioned above, the estimates of spatial tactile acuity in younger sighted and blind range from 1 to 1.7 mm, thus being roughly half the center-to-center dot spacing in a Braille cell (see Legge, Madison et al. 2008 for a review), suggesting that recognition of Braille characters operates close to the tactile acuity threshold. Importantly, each single Braille cell can be entirely covered by the fingertip, without requiring any sequential exploration, although Braille is usually read in an active scanning mode. In fact, as noted by Millar (1997), proficient Braille reading also requires the choice of appropriate scanning strategies with the fingers and the two hands.

Goldreich and Kanics (2003, 2006) did not find differences between blind Braille readers and non-readers in their tactile tasks; nor did they find differences among the Braille readers due to the amount of daily practice, the age at which Braille was learned or number of years since learning Braille. Similarly, Van Boven et al. (Van Boven, Hamilton et al. 2000) did not find a correlation between enhanced tactile acuity of the Braille-reading finger and Braille-reading experience in their sample of blind participants, although reporting that 9 of 13 Braille readers with a preferred reading finger had greater acuity on that finger than on the three other fingers. Legge and colleagues (Legge, Madison et al. 2008) again did not report a significant correlation between tactile acuity of their blind participants, age at which Braille was learned, and the amount of daily or weekly reading, whereas a weak correlation was found between tactile acuity and the number of years reading Braille. Stevens et al. (Stevens, Foulke, and Patterson 1996) found only a weak correlation between tactile acuity and Braille-reading speed among blind subjects. According to Goldreich and Kanics (2003), blindness per se rather than prolonged tactile experience may be responsible for enhanced tactile acuity in blind individuals. However, there is evidence that practice may indeed affect sensory threshold: piano players have been found to have lower two-points threshold than controls, and their threshold inversely correlated with daily piano practice time (Ragert, Schmidt et al. 2004). The amount of practice needed to induce such effects remains to be established: in fact, even a brief practice allowed sighted participants to perform as well as blind Braille readers in a Braille-dot pattern test in the study by Grant et al. (Grant, Thiagarajah, and Sathian 2000) discussed above. Conversely, it has been reported that passive tactile acuity on the right index finger was unaffected by five days of intense daily Braille training in a group of sighted individuals, whereas enhanced tactile acuity on this finger was significantly enhanced by a five-days period of blindfolding (Kauffman, Théoret, and Pascual-Leone 2002). Even a shorter blindfolding (90 minutes) has been found to induce passive tactile-acuity gains (Facchini and Aglioti 2003).

A critical study by Sterr et al. (Sterr, Green, and Elbert 2003) has demonstrated that Braille reading practice might even be detrimental for accurate tactile localization. In particular this study, confirming some earlier observations (Sterr, Müller et al. 1998b), showed that blind Braille readers encountered more difficulty in identifying the finger to which a light tactile stimulus was administered than sighted subjects. Critically, mislocations errors mainly occurred at the right (reading) hand, affecting all fingers (reading fingers were less prone to mislocation but tended to attract most of the misperceived stimuli) and suggesting that mislocations were related to Braille reading rather than the loss of vision per se. As suggested by Sterr et al. (Sterr, Green, and Elbert 2003), it is likely that Braille reading leads to enlarged finger representations with greater overlap of the respective neural networks (see Braun, Schweizer et al. 2000), thus inducing mislocation errors between the different fingers. Furthermore, Braille reading might also strengthen the connections to more distant regions in the hand area, so that the neural network activated by a weak tactile stimulus is less circumscribed in the blind that in the sighted, leading to localizing errors.

The specific role played by visual deprivation per se and by tactile practice (e.g., Braille reading, but also texture discrimination and so forth) in leading to enhanced tactile performances in blind individuals still remains to be fully clarified. As we will see in chapter 8, training and visual deprivation might lead to different cortical plasticity phenomena (unimodal vs. crossmodal) resulting in different behavioral outputs.

2.10 Passive versus Active Touch

Most of the studies reviewed above concerned "passive" touch. According to Gibson (1962), "passive touch" refers to the perception of a tactile stimulus by a passive observer. Conversely, "active touch" refers to the "active" exploration of objects by the subject, thus including both bottom-up tactile stimulation and kinesthetic signals from movements of the hands or fingers. In active touch, the agent plans and executes finger movements to explore the target, also adopting the scanning strategy most suitable to reach the required goal (see Lederman and Klatzky 1987). It is worth noticing that, in some circumstances, moving tactile stimuli have been presented to the static fingers of the subjects: this experience still pertains to passive touch, since the subject cannot exert control over the movement.

Previous experimental evidence with sighted individuals has demonstrated that active touch may be advantageous compared to passive touch in tactile recognition (cf. Loomis 1985; Heller 1986). The almost complete lack of correlation between Braille reading and tactile (passive) acuity reported in many studies (e.g., Stevens, Foulke, and Patterson 1996; Goldreich and Kanics 2003, 2006; Legge, Madison et al. 2008) points to the importance that the "active" component of haptic experience may have in determining superior tactile abilities in blind individuals. In fact, as noticed by Legge and colleagues (Legge, Madison et al. 2008), blind individuals continuously have to rely on tactile shape or texture discrimination in their everyday activities (choosing the right dress by recognizing its fabric texture, recognizing coins, selecting keys, etc.). These active tactile experiences when prolonged over time may result in an enhanced capacity to recognize objects or features of objects at touch. In this section, we present a few studies that have specifically investigated possible differences between blind and sighted individuals in more "active" tactile tests.

Early reports found that blind individuals were better than sighted controls in the haptic estimation of macro-curvature (Hunter 1954; Pick, Pick, and Thomas 1966). Davidson (1972) found blind participants to be superior in a task requiring that they categorize macro-curvatures as straight, concave or convex, and argued that the higher accuracy of blind participants in curvature judgments depended on differences in the active exploratory strategies they used.

Alary et al. (Alary, Goldstein et al. 2008) have compared blind and sighted individuals in a haptic angle-discrimination task, depending on both cutaneous and proprioceptive feedbacks. Participants had to actively scan with their right index finger pairs of two-dimensional angles, identifying the larger one. The same exploratory strategy (a single contour-following movement over the angles) was imposed on all subjects to ensure that all relied on the same information in making their sensory decisions. Alary et al. (Alary, Goldstein et al. 2008) found that blind individuals performed significantly better than sighted individuals; however, this advantage was only evident when the angles were scanned with the right index finger of the outstretched arm (with cutaneous feedback arousing from the finger and proprioceptive feedback from the shoulder). Conversely, when the arm was flexed at the elbow so that the resulting joint movement was distal (wrist, finger) no differences between blind and sighted controls were reported. As suggested by Alary et al. (Alary, Goldstein et al. 2008), this difference in results between the proximal and distal movement conditions might have partially depended on blind subjects being better trained for proximal movements, due to their level of practice with Braille reading (that typically involves movement of the whole arm, particularly rotation of the shoulder, as the finger is scanning over the lines of the text). If these results overall show that blind subjects develop a greater sensitivity to haptic inputs, they do not clarify the role played by cutaneous and proprioceptive feedback in leading to higher haptic accuracy in the blind group. A subsequent study (with the same blind participants) was carried out by Alary et al. (Alary, Duquette et al. 2009) to separately look at the cutaneous and proprioceptive components: in this second study, blind subjects outperformed a new sighted control group (but not the old sighted control group) in a texture-discrimination task, whereas no difference between the blind and the two sighted control groups were reported in a grating-orientation judgment and in a vibrotactile frequency-discrimination task. Hence, it is difficult to establish whether better haptic performance of blind individuals as reported by Alary et al. (Alary, Goldstein et al. 2008) in haptic discrimination was due to superior cutaneous sensitivity, to the feedback component or to other factors.

Heller and colleagues (Heller, Kappers et al. 2008) have investigated the effects of curvature on haptic judgments of length in sighted and blind individuals. Although the focus of their paper was on assessing whether visual experience is determinant for the psychophysical effect for which curved lines are usually perceived as shorter than straight lines, their findings in it are also relevant in the context of possible differences in haptic perception between blind and sighted individuals. Similar performances were reported for sighted and blind subjects, although early blind subjects show a smaller systematic underestimation of greater extents. Subjects were required to explore the lines with their right index finger, but no control on exploratory strategies (time of exploration, number of scans, etc.) was given; hence, it is not possible to establish whether blind and sighted subjects did indeed rely on the same exploratory strategies.

2.11 Tactile Attention

As we have already discussed when dealing with enhanced auditory capacities in blind individuals, attention mechanisms may influence tactile perception, likely by means of top-down processes, which modulate information processing in primary sensory regions (e.g., Ahissar and Hochstein 1993). Hence, it might be that superior tactile capacities of blind individuals depend on improved attentional mechanisms developed through continuous practice or on the use of more efficient sensorimotor strategies (see Hollins 1989; Shimizu, Saida, and Shimura 1993; D'Angiulli, Kennedy, and Heller 1998) rather than on changes of sensory processing at low-level sensory stages.

In the study by Sterr et al. (Sterr, Green, and Elbert 2003) discussed above (requiring to identify the finger on which a light tactile stimulus was administered), mislocation errors were greater in Braille blind readers than in sighted controls for the

Braille-reading hand; in particular, stimuli tended to be mislocated toward the reading fingers. As suggested by Sterr et al. (Sterr, Green, and Elbert 2003), this "stimuli attraction" by the reading fingers might reflect attentional mechanisms; in other words, the reading finger of the blind Braille readers is likely to "automatically" attract attention when stimuli are presented to the hand, since those fingers are the ones usually "relevant" when stimulation occurs. These findings suggest that blind individuals may pay more attention to specific regions of their hands, and this might result in higher performance in some tactile-discrimination tasks (while negatively affecting others: Sterr, Green, and Elbert 2003).

In the study by Collignon et al. (Collignon, Renier et al. 2006)—which we discussed when dealing with attentional versus sensory explanations for enhanced auditory abilities in blind individuals (see section 2.6)—the authors compared performances of blind and sighted individuals in selective and divided attention tasks with individually adjusted tactile stimuli: by adjusting stimuli according to each individual's sensory threshold, the authors could assess attentional performance independently of sensory influence. Tactile nociceptive sensitivity was not found to be different between blind and sighted subjects; moreover, no differences in tactile detection threshold were found between the two groups in a task measuring intermanual intensity differences where stimuli consisted of short charge biphasic square wave pulses. In selective and divided attention tasks, participants were faced with four auditory-tactile stimulus combinations that depended on their spatial origin (left or right); subjects had to respond to specific stimuli depending on the task (left-sided tactile pulses in the selective attention condition or the combination of a right-sided sound and a left-sided pulse in the bimodal divided condition). Critically, Collignon et al. (Collignon, Renier et al. 2006) reported faster reaction times for blind subjects, thus suggesting a more efficient modulatory role of attention in the blind when stimuli have to be selected according to modality and spatial features.

Evidence from altered tactile spatial attention mechanisms in blind individuals come also from studies using event-related brain potentials (ERPs). Shorter latencies for somatosensory ERPs (Feinsod, Bach-y-Rita, and Madey 1973) have been reported in blind individuals compared with sighted individuals—a result that is replicated by Röder et al. (Röder, Rösler et al. 1996), who also reported shorter discrimination times in blind individuals. Forster, Eardley, and Eimer (2007) found differences in the ERPs pattern of early blind and sighted individuals by employing a relatively difficult spatial selection task that required subjects to attend to one of three locations on their index finger (on the palm side and including the top and part of the middle phalanx, i.e., the part of the finger used in Braille reading) and to respond vocally when they detected infrequent tactile targets (weak vibrations) at this location, while ignoring stronger non-target tactile vibrations at the attended location, and all tactile events presented to the two unattended locations. Forster et al. (Forster, Eardley, and Eimer

2007) found that blind participants were faster and more accurate than sighted controls in detecting infrequent tactile targets at currently attended location. This behavioral effect was associated with an early attentional modulation of the somatosensory P100 component that was not present in the sighted group: moreover, the P100 occurred earlier in blind compared to sighted subjects, indexing faster tactile processing speed (see also Feinsod, Bach-y-Rita, and Madey 1973; Röder, Rösler et al. 1996). The compensatory enhancement of attentional selectivity was present in the blind subjects regardless of which hand was stimulated; since all those blind participants reportedly read Braille with two hands (reading with one index finger while using the other index finger as a guide between lines), the results by Forster et al. (Forster, Eardley, and Eimer 2007) do not establish whether the enhanced capability of focusing attention on small regions of the finger and ignoring stimuli at nearby locations depends on Braille reading or rather reflects a general enhancement of discriminating fine spatial patterns in blind individuals.

Nonetheless, results are not always consistent, and evidence against enhanced attentional mechanisms in blind individuals has also been reported. For instance, in a tactile-detection task requiring blind and sighted participants to shift attention to either the left or the right hand (as indicated by an auditory cue presented at the start of each trial) in order to detect infrequent tactile targets delivered to this hand, no overall differences were reported in reaction times between the blind and the sighted groups (Van Velzen, Eardley et al. 2006). Moreover, the pattern of ERP lateralization was remarkably similar in the two groups (Van Velzen, Eardley et al. 2006). Hötting et al. (Hötting, Rösler, and Röder 2004) failed to find electrophysiological evidence for differences in the spatial tuning of tactile attention between sighted and blind participants (although at the behavioral level the blind demonstrated enhanced tactile discrimination). As underlined by Forster et al. (Forster, Eardley, and Eimer 2007), specific task requirements may partially explain the discrepancies in different ERPs findings: in fact, tasks that call for attending to one finger or hand while ignoring tactile events at other fingers or on the other hand may be too easy to reveal systematic differences between the blind and the sighted.

2.12 Olfactory and Taste Perception

Although in principle sensory compensation cannot be confined to the auditory and tactile domains, there is very limited behavioral research on olfactory and gustatory perceptual capacities in visually impaired individuals. This likely depends both on the sense of smell and taste playing a less prominent role in humans (compared to touch and audition), and on intrinsic methodological limits related to the use of self-reports as measure. Nevertheless, smell and taste are useful in many everyday situations—for instance, to recognize spoilt food, to detect toxic substances or the presence of smoke originating from an unseen fire—and olfaction is even more commonly used by blind individuals to recognize objects and other people (Hatwell 2003).

Available behavioral evidence is controversial with regard to the possibility that blind individuals develop enhanced olfactory capacities. Early reports suggested that blind individuals may be better than sighted individuals at identifying odors (Murphy and Cain 1986). However, other studies do not support this view. For instance, Schwenn, Hundorf, Moll, Pitz and Mann (2002) compared the smelling abilities of blind and sighted participants using both subjective tests (threshold, discrimination and identification) and objective tests (olfactory-evoked potentials and trigeminal-evoked potentials) without reporting any difference between the two groups. In a large-scale study carried out on 50 blind individuals (Smith, Doty et al. 1993), basic chemosensory functions were compared in blind and sighted individuals, through a series of olfactory and gustatory tests. Blind subjects did not outperform sighted controls in any test of chemosensory function. Conversely a sub-group of sighted participants that were highly trained for the sense of smell (all being employed for a governmental water department and trained to serve on its water quality evaluation panel) outperformed all the other subjects in odor detection, odor discrimination and taste identification test. These findings suggest that blindness per se has little influence on chemosensory functions and support the notion that specialized training enhances performance on a number of chemosensory tasks. Similar conclusions have been reached by studies with blind children. Rosenbluth, Grossman and Kaitz (2000) tested olfactory sensitivity, odor recognition and odor labeling in blind children and sighted controls. Blind children were more proficient at correctly labeling 25 common odors, compared to the sighted. However, blind children were neither more sensitive to a target odor, nor more proficient at choosing the correct odor label from a list of four. Similarly, Wakefield and colleagues (Wakefield, Homewood, and Taylor 2004) found that early blind children did not perform better in an odor-sensitivity task compared to the sighted, although they did significantly better on an odor-naming task. These findings suggest that a limited but still present compensatory cognitive function may lead to a circumscribed advantage of blind children: in other words, the cognitive skills of blind children (e.g., the ability to self-generate and retrieve odor labels) may facilitate performance in a top-down fashion in perceptual tasks that involve some sort of attentional/cognitive skill. Hence, the advantage of blind individuals in olfactory perception is likely to be more "cognitive" than "perceptual."

Nonetheless, it is possible that the specific task used and the sample and subjects' characteristics have masked subtle differences in olfactory acuity between blind and sighted individuals. In fact, Cuevas et al. (Cuevas, Plaza et al. 2009) noted how previous studies included early blind and late blind subjects as a unique group, and did not control for participants' gender (whereas gender is a critical variable in determining olfactory capacity, since women usually outperform men in olfactory tests: see

Landis, Konnerth, and Hummel 2004). In light of this, Cuevas and colleagues (Cuevas, Plaza et al. 2009) assessed the capacity of a group of congenitally male blind individuals and a group of male sighted subjects to discriminate (perceptual task) and identify (semantic task) familiar odors (of flower, fruit or domestic elements). In the perceptual discrimination task, two odors were presented for three seconds each and subjects had to tell whether the odors were the same or different. In the identification/semantic task, subjects had to smell a series of single odors and to identify them (by naming them or classifying them into a category given by the experimenter or selecting a label among multiple choices). Early blind subjects were found to perform better than sighted subjects in both the odor-discrimination task and in identifying the odors—both when no cue was provided and when the semantic category was given (no differences were found in the multiple-choice discrimination tasks, probably due to ceiling effects in both groups). No studies have so far investigated whether cross-modal reorganization of de-afferented visual brain areas contributes to odor processing in the early blind.

2.13 Effect of Blindness on Multisensory Interaction

In the previous sections of this chapter we have discussed findings regarding how blindness affects the functioning of the other sensorial channels independently from each other. Here we will consider data suggesting that blindness also affects the way the other senses interact and the multisensory control of action (for review, see Hötting and Röder 2009). A series of experiments carried out by Brigitte Röder and colleagues (see Putzar, Goerendt et al. 2007; Röder, Kusmierek et al. 2007; Röder, Föcker et al. 2008) suggests that different sensory inputs can be efficiently integrated only when remapped into an external spatial reference frame, and this—according to Röder and colleagues—requires vision to properly develop (see also Collignon, Voss et al. 2009). Röder et al.'s hypothesis is supported by a series of experimental findings. For example, in one study (Röder, Rösler, and Spence 2004) sighted and congenitally blind subjects had to judge the temporal order in which two tactile stimuli were delivered to their left and right hands; and in some conditions their hands were crossed. As expected, temporal order judgments of sighted subjects were less accurate with crossed than uncrossed hands, indicating the existence of a conflict between external and somato-topic spatial codes. By contrast, congenitally blind individuals were not affected by this manipulation. Hence, whereas sighted individuals likely rely on a visually defined reference frame to localize tactile events in external space, thus being impaired by conflicting external and somato-topic spatial information, blind subjects do not seem to rely on external spatial coordinates but solely on somato-topic ones. In a similar study using ERPs, subjects were instructed to attend to one hand (a tone was presented indicating which hand had to be attended to) and to detect rare double tactile stimuli on that hand while ignoring double touches presented to the unattended hand and single touches presented to the attended hand, while adopting either a parallel or crossed-hands posture (Röder, Föcker et al. 2008). Critically, again no hand-posture effect was reported in the blind, whereas the sighted performed more accurately with uncrossed than with crossed hands (ERPs data confirmed the behavioral evidence), supporting the view that blind individuals do not automatically remap sensory inputs into external (eye-centered) space. Hötting and colleagues (Hötting, Rösler, and Röder 2004) studied the strength of an auditory-tactile illusion in sighted and congenitally blind individuals. In Hötting et al.'s task, subjects were required to judge the number of a series of rapidly presented tactile stimuli which were presented together with one or multiple task-irrelevant tones. Critically, although all participants showed the illusory effect for which they reported perceiving more than one touch when the tactile stimulus was accompanied by multiple tones, the effect was significantly stronger in the sighted than in the blind, indicating that audiotactile temporal interaction was more pronounced in the sighted than in the blind. In a further study, Röder et al. (Putzar, Goerendt et al. 2007) found that a group of eleven sighted individuals that had been deprived of vision for at least five months of their life as a result of congenital binocular cataracts, showed reduced audiovisual interaction compared to a sighted control group.

Notably, the lower incidence of using an external reference frame as the default coordinate system in congenitally blind individuals has also been observed in tasks investigating multisensory control of action. For instance, Röder et al. (Röder, Kusmierek et al. 2007) found that when late blind, early blind and sighted subjects were required to answer with their hands to a series of tones (whose location was irrelevant to the task), all participants responded faster with uncrossed hands when the sound was presented from the same side as the responding hand ("Simon effect," see Simon, Hinrichs, and Craft 1970), however, this effect reversed with crossed hands in the congenitally blind only. In light of their results, Röder et al. (Röder, Kusmierek et al. 2007) argued that developmental vision induces the default use of an external coordinate frame for multisensory action control, which facilitates not only visual but also auditory-manual control. Similar results were obtained by Collignon and colleagues (Collignon, Voss et al. 2009) in a task requiring early blind, late blind, and sighted participants to lateralize auditory, tactile, or bimodal audiotactile stimuli by pressing the appropriate response key with either the left or the right hand. Participants had to perform the task either with uncrossed hands (pressing the right button with their right hand in response to right-sided auditory stimuli and tactile stimulation of the right hand) or in a crossed-hands posture (pressing the right button with their left hand in response to right-sided auditory stimuli and tactile stimulation of the left hand). In this task, crossing the hands clearly generates a conflict between a proprioceptive/peripersonal representation of space and extrapersonal/external coordinates (i.e., visual space). Interestingly, both late blind and sighted subjects were affected by such a conflict in localizing sounds or tactile stimuli. Conversely, the crossed-hands posture affected the early blind's performance only when required to detect auditory stimuli and not tactile ones. This is consistent with the view that early blind individuals do not automatically remap proprioceptive space into external coordinates, so that in the crossed-hands posture there is no conflict between these two spatial systems. Conversely, responding to sound positions with crossed hands requires an explicit matching of the external sound location with the anatomical coordinate of the responding hand for sending the correct motor command, thus explaining why the early blind are slower in this condition. This view is also supported by the finding that both late blind and sighted subjects were faster in bimodal than in unimodal conditions, suggesting that they combined audiotactile stimuli in an integrative way. Conversely, early blind subjects were faster in bimodal than in unimodal conditions only in the uncrossed-hands positions. These data indicate that audition and touch initially code space in different reference frames—external for audition and body-centered for touch. They also indicate that the early blind do not automatically remap tactile spatial representations into external spatial coordinates: the crossed-hands posture may induce a conflict between the auditory and tactile frames of reference, thus preventing efficient multisensory integration. Finally, the fact that early blind subjects do not make an automatic correspondence between a non-visual reference frame and a visual one could also explain why early blind participants were significantly faster than sighted controls in all experimental conditions apart from the crossed-hands bimodal condition.

Sighted individuals would by default activate an external spatial reference-frame system for sensory perception and action control even when the use of a modality-specific reference frame would be sufficient to perform a particular task: early blind individuals do not activate such representations and, in turn, they are faster in processing non-visual spatial information when such correspondence is not required to carry out the task. This hypothesis found support in other findings: Occelli et al. (Occelli, Spence, and Zampini 2008) reported stronger audiotactile interaction in the blind than in the sighted, in a task that required responding with the right and the left hand to tactile and auditory lateralized stimuli with subjects maintaining an uncrossed-hands posture. More specifically, in the study by Occelli and colleagues (Occelli, Spence, and Zampini 2008), pairs of auditory and tactile stimuli were presented on the left or right of participants at varying stimulus-onset asynchronies and subjects had to make temporal-order judgments regarding which sensory modality had been presented first on each trial. Critically, early and late blind subjects were more accurate when tactile and auditory stimuli were presented in different locations than from the same position, while this effect was not present in the sighted. According to Occelli et al. (Occelli, Spence, and Zampini 2008) these findings suggest that the absence of visual cues results in the emergence of more pronounced audiotactile *spatial* interactions.

Overall, the results discussed above indicate that the mapping of sensory inputs into external coordinates is not innate, but occurs as a consequence of visual input during ontogeny. Importantly, as noted by Hötting et al. (Hötting, Rösler, and Röder 2004; see also Collignon, Renier et al. 2006), reduced multisensory interactions in blind subjects could also be explained by enhanced skills of the blind in processing unimodal inputs (Hötting and Röder 2004; Hötting, Rösler, and Röder 2004).

3 The Relationship between Visual Perception, Imagery, and Cognitive Functions

For what is there so unreal and unheard of that we cannot form a mental picture of it? We even shape things which we have never seen—as the sites of towns and the faces of men. Then, by your theory, when I think of the walls of Babylon or of the face of Homer, some "phantom" of what I have in mind "strikes upon my brain"! Hence it is possible for us to know everything we wish to know, since there is nothing of which we cannot think.
—Cicero, *De divinatione*

3.1 *The Soul Never Thinks without a Mental Image . . .* or Does It?

Mental imagery is a familiar aspect of most individuals' mental lives, and is conceivable as a quasi-perceptual experience which occurs in the absence of actual stimuli for the relevant perception (cf. Finke and Freyd 1989; Rinck and Denis 2004). It has been demonstrated to be of critical importance in domains such as learning and memory (cf. Yates 1966; Paivio 1986), reasoning and problem solving (cf. Denis and Boucher 1991; Schwartz and Black 1996), inventive or creative thought (cf. LeBoutillier and Marks 2003 for a review), rehabilitation (for instance, with post-stroke patients: cf. Zimmermann-Schlatter, Schuster et al. 2008), and even for athletes' performances (cf. Hall, Mack et al. 1998; Fournier, Deremaux, and Berniera 2008). On the basis of functional analogies with the properties of visual perception, imagery has often been associated with sensory mechanisms or considered as an "interface" between sensorial and higher-level structures (Kosslyn 1980; Kosslyn and Ochsner 1994). As we will see in chapter 4, the relationship between imagery and perception—specifically, their functional analogies and the neural mechanisms that underlie both functions—has been broadly investigated in blind individuals. In fact, blindness offers the rare opportunity to study whether imagery abilities strictly depend on a normal visual experience or can develop in the absence of any visual input, and what this implies for the underlying cortical networks. In this chapter, we will illustrate the basic characteristics of imagery and its relationship to perception and other cognitive functions; and after reading this chapter, it should be clear why investigating imagery abilities in the blind is extremely important in order to get a better idea of how their cognition works, as well as to develop new training programs which support the blind in their everyday activities.

Ancient philosophers asserted that "the soul never thinks without a mental image" (Aristotle, *De anima*, 431a 15–20), and mental images were originally likened to impressions stamped on a wax block by perceptions and thoughts (cf. Plato, *Theatatus*, 191c–d) or pictures painted in the soul by an inner artist (Plato, *Philebus*, 39c). Nevertheless, the existence—or at least the functional importance—of mental images in cognitive life has been questioned many times since the rise of philosophy of mind and psychology. At the end of the nineteenth century, for instance, the eclectic scientist Francis Galton thought to have found an important exception to the common use of images in mental processes—namely, scientists. In fact, in describing his work on mental imagery, Galton (1880, 1883) claimed to have first carried out a pilot study with his "friends in the scientific world." He observed: "to my astonishment, I found that the great majority of the men of science to whom I first applied, protested that mental imagery was unknown to them. . . . They had no more notion of its true nature than a color-blind man who has not discerned his defect has of the nature of color" (Galton 1880, 302). However, he continued, when he used his questionnaire on individuals from "general society," they reported commonly experiencing visual imagery phenomena. On the basis of these results, Galton concluded that "scientific men as a class have feeble powers of visual representation. There is no doubt whatever on the latter point, however it may be accounted for" (Galton 1880, 304). Although Galton's conclusion here has been denied (cf. Brewer and Schommer-Aikins 2006), his studies yet demonstrate that individuals can differ enormously in how they experience and describe their mental images, with some describing images of photographic clarity, rich in detail, while others report very sketchy images, in which visual qualities are missing—or indeed, no images at all (Galton 1883).

One of the first "classical" empirical investigation on imagery processes was carried out in Edward B. Titchener's laboratory at Cornell University by one of his postgraduate students—a woman—the psychologist Cheves West Perky (Perky 1910). Basically, in Perky's experiment, participants had to stare fixedly at a point on a ground glass screen in front of them and "mentally" visualize various objects there (e.g., a blue book, a banana, a leaf, a lemon). Simultaneously, a faint patch of color—of an appropriate size and shape, and just above the normal threshold of visibility—was back-projected (in soft focus) onto the screen, without participants being advised of this. In almost all cases the observers reported images only after the illumination had been increased well above the threshold at which these stimuli were perceived by a control group of viewers (who were not asked to vividly imagine any objects). This was the case even if the projections unconsciously influenced their mental images as revealed by the fact that some subjects reported that what they eventually imagined did not entirely correspond to what they thought they were trying to imagine (for instance, a banana in an upright position rather than one lying on a horizontal plane). Perky's findings have been regarded as a type of visual *masking* by imaginary mental images, thus clearly suggesting that perception and imagery processes are inherently related.

A century after Perky's experiment, the interrelation between imagery and perception continues to attract the interest of researchers. For instance, in order to investigate the effects of imagery on perception, Pearson et al. (Pearson, Clifford, and Tong 2008) presented participants with a green vertical grating to the left eye and a red horizontal grating to the right eye and hypothesized that imagery would have altered the balance of competitive visual interactions, possibly facilitating the imagined pattern. In fact, in binocular rivalry paradigms, individuals are more likely to perceive a given pattern if the same pattern appeared dominant on the preceding trial: this effect is known as *perceptual stabilization* (i.e., the persistence of rivalry dominance across successive presentations), and is interpreted as reflecting the automatic formation of a sensory memory that facilitates subsequent perception (Leopold, Wilke et al. 2002; Pearson and Brascamp 2008). Pearson and colleagues (Pearson, Clifford, and Tong 2008) asked participants to imagine one of the two rivalry patterns during the interval between the presentation of the stimuli—either the pattern that resulted in being dominant, or the pattern that was suppressed on the preceding rivalry presentation. In this study, they found that imagery biased subsequent perception in favor of the imagined pattern (see figure 3.1). Interestingly, similar facilitatory effects were also obtained by presenting (instead of asking subjects to imagine) the pattern that was perceived as dominant, at 40 percent of its original luminance—that is, in a "weakened" perceptual form (Pearson, Clifford, and Tong 2008: experiment 2)—thus suggesting that imagery could be regarded as a "degraded" actual visual experience. Moreover, both longer periods of imagery and longer periods of actual (weakened) perception resulted in stronger facilitatory effects, further suggesting that prolonged mental imagery leads to the gradual accumulation of a perceptual trace resembling the effect of a weak perception. After this trace is formed, it can persist for short periods during which observers can also be actively engaged in another visual task, such as a letter-discrimination task (Pearson, Clifford, and Tong 2008: experiment 3).

These findings have been taken as compelling evidence that imagery is indeed "pictorial" (cf. Slotnick 2008). In fact, whether mental images have a pictorial format or not has been the object of the well-known *imagery debate* in which two main theoretical positions have been challenging each other over the last several decades: the *pictorial (or depictivist) theory* (Kosslyn 1973, 1980, 1994, 2006) and the *propositional (or descriptivist) theory* (Pylyshyn 1973,1981, 2003). It would take an entire book to describe these approaches in detail; still, it is worth giving at least a brief sketch of them here. According to the depictivist theory of mental imagery (cf. Kosslyn 1980, 1994, 2006), mental images consist in representational brain states that are genuinely

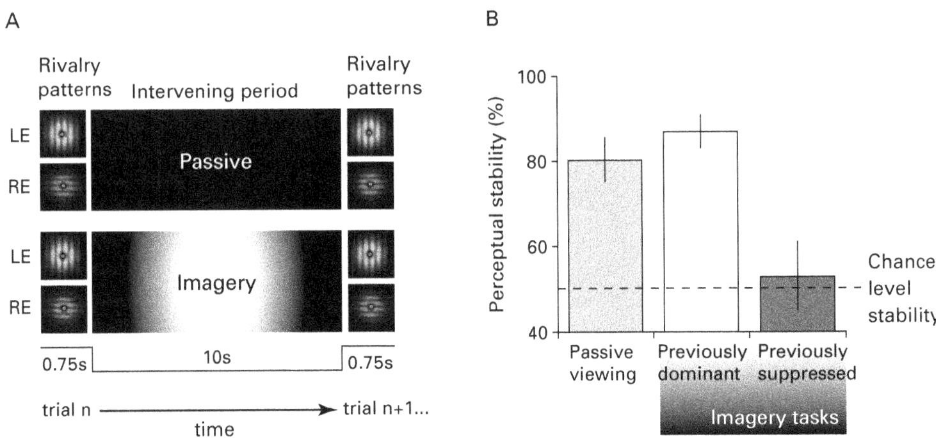

Figure 3.1

Effects of mental imagery on subsequent perceptual dominance in rivalry as investigated by Pearson, Clifford, and Tong (2008). (A) *Visual stimuli and timing of events.* A rivalry display was presented every 10.75 seconds (s), and observers reported which of the two rival patterns appeared dominant. During the 10 s blank interval following each presentation, observers were instructed either to maintain fixation passively or to imagine the pattern that was dominant or suppressed on the previous rivalry presentation. (B) *Results showing perceptual stability across successive rivalry presentations (N = 7).* Observers tended to perceive the same pattern across successive presentations during passive viewing (perceptual stability 80 percent, chance level 50 percent). Imagery led to significant changes in perceptual stability. Whereas imagery of the previously dominant pattern led to somewhat higher levels of perceptual stability than passive viewing, imagery of the previous suppressed pattern led to significantly lower levels of perceptual stability. Error bars represent ±1 SEM.

Reprinted from Pearson, Clifford, and Tong, "The functional impact of mental imagery on conscious perception," *Current Biology* 18 (13) (2008): 982–986. (© 2008. Reprinted by permission of Elsevier)

"picture-like." This position finds support in well-known experiments on mental rotation (Shepard and Metzler 1971; Shepard and Cooper 1982) and mental scanning (Kosslyn 1973, 1980). In particular, Shepard and Meztler (1971) measured subjects' reaction times in answering whether pairs of figures presented to them were the same or not. The pairs of figures varied in the degrees of rotation they differed by: results indicated that reaction time of the "same" pairs correlated with the angle of rotation for which the two objects differed. These results were explained by assuming that individuals imagine the pictures and mentally rotate them. Similarly, in mental scanning experiments, participants had to memorize particular maps or figures and were subsequently asked to mentally scan the pathway from one location to another of the map, pressing a button once the indicated destination point was reached (for a review, see Denis and Kosslyn 1999). The results demonstrated that shifting attention between different parts of the image required an amount of time directly proportional to the distance between the two indicated points, as if the participants were scanning a physical map with their eyes (cf. Kosslyn, Ball, and Reiser et al. 1978; see also Borst and Kosslyn 2008). On the basis of such findings, images in the mind were considered to be functionally equivalent to inner pictures, a sort of copy of previous sensory impressions. Notably, this would also be beneficial—according to supporters of the depictivist view—in an evolutionary perspective, since maintaining information in the form of an image (where a lot of information can be simultaneously combined) is more parsimonious than maintaining it in the form of a propositional description (Thompson, Kosslyn et al. 2008).

Conversely, on the descriptivist account of mental imagery (cf. Pylyshyn 1973, 1981, 2003), there is nothing specifically perceptual in the mental images' format: of course, mental images are real since they could be experienced as percept-like pictures, but they are an epiphenomenon since they are not indispensable for having a representation of a specific object or scene. Pylyshyn argues that reasoning with mental images activates the same processes and forms of representation as reasoning in general—that is, propositional representations consisting of an abstract symbolic system which can be used to express the contents of the mind via predicate calculus. According to this view of mental imagery, many phenomena cited in favor of the pictorial view can be accounted for by referring to the "tacit knowledge" that individuals have of the external world. In fact, according to Pylyshyn, "nearly all experimental findings cited in support of the picture theory can be more naturally explained by the hypothesis that when asked to imagine something, people ask themselves what it would be like to see it, and they then simulate as many aspects of this staged event as they can and as seem relevant. I refer to this explanation as the 'null hypothesis,' because it makes no assumptions about format—it appeals only to the tacit knowledge that people have about how things tend to happen in the world, together with certain basic psychophysical skills" (Pylyshyn 2003, 1). For instance, the stimulus-response compatibility effect—that is, the fact that individuals are usually slower in giving left-side responses to things appearing on their right side—has been reported also in mental images (Tlauka and McKenna 1998), supporting the view that mental representations have a strong spatial nature. However, according to Pylyshyn (2003), these findings do not necessarily call for the existence of picture-like representations in memory, but can be explained by assuming that what people do when they image something is to superimpose the mental image to the actual real space and hence use the real world's spatial properties as a "reference" for the generated mental image. According to Pylyshyn (2003), this is possible even when keeping the eyes closed by relying on the perception of space via other sensory modalities (e.g., proprioception, audition).

Yet the depictivist view is supported by many novel findings. For instance, Thompson, Kosslyn and colleagues (2008) have demonstrated that participants could re-explore mental images with the same ease as an actual visual percept when required to extrapolate a physical attribute of the (imagined or perceived) stimulus that was previously unnoticed. In particular, using alphabetic letters as stimuli, the authors first showed that most people tend to spontaneously report "explicit" attributes (such as the presence of a diagonal line) that are likely to be encoded in memory "by default." Conversely, other attributes (such as whether letters are symmetrical, or the presence of a triangle in the letter "A") appear to be more "implicit"—that is, they are less evident at first glance and have to be indirectly derived by reorganizing what has been encoded explicitly. Critically, Thompson et al. (Thompson, Kosslyn et al. 2008) found that naïve participants were able—when explicitly required by the experimenter—to report implicit properties with the same ease when the letters were perceived as when they were just imagined. These findings are in contrast with Pylyshyn's propositional or descriptivist theory, according to which longer reaction times should have been reported in the imagery condition compared to the perceptual condition as a result of the "computation" needed to derive less-evident properties (i.e., "implicit" attributes) from the more evident properties. Conversely, the results fit well with the depictivist account, and suggest that mental imagery makes implicit properties explicit and accessible much (if not just) as when individuals are actually exploring a picture in front of them.

From the examples described above, it should be evident that the imagery debate is far from being concluded. And maybe Pylyshyn is right when he claims that the issue about the format of mental images—in particular, "why do our mental images resemble what we are imagining?"—"might not have a scientific answer because it concerns the relation between brain processes and conscious experience—nothing less than the intractable mind-body problem" (Pylyshyn 2003, 117). Whatever the format of a mental image may be, in the next paragraphs and chapters we will discuss the importance of mental images in many different domains (from learning and memory to reasoning, problem solving, etc.). And furthermore, although attention has been mainly focused on *visual* imagery—hence the designation "pictorial"—imagery phenomena are also possible in other sensory modalities (i.e., auditory, olfactory, haptic). This is particularly important when considering the case of blind individuals (see chapter 4), whose mental representations are generated on the basis of non-visual sensory information.

3.2 Imagery in Cognitive Abilities

When considering studies on mental imagery, it is important to highlight that, within the last thirty years, imagery functions have been associated either to perceptual or to memory structures. In the previous section, we mainly discussed the idea that imagery is a "quasi-perceptual" experience that shares properties (and also neural structures, as we will see later in this chapter) with visual perception (see Kosslyn 1980, 1994). This approach focuses on the pictorial properties of mental images, and on the subjective experience of dealing with mental representations. However, images are also a critical *medium* for memory, reasoning, numerical and other cognitive functions. Baddeley and Hitch (1974; Baddeley 1986, 2007) proposed that we consider mental imagery as a peculiar function of the working memory network (see also Logie 1995; Cornoldi and Vecchi 2003).

Several tasks require the generation and processing of mental images and these functions can be interpreted within the visuo-spatial working memory system (VSWM): "The theoretical concept of working memory assumes that a limited capacity system, which temporarily maintains and stores information, supports human thought processes by providing an interface between perception, long-term memory and action" (Baddeley 2003, 829; for recent discussions of working memory see Baddeley 2007; Quinn 2008; Zimmer 2008).

In the multi-component model of working memory (WM), originally proposed by Baddeley and Hitch (1974), the adjective "working" was meant to emphasize the operational capacity of the system, contrary to previous models that tended to depict memory as simply having a "storage" character. In turn, WM came to be regarded as a system of critical importance not just in retaining and retrieving information, but also in mediating important cognitive functions such as reasoning, learning and comprehension. Baddeley (1986) proposed that visuo-spatial information is stored in a specialized subsystem, which has been further divided into separate components for *visual* and *spatial* information (cf. Logie 1995).

More recently, Baddeley (2007) proposed that VSWM can be functionally, and possibly anatomically, divided into three distinct components: a spatial, an object-based and a sequential component. This hypothesis is based on data coming from different traditions of research. Specifically, the distinction between spatial and object-based processes refers to the seminal work of Ungerleider and Mishkin (1982), who identified distinct visual pathways in monkeys, which are specialized in processing the identity of an object (the ventral pathway, also known as the "what" stream) and objects' spatial features (the dorsal pathway, also known as the "where" stream). A similar distinction was later observed in humans, by Farah and colleagues (Farah, Hammond et al. 1988) and many others (e.g., Luzzatti, Vecchi et al. 1998). Further, the distinction between sequential and simultaneous processes in VSWM has been proposed both to match a dissociation reported in verbal memory (see Pazzaglia and Cornoldi 1999; Mammarella, Cornoldi et al. 2006; Mammarella, Pazzaglia, and Cornoldi 2008) and to explain results obtained in visuo-spatial tasks tapping specific motor components (e.g., the Corsi task). Sequential motor processes within the VSWM system have also been postulated by Milner and Goodale (1995) to account for actions-memory, planning and execution. Each of these components has been separately investigated and further distinctions between sub-processes have been proposed. (See for example the definitions of visual characteristics such color, shape or texture—e.g., Logie 1995—or the distinction between categorical or coordinate spatial relationships—cf. Kosslyn 1994—or the nature of different motor actions such as reaching, grasping and so forth—cf. Goodale and Milner 1992; Jeannerod, Decety, and Michel 1994; Jeannerod, Arbib et al. 1995; Goodale, Westwood, and Milner 2004.) Overall, there is now strong converging evidence which indicates that the VSWM is a complex and articulated structure capable of linking perceptual and long-term memory information during the execution of different tasks. In fact, regardless of the different possible theoretical interpretations of the VSWM (cf. Cowan 1995; Logie 1995; Baddeley 2000; Cornoldi and Vecchi 2003; Barrouillet, Bernardin, and Camos 2004; Cowan 2005; Baddeley 2007; Vergauwe, Barrouillet, and Camos 2009), it is clear that cognitive processes such as learning, memory or reasoning do require that we "operatively" combine perceptual and long-term information: the working-memory system is likely to be the functional structure that allows for this.

Learning and Memory

The importance of mental images in learning and memory processes has been known for centuries, as is demonstrated by the use of mnemonic techniques already in ancient times (for research on imagery mnemonics, cf. Yates 1966; Bower 1972). According to a legend reported by Cicero (106–43 BCE), the Greek poet Simonides (ca. 556–ca. 468 BCE) first discovered the powerful mnemonic properties of imagery. As the story goes, Simonides was attending a banquet in Thessaly in order to present a lyric poem written in praise of the host. After his speech, Simonides was called outside and during his short absence the roof of the banqueting hall suddenly collapsed, killing all the guests inside. Simonides was able to identify the bodies of the dead guests (important for proper burial) on the basis of where they were found by retrieving from memory the visual image of the diners sitting around the banqueting table. From this tragic event, the legend suggests that Simonides inferred that forming an image, in which the to-be-remembered objects are linked to well-known places, is a very efficient way of improving memory, with the order of the places preserving the order of the things themselves (Cicero, *De oratore*, II). This technique was taken up in ancient rhetoric and became known as the *method of loci*. Described at greatest length by Roman rhetoricians such as Cicero and Quintilian (ca. 35–ca. 95 CE), this originally Greek technique was mainly employed by orators to retrieve the different passages of a speech in their proper order (Carruthers 1990, 1998; Small 1997; Rossi 2000). The common English phrases "in the first place," "in the second place," and so on are still reminisces of this technique. And the extraordinary abilities of George Koltanowski

(d. 2000), a famous chess player, in his version of the ancient exercise known as the Knight's Tour—in which a lone knight has to traverse an otherwise empty board visiting each square only once—can be regarded as a curious modern application of the method of loci. Before starting a performance, Koltanowski encouraged members of the audience to enter words and numbers into the squares of a large chalkboard divided into 64 cells (to mirror his board). After examining this chalkboard for a few minutes, Koltanowski would sit with his back to it and ask the audience to call out a square: making imaginary knight-moves through his re-entry sequence, Koltanowski was able to recite the contents of each square as the knight landed on it.

Going back to more scientific contexts, the dual coding theory of memory proposed by Allan Paivio (1971, 1986, 1991) represents a paradigmatic demonstration of the powerful mnemonic effects of imagery. According to Paivio, memory comprises two distinct (although interacting) systems with peculiar structural and functional properties. The first system consists of verbal representations and derives from language experience, whereas the second, the "imagistic" system, derives from perceptual experience. In Paivio's view, imagery facilitates recall of verbal material because, whenever a word evokes an associated image, two separate but linked memory traces, a verbal one and an iconic one, are retrieved. This explains why concrete words are usually more successfully recalled than abstract words: it is easier to associate a pictorial mental code with the former than with the latter (Paivio 1991). In fact, if all verbal stimuli initially activate a representation in a verbal/linguistic semantic system, concrete words, but not abstract words, may also activate information in a nonverbal imagistic system through referential connections to that system. Subsequent studies have extended investigations of language concreteness to sentences, paragraphs and texts of various lengths and contents, overall finding that concrete language is—according to Paivio's predictions—more imageable, comprehensible and easy to memorize than abstract language (e.g., Anderson, Goetz et al. 1977; Sadoski and Quast 1990; Sadoski, Paivio, and Goetz 1991; Sadoski, Goetz, and Rodriguez 2000; Sadoski and Paivio 2001, 2004). Interestingly, concrete, highly imageable words increase the likelihood of use of imagery as a strategy in the *production* of written definitions, leading also to definitions of higher quality (Goetz, Sadoski et al. 2007).

Blindfold chess, where the game is conducted without the players having sight of the positions of the pieces or any physical contact with them, is another paradigmatic example of how imagery can be used to support reasoning. Given that it seems to require extraordinary visuo-spatial abilities and memory, this form of chess has led to considerable research in psychology. In fact, in order to go ahead with the game, players have to maintain a mental representation of the positions of the pieces and moves are communicated via a recognized chess notation. One of the first psychological studies on the importance of mental imagery in blindfold chess dates back to 1894 by the French psychologist Alfred Binet (remembered as the inventor of the first modern intelligence test, the Binet–Simon intelligence scale). Binet hypothesized that chess-playing abilities might depend upon phenomenological qualities of the players' visual memory: to prove this idea, Binet assessed the ability of chess players to play while blindfolded, thus having to rely solely on memory. Binet discovered that only masters could play successfully in absence of vision, while the task proved impossible for amateur or intermediate players (Binet 1894). Overall, skilled players reported that they did not encode the physical features of the chess pieces and board (such as color or style of the pieces) but relied on a more abstract type of representation. These results suggest that the ability of blindfolded players seem to be mediated by *spatial* imagery more than *visual* imagery. In fact, replacing chess pieces with dots did not significantly affect memory performance for both masters and medium-class players, confirming abstract representation in blindfold chess (Saariluoma and Kalakoski 1998). These findings are critical in showing that spatial features are likely to be the structural elements characterizing mental images, as we will see many other times in this book.

Reasoning and Mental Models

Mental imagery and reasoning are strongly interconnected (e.g., De Soto, London, and Handel 1965; Kosslyn 1994). Reasoning means to make inferences about something, where an inference is a cognitive process in which new information is derived from given information. Two major theories have dominated the cognitive literature on deductive reasoning: on one hand, the *mental logic theory* assumes that deduction is underwritten by a system of (linguistic) rules sensitive to the logical form of the argument (Rips 1994), and on the other hand, the *mental model theory* assumes that a visuo-spatial representation of the argument is constructed and evaluated (Wason and Johnson-Laird 1972; Johnson-Laird 1983, 1994). According to the mental model's view, many problems can be solved in an analogical, "pictorial" format: in fact, a mental model can be conceived as a representation *isomorphic* to the physical situation that it represents and in which the inference processes simulate the physical processes being reasoned about (cf. Johnson-Laird 1998; Zwaan and Radvansky 1998). Imagery seems to be particularly critical in *relational reasoning*, in which the problem information is usually given by two statements which are called premises, and the task is to find a conclusion that necessarily follows from these premises. A typical hyper-simplified example of relational reasoning (or linear syllogism requiring a transitive inference) is: "A is taller than B"; "B is taller than C"; "Is C shorter than A?" (cf. Wason and Johnson-Laird 1972; Sternberg 1980). Several studies suggest that the entities of a relational reasoning problem can be represented as a mental image where the conclusion can then be "read off" by inspecting the image (cf. Vandierendonck, Dierckx, and De Vooght 2004; Goodwin and Johnson-Laird 2005). According to this approach, the information given in the premises is integrated in a single spatial representation, which usually takes the form of a linear array (for a review, see Evans, Newstead, and

Byrne 1993), generally left-to-right oriented as a result of a cultural bias in visual scanning (Bergen and Chang 2005; Spalek and Hammad 2005). As computational models suggest, the inspection process can be functionally described as a shift of a spatial focus that checks the various cells of the spatial array and infers from the scan-direction the relation between two objects in the array (Schlieder and Berendt 1998; Ragni, Knauff, and Nebel 2005). This type of representation can be used to derive novel conclusions or to check given conclusions even if the relation is temporal or abstract (Boroditsky 2000; Goodwin and Johnson-Laird 2005).

Although previous research found that reasoning is faster with problems that are easy to envisage than with problems that are hard to envisage (e.g., Shaver, Pierson, and Lang 1975; Clement and Falmagne 1986), other studies have failed to detect any effect of imageability on reasoning (cf. Newstead, Pollard, and Griggs 1986; Johnson-Laird, Byrne, and Tabossi 1989). These controversial results may be explained by considering the distinction between *visual imagery* and *spatial imagery* (Knauff and May 2006). *Visual imagery* refers to the representation of the visual appearance of an object, such as its shape, color or brightness, whereas *spatial imagery* refers to the representation of the spatial relationships between the parts of an object and the location of objects in space or their movement. According to Knauff and May (2006), *spatial* mental models are critical for reasoning while the generation of visual images can occur when the generation of the appropriate spatial mental model requires that we retrieve spatial information from a visual image: in these situations, additional processes come into play and can even impede the process of reasoning (Knauff and Johnson-Laird 2002). Hence, the "structure" of the reasoning process is likely made of spatially organized mental models that cannot be identified with visual images (cf. Farah, Hammond et al. 1988; Logie 1995).

Imagery is also extremely important in making mechanical inferences (for a review, see Hegarty 2004). Also in *mechanical reasoning*, the *spatial* aspects of the representation are the most critical, as is quite intuitive since mechanics is the science of motion and motion is a spatial property. Of course, mechanical reasoning is also possible by relying on descriptivist/propositional models, but inferences from spatial and descriptive representations involve different cognitive processes (Hegarty 2004). Inferences from spatial representations result from spatial transformations, such as mental rotation and translation. For instance, Hegarty (2004) makes the case of a person that has to infer the motion of the gears in a gear chain: he can do that by mentally rotating the successive gears (that is, by means of a mental simulation) or by referring to inference rules (e.g., "gears that mesh with each other turn in opposite directions"). Mental simulation in mechanical reasoning problems (such as this gear-motion one) seems to be the default strategy preferred by most individuals, where the inference processes are *analogous* to the physical processes that they simulate. Accordingly, a study by Schwartz and Black (1996) has shown that the time taken by participants in inferring the rate of rotation of two interlocking gears varied proportionally to the angle of rotation, thus suggesting that participants were relying on analogical representations. Nonetheless, mechanical simulation does not simply coincide with spatial mental imagery (Hegarty 2004), but also involves semantic knowledge (for instance, of the law of gravity) and verbal descriptions (many rules of mechanical reasoning can be easily verbalized; see Hegarty, Just, and Morrison 1988).

Mathematics and Numerical Cognition

Mental imagery is extremely important for learning and developing mathematic abilities and it has been suggested that all mathematical tasks require *spatial* thinking (Fennema 1979). Also in the case of mathematics, the distinction between spatial imagery and visual imagery is particularly critical (Hegarty and Kozhevnikov 1999; Kozhevnikov, Hegarty, and Mayer 2002). Similarly to Knauff and May's (2006) findings of imagery effects on reasoning, Hegarty and Kozhevnikov (1999) found that in sixth-grade students the use of schematic images (i.e., images that encode the spatial relations described in a problem) was positively related to success in mathematical problem solving, whereas the use of pictorial images (i.e., images that encode the visual appearance of objects or people) was negatively related to success in mathematical problem solving. Presmeg (see Presmeg 1986a,b,2006) has identified five types of visual imagery that students may use to solve mathematical problems: (a) concrete pictorial imagery, namely, pictures in the mind; (b) pattern imagery, that is, pure relationships depicted in a visual-spatial scheme; (c) kinesthetic imagery, which involves hand movement and other gestures; (d) dynamic imagery, which involves dynamic transformations of geometric figures; and (e) memory of formulas, wherein visualizers typically imagine a formula written on a blackboard or in their notebook. Presmeg (1986a,b 1992) argued that not all types of imagery can improve mathematical learning and performance: for instance, the use of concrete pictorial imagery may focus the reasoning on irrelevant details that distract the problem solver's attention from the main elements in the original problem representation. According to Presmeg (1997), pattern imagery (i.e., imagery where pure relationships are depicted in a visual-spatial scheme) is likely to be the most useful in mathematical reasoning because it shows the *relational* aspects of a problem, thus being better suited to abstraction and generalization (dynamic imagery is also quite effective, cf. Wheatley 1997). Data obtained with gifted students and with those affected by learning disabilities confirm this view. For instance, van Garderen (2006) found that gifted students performed better in spatial visualization tasks than students with learning disabilities and average-achieving students, and the use of schematic imagery in problem solving significantly and positively correlated with higher performance on each spatial visualization measure.

Numerical cognition also seems to be highly related to spatial imagery. A clear mapping between numbers and space has been reported in many studies: the so-called

SNARC effect (i.e., spatial numerical association of response codes) for instance refers to the tendency to respond faster with the left hand to relatively small numbers and faster with the right hand to relatively large numbers, and has been interpreted as an automatic association of spatial and numerical information, that is, as a congruency between the lateralized response—the left and right side of the egocentric space—and the relative position of the numbers on a left-to-right oriented spatial mental number line (Dehaene, Bossini, and Giraux 1993). The correspondence between numerical space and visuo-spatial space is well documented by experiments demonstrating that numbers can bias the allocation of visuo-spatial attention in different paradigms, such as in target detection or line bisection (see Fischer 2001; de Hevia, Girelli, and Vallar 2006; Cattaneo, Merabet et al. 2008).

Creative Thought, Motor and Skilled Performances

Mental imagery is known to have played an important role in the thinking of many great scientists (e.g., Ferguson 1977; Shepard 1978; Tweney, Doherty, and Mynatt 1981; Miller 1984); as, for instance, in Galvani's path of discovery of "animal electricity" (i.e., the electricity present in a condition of disequilibrium between the interior and the exterior of excitable animal fibers) (cf. Piccolino 2008). However, most of the available data are based on the self-reports of major figures in the history of science describing the role of imagery in their thinking, and not derived by systematic empirical studies. In fact, a meta-analytic review carried out by LeBoutillier and Marks (2003) has shown that imaging capacity may account for only 3 percent of the total variance in divergent thinking (i.e., creative thought) measures.

Mental imagery has also been widely investigated in the psychology of sport, where its use has been demonstrated to improve athletes' performances (see Smith and Wright 2008), and in skilled abilities training, such as medical practice (for instance, it is frequently used by surgeons when preparing to operate: Hall 2002; Sanders, Sadoski et al. 2008).

3.3 Beyond the Inner Mirror Approach

The seminal work of George Sperling (1960) on iconic memory originally demonstrated that the brain can store a large amount of visual information for a few hundred milliseconds. However, these immediate iconic memory traces, which depend upon a very recent visual experience and are thus very close to perceptual processes, should not be confused with mental images (for a review, see Cornoldi, De Beni et al. 1998). In fact, mental images often represent the output of top-down processes involving long-term memory; therefore, mental images are not just a derivate of perception but "could be fed into working memory through either perception or long-term memory" (Baddeley and Andrade 2000, 128). Indeed, this is quite intuitive since one can obviously mentally visualize a dog simply after reading the word "dog" or after hearing a dog barking (cf. Intons-Peterson 1996). However, some differences seem to exist between images generated on the basis of just-experienced stimuli or on the basis of information retrieved by long-term memory, as for instance demonstrated by Hitch et al. (Hitch, Brandimonte, and Walker 1995) in a "mental synthesis" experiment. Mental synthesis refers to a process by which individuals have to mentally manipulate and transform visual mental representations to produce new configurations or discover emerging properties. Hitch et al. (1995) required participants to mentally synthesize a pattern based on two sequentially presented line drawings, and found that although mental synthesis was also possible when elements were verbally rather than visually presented, mental visual images generated from visually presented stimuli maintained surface perceptual properties to a greater extent than images generated from verbal information. In fact, performance was impaired if the stimulus-background contrast was incongruent in the two drawings (that is, when one drawing was made of black lines on a white background and the other one of white lines on a black background), but only when mental synthesis was based on visual traces maintained in short-term memory. No effect of contrast congruity was reported when images had to be generated from long-term memory (Hitch, Brandimonte, and Walker 1995). Contrast—compared to shape—is considered a "surface" property: the fact that differences in contrast affected mental images generated from short-term memory but not from long-term memory suggests that representations from long-term memory have a more "schematic" or abstract nature (Hitch, Brandimonte, and Walker 1995). Similar results were obtained by Pearson and Logie (Pearson and Logie 2003/2004), who investigated the ability of combining alphanumeric and geometrical symbols, either verbally or visually presented in sequence, into meaningful images: in the sequential visual presentation condition, subjects were able to produce patterns with a significantly higher degree of mental transformation and manipulation than in the sequential verbal condition. According to Pearson and Logie (2003/2004), these findings support the view that although visual mental images can be generated from long-term memory in response to verbal cues, such images are cognitively different from those generated directly from visual traces. The process behind the generation of the mental image is also different: a visual presentation of the stimuli allows the generation of a visual mental image directly into the visuo-spatial working-memory system, while in the case of a verbal presentation of the symbols to be combined, images need first to be generated from long-term memory using verbal representations within the phonological loop (cf. Baddeley 2007; Pearson, Logie, and Gilhooly 1999). Accordingly, Cornoldi and colleagues (Cornoldi, De Beni et al. 1998) distinguished between visual traces and generated images on the basis of the degree of attentional requirements, voluntary manipulation, rehearsal mechanisms and capacity limitation associated to them.

Converging behavioral evidence supports this view. For instance, Borst and Kosslyn (2008) investigated whether information is represented in the same way either in a real visual percept, in an iconic image and in a mental image (i.e., involving long-term memory) of the same stimuli, using the mental scanning paradigm. The results showed that although the time to scan increasing distances increased at comparable rates in the three situations, when mental images were created from information stored in long-term memory, participants scanned more slowly compared to the other two conditions. Nevertheless, the rates of scanning in the perceptual task highly correlated with the rates of scanning in the imagery tasks. These results support the view that visual mental images and visually perceived stimuli are "structurally equivalent," that is, they are represented similarly and can be processed in the same way (Borst and Kosslyn 2008). However, when participants created the to-be-scanned image from long-term memory, the task was more difficult (as demonstrated by longer response time) than when the pattern was encoded immediately prior to generating the image. In a way, mental images generated on the basis of information stored in long-term memory (LTM) may be akin to degraded iconic images: slower scanning process with images generated from LTM would thus be justified by this difference in vividness between images generated from LTM that are likely to be degraded and those generated on the basis of perceptual input that has just been encoded. Also, mental images generated from LTM may be more fragmented than those generated on the basis of a just-seen stimulus, with part of the scanning process involving filling-in missing material (Borst and Kosslyn 2008).

A similar dissociation between images generated on the basis of a recent perceptual experience and images generated from long-term memory has been reported at the neurophysiological level. In particular, Moro et al. (Moro, Berlucchi et al. 2008) reported the case of two brain-damaged patients with a visual system apparently enabling a largely normal visual perception and including an anatomically intact primary visual cortex (V1), but with deficits at the imagery level. Interestingly, the visual imagery impairment in these patients was mostly restricted to an inability to generate mental visual images from semantic knowledge such as a detailed image of a dog upon hearing or reading the corresponding word. Conversely, the generation of visual images in response to visual inputs appeared to be spared. At a neurophysiological level—as we will better discuss later in this chapter—these findings can be accounted for by considering that visual perception (and possibly imagery for just-perceived items) is mediated by bottom-up mechanisms arising in early visual areas, whereas top-down influences from prefrontal cortex and superior parietal areas appear to be at play during imagery of the same items when these have to be retrieved from long-term memory (e.g., Mechelli, Price et al. 2004). What is important to stress here is that at the pure "representational" level, mental images are not exactly the same as iconic memory traces.

In fact, Kosslyn (1980, 1994) suggested that potential images are stored in long-term memory as "deep representations," structural descriptions not directly accessible to awareness, that are used to generate the actual depictive-analogical images in the "visual buffer." The process of generating a mental image may be exemplified by thinking of what happens in a computer graphic program: data are saved in particular files (analogous to the "deep representations" stored in LTM), on which basis visual pictures can then be generated on the computer screen. In the human cognitive system, the screen is the "visual buffer"; here information becomes available to consciousness and could be analyzed by the "mind's eye" function. From a different theoretical perspective, Logie (1995) hypothesized a major involvement of LTM in imagery processes and considered the visuo-spatial working-memory system —the "visuo-spatial sketchpad" in Baddeley's terms—as the underlying cognitive medium. The visual buffer or the VSWM are then the interfaces that support depictive representations: from here, signals are sent to areas that store visual memories with which the transmitted input is matched in order to be interpreted (for a more extensive discussion on Kosslyn' s and Logie's models, see Cornoldi and Vecchi 2003). Kosslyn (see Kosslyn, Shephard, and Thompson 2007) argues that visual perception should be conceived in terms of two phases: *early* visual processing relies solely on signals from the retina; *late* visual processing relies partially on information stored in LTM. According to Kosslyn (Kosslyn, Shephard, and Thompson 2007) visual mental imagery, which arises from stored knowledge in LTM, relies on the same mechanisms as late *visual* perception.

Moreover, when generating a mental image of an object from long-term memory, different types of image can be produced. Cornoldi et al. (Cornoldi, De Beni et al. 1989) suggested a taxonomy of mental images making a clear distinction between *general* and *specific* images. According to Cornoldi et al. (Cornoldi, De Beni et al. 1989), a general image can be regarded as a skeletal, basic and prototypical representation of an object; conversely, a specific image refers to a visual representation of a particular exemplar of an object with its distinctive details. Different neuronal pathways support the generation of general and specific mental images (cf. Gardini, De Beni et al. 2005; Gardini, Cornoldi et al. 2009; for a discussion see later in this chapter).

The hypothesis of a mental image as a sort of "weakened" perception is particularly intriguing when considering the case of individuals affected by a partial visual impairment (i.e., low vision, see chapter 6). Are visually impaired individuals' mental images more degraded than those of normally sighted individuals? That is to say, are differences in mental imagery abilities just a matter of "degree"? These questions will be considered later in the book. What matters here is that, regardless of the difference in visual quality (vividness, presence of detailed surface attributes, etc.) of the images generated from long-term memory or from recent visual percepts, the reported findings seem to converge in suggesting that image representations "depict" information. In the next section we will discuss similarities and differences between visual imagery and visual perception from a neuropsychological and neurophysiological perspective.

3.4 Imagery and Perception: Where in the Brain?

It is generally accepted that there is a degree of modularity in brain organization; hence, some brain regions are involved in processing language, others are specialized for processing of visual and spatial information and so forth. One critical issue concerns whether the same brain areas that are involved in perceptual processing are also involved in imagery (this issue being especially important when considering individuals who lack all visual experience). The parallelism between visual perception and visual imagery likely becomes clearer if one considers that perception is itself a sort of *predictive hypothesis* entailing many stages of physiological signaling and complicated cognitive computing, and is therefore only *indirectly* related to external reality (Gregory 1980, 1981). In the following paragraphs, we will briefly see how visual information is processed by the brain and how the cortical networks devoted to process perceptual information also subserve (at least to a certain extent) imagery processes.

Information Processing in the Visual Cortex

The majority of fibers in the optic nerve converge—after passing through the lateral geniculate nucleus of the thalamus—in the primary visual cortex (or V1, also called "striate cortex" because of the distinctive stripes it bears). The primary visual cortex has been shown to contain a retinotopic map of the world in which each point is represented by neurons with specialized receptive fields that encode basic visual features, such as orientation of light bars or edges (cf. Felleman and Van Essen 1991). Initially, the visual system was considered to be a hierarchically organized system, with V1 basically having the merely "passive" function of extracting information from the retinal image, while successive levels were thought to subserve progressively higher functions. Recently though, the understanding of the neuronal mechanisms underlying vision has changed from a passive role of the analysis of the retinal image to one of inference and the construction of constancy (see Kennedy and Burkhalter 2004). In fact, there is increasing agreement that the visual system is a dynamic one in which the individual stations are involved together in a computational process directed at determining the probabilities of feature combinations in the visual environment (cf. Zeki 1993; Young 2000). Once basic processing has occurred in V1, the visual signal enters the other higher cortical areas generally referred to as extrastriate areas. At this level, the visual brain is highly functionally specialized (cf. Livingstone and Hubel 1988; Zeki, Watson et al. 1991; Zeki 2008): for instance, the color system (area V4) and the visual motion system (area MT/V5) occupy distinct locations in the visual cortex (e.g., Wade, Brewer et al. 2002). Extrastriate areas also perform the two broad tasks of perceiving "what" forms are in the visual image and "where" objects are in space. In particular, the occipito-temporal pathway (ventral or "what" stream) is specialized in object recognition, and the occipito-parietal pathway (dorsal or "where" stream) is devoted to processing spatial features and is important in motion-coding related to the control of action (Ungerleider and Mishkin 1982; Goodale, Meenan et al. 1994; Milner and Goodale 1995). Together, through simultaneous activity, these cortical networks allow us to very quickly see, understand and respond to an enormous range of visual scenes. "Chronoarchitectonic" maps of the human cerebral cortex generated when subjects view complex scenes have also been identified (cf. Bartels and Zeki 2004): for instance, it has been demonstrated that color is perceived before motion by around 80 ms, and locations are perceived before colors (Pisella, Arzi, and Rossetti 1998); further, colors are perceived before orientations (Moutoussis and Zeki 1997).

Moreover, the physiology of the visual system is increasingly interpreted in terms of feedforward (i.e., from the thalamus to the cortex) and feedback (i.e., cortico-cortical connections) mechanisms underlying the hierarchical organization of the cortex (cf. Felleman and Van Essen 1991; Shao and Burkhalter 1996; Lamme and Roelfsema 2000). Hence, visual perception results from both bottom-up and top-down processes. Feedforward inputs terminate principally in layer 4 of the visual cortex in a topographically organized fashion (cf. Price, Ferrer et al. 1994). Pathways leading from higher to lower areas are provided by feedback connections—estimated to be at least as numerous as the feedforward connections (cf. Kennedy and Burkhalter 2004)—that terminate outside layer 4 and distribute their outputs over more extensive parts of the visuotopic map than do feedforward connections (cf. Perkel, Bullier, and Kennedy 1986). The physiological role of feedback connections has been traditionally studied by reversible cooling of higher cortical areas and by recording the cooling-induced effects on neuronal response in lower areas: using this technique it has been discovered, for instance, that feedback inputs from both V3 and V2 to V1 facilitate responses to stimuli moving within the classical receptive field (Sandell and Schiller 1982). More recently, studies using transcranial magnetic stimulation have shown that the fronto-parietal network exerts top-down modulation on visual cortical activity, as demonstrated for instance by the finding that stimulation of the frontal eye fields increased the excitability of the visual cortex (Silvanto, Lavie, and Walsh 2006; see also Ruff, Blankenburg et al. 2006; Ruff, Kristjánsson, and Driver 2007; Taylor, Nobre, and Rushworth 2007; Silvanto, Muggleton, and Walsh 2008). Feedback connections are likely to mediate top-down influence that results from attention, memory retrieval and imagery (cf. Motter 1994; Ishai and Sagi 1995; McAdams and Maunsell 2000; Chelazzi, Miller et al. 2001; Naya, Yoshida, and Miyashita 2001). Top-down influences are likely to be involved in processing a large variety of categories, including features, surfaces, objects, object categories, temporal context and virtually any other perceptual group (see Gilbert and Sigman 2007 for a recent review). Similarly, early visual areas in the ventral stream are likely to be involved not only in lower-level visual processing, but also in higher-level cognitive processing with a later time course (e.g., Lamme and Roelfsema 2000), where this late engagement is likely to be exerted by top-down reactivation onto low-level visual areas by more anterior temporal and prefrontal areas (over an extended processing time). Hence, the process of "seeing" should be conceived as an active process in which top-down mechanisms are constantly at play (see also Findlay and Gilchrist 2003).

The Neural Bases of Imagery

Neuroimaging techniques (such as PET and fMRI) and non-invasive brain techniques (such as TMS) offer critical contributions to the understanding of the brain circuits involved in imagery processes. In particular, functional connectivity analyses in fMRI allow us to look at the interplay within and across the widely distributed cortical networks of activated brain regions, and new paradigms combining different techniques may help to clarify the similarities between cortical activations that subtend perception and imagery.

Several neuroimaging studies have reported that visual imagery is associated with activity in striate and extrastriate cortices (for reviews, see Kosslyn, Ganis, and Thompson 2001; Kosslyn and Thompson 2003), and there is evidence for a positive correlation between visual cortex activity and vividness of visual imagery (Amedi, Malach, and Pascual-Leone 2005; Cui, Jeter et al. 2007). By stimulating the occipital cortex with repetitive transcranial magnetic stimulation (rTMS), which can temporarily interfere with local cortical processing, Kosslyn et al. (Kosslyn, Pascual-Leone et al. 1999) found impaired performance on a visual imagery task. These results showed that activity in the occipital cortex is not epiphenomenal during visual mental imagery, but rather plays a critical functional role. Similarly, Sparing et al. (Sparing, Mottaghy et al. 2002) showed, using the phosphenes threshold as an indicator of visual cortical excitability, that visual imagery increases excitability of early visual cortical neurons involved in the imagery task. Specifically, visual imagery decreased the intensity of TMS required for phosphene induction when the imagined stimulus spatially overlapped with the phosphene. Yi et al. (Yi, Turk-Browne et al. 2008) have combined the adaptation paradigm with fMRI to investigate imagery impact on perception. In fMRI context, adaptation (or repetition suppression) refers to the reduced BOLD signal observed for repeated as opposed to novel stimuli, which is believed to reflect the sharpening of perceptual representations with experience or a reduction in the visual processing that is necessary for object identification (Desimone 1996; Wiggs and Martin 1998; Grill-Spector, Henson, and Martin 2006). Using this paradigm, Yi et al.

(Yi, Turk-Browne et al. 2008) found that briefly mentally visualizing a recent perceptual stimulus was comparable to seeing it again, suggesting that the same population of neurons in the inferior temporal cortex is responsible for both bottom-up and top-down object representations (cf. Kosslyn 1994).

Notably, activation of visual brain regions by imagery processes seems to be object-category specific: in fact, perceptual-specific areas were activated when participants imagined faces, houses or chairs (Chao, Martin, and Haxby 1999; Ishai, Ungerleider et al. 1999; Ishai, Ungerleider, and Haxby 2000; O'Craven and Kanwisher 2000; Ishai, Haxby, and Ungerleider 2002; Mechelli, Price et al. 2004). Similarly, Goebel et al. (Goebel, Khorram-Sefat et al. 1998) found activity in perceptual motion area MT/V5 when participants were required to imagine movements. Notably, the spatial extent of the imagined objects has been found to match the known spatial organization of early visual areas, with objects that subtend smaller visual angles producing activity near the occipital pole (where stimuli falling in the central visual field are represented), and objects that subtend larger visual angles inducing more anterior activity (where stimuli falling in the peripheral visual field are represented) (cf. Kosslyn, LeSueur et al. 1993; Kosslyn, Thompson et al. 1995; Tootell, Mendola et al. 1998).

Although most of the available studies have been carried out on visual imagery, partially overlapping networks for perception and imagery have also been reported for tactile, auditory, olfactory, gustatory and motor imagery (see Jeannerod, Arbib et al. 1995; Kosslyn, Ganis, and Thompson 2001; Kobayashi, Takeda et al. 2004; Stevenson and Case 2005; Goyal, Hansen, and Blakemore 2006). For instance, auditory imagery of a simple monotone-induced bilateral activation in the primary and secondary auditory areas (Yoo, Lee, and Choi 2001), and tactile imagery of gentle brushing of the hand activated part of the primary and secondary somatosensory that were also active during actual tactile stimulation (Yoo, Freeman et al. 2003). Motor imagery has been found to activate the supplementary motor area and the premotor cortex (Dechent, Merboldt, and Frahm 2004), and notably, olfactory imagery has also been found to be accompanied by similar brain activations as actual odor sensation, though once more to a lesser extent (Stevenson and Case 2005).

In fact, the overlap between cortical networks subtending perception and those mediating imagery is not complete, as suggested by studies with brain-damaged patients. For instance, Moro et al. (Moro, Berlucchi et al. 2008) reported the case of two patients with a severely disordered ability for generating and using visual images but with a visual system apparently enabling normal visual perception and including an anatomically intact primary visual cortex (V1). Bartolomeo et al. (Bartolomeo, Bachoud-Lévi et al. 1998) reported the case of a young woman with bilateral brain lesions in the temporo-occipital cortex with impaired object recognition, reading, color and face processing but with a perfectly preserved imagery for the same visual entities (see also Chatterjee and Southwood 1995; Goldenberg, Müllbacher, and

Nowak 1995). According to Kosslyn (Kosslyn 1994), the similar cortical activation observed during visual imagery and perception reflects the fact that—at the functional level—they both share the same structure, that is the "visual buffer." Visual mental images would derive from top-down activation of early visual cortices from more anterior areas; in other words, imagery would result from memory retrieval through the "re-activation" of the same cortical areas that had processed the relevant information during perception. Such a reactivation mechanism of visual cortices by means of top-down projections from other cortical areas explains why patients with lesions in the temporal areas but relatively spared early visual areas are still able to perform imagery tasks (see Bartolomeo, Bachoud-Lévi et al. 1998). Accordingly, traumatic brain injuries, like those suffered by the patients in Moro et al. (Moro, Berlucchi et al. 2008), typically provoke diffuse axonal injury, which is likely to disrupt large-scale brain networks extending beyond early visual cortices that are nonetheless involved in imagery processes. In this regard, it is worth noting that it is a controversial question whether visual imagery activates primary visual cortices (V1) or only extrastriate areas. Slotnick and colleagues (Slotnick, Thompson, and Kosslyn 2005) reported that a high-resolution visual mental imagery task evoked topographically organized activity in the extrastriate cortex, but activated striate cortex in only half of participants. According to a meta-analysis of imagery studies carried out by Kosslyn and Thompson (2003) two task variables, in addition to the use of a sensitive technique, can predict whether early visual areas are activated during visual mental imagery: first, the imagery task has to require that subjects visualize shapes with high resolution (with details subtending 1 degree of visual angle or less); and second, the task does not have to rely on the processing of purely spatial relations.

Moreover, fMRI findings supporting a perfect parallelism between perception and imagery should be interpreted with caution. In fact, because of the scarce temporal resolution of neuroimaging techniques based on hemodynamic signals, fMRI data cannot conclusively determine whether the effects of visual mental imagery observed in perceptual processing areas actually reflect early perceptual processes, as opposed to later processes, also taking place in these same cortical areas (cf. Lamme and Roelfsema 2000; Ganis and Schendan 2008). Moreover, the same neural populations may exhibit the same average activation but be in different functional states, due to their participation in different processes (Gilbert and Sigman 2007; Schendan and Kutas 2007). In other words, the fact that the same area is active in two situations doesn't automatically imply that the process going on in the two cases is identical. Luckily, part of these problems may be overcome by combining different paradigms. For instance, different functional states can be revealed by using an adaptation paradigm and measuring how a specific neural population responds to subsequent probe stimuli; in such paradigms, adaptation effects can be determined as the difference between the response elicited by non-adapted and by adapted stimuli. Combining

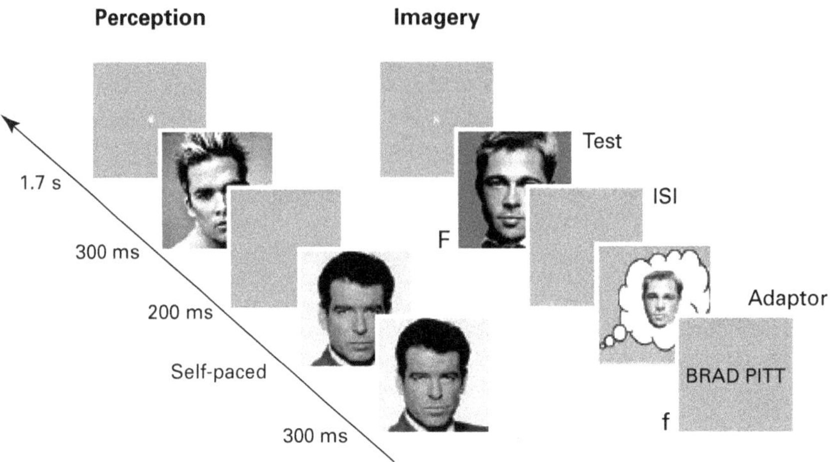

Figure 3.2
Diagram of an experimental trial for the visual mental imagery and perception conditions used by Ganis and Schendan (2008). Perception and imagery trials had a parallel structure. In the perception trials, left side of the figure, an adaptor face was perceived and subjects pressed a key as soon as they recognized it. The test face appeared 200 ms after the key-press. In the imagery trials, right side of the figure, an appropriate face (the adaptor) was visualized upon seeing the corresponding word (which was on the screen for 300 ms). Subjects pressed a key as soon as they had generated a vivid mental image, and the test face appeared 200 ms after this key-press, as in the perception trials. There was no task on the test faces.
Reprinted from Ganis and Schendan, "Visual mental imagery and perception produce opposite adaptation effects on early brain potentials," *NeuroImage* 42 (4) (2008): 1714–1727. (© 2008. Reprinted by permission of Elsevier)

adaptation with ERPs recording, Ganis and Schendan (2008) have measured neural adaptation effects on face-processing induced by visual mental imagery and visual perception (see figure 3.2). Their aim was to investigate whether the visual mental imagery of faces activated similar neural populations as the perceptual categorization of faces, and whether the "functional" effect of engaging these neural populations was the same in both cases. Ganis and Schendan (2008) found similar responses in the N170/VPP complex (where N170 and VPP are potentials elicited in ventrolateral temporal regions by faces peaking between 140 and 200 ms post-stimulus and considered as an index of the perceptual categorization of faces; cf. Schendan, Ganis, and Kutas 1998) both when real faces and imagined faces were used as "adaptors." Hence, visual mental imagery of faces recruited the same general neural populations in the ventral stream that were activated during early face perception (e.g., the fusiform gyrus, extending into the inferior, middle, and superior temporal gyri and into the middle occipital gyrus), and with a similar time-course. However, a difference was observed between the perceptual and the imagery condition: whereas perceived faces induced a reduction in the amplitude of the N170/VPP complex, an established effect depending on neural fatigue or on synaptic depression (see for reviews, Kourtzi and Grill-Spector 2005; Grill-Spector, Henson, and Martin 2006), imagined faces determined an enhancement of the amplitude of the N170/VPP complex. According to Ganis and Shendan (2008), the enhancement effects found in the imagery condition reflected the mechanism of working memory necessary to maintain infero-temporal neural representations active over time by means of top-down signals, possibly originating in the prefrontal cortex (Miller, Erickson, and Desimone 1996; Tomita, Ohbayashi et al. 1999). In summary, Ganis and Shendan's (2008) findings indicate that perceived adaptors influenced neural populations that support early perceptual processing of faces by means of *bottom-up* mechanisms, whereas imagined faces influenced these same neural populations *but* via *top-down* mechanisms. Interestingly, these findings may also clarify why the brain does not routinely confuse visual percept and visual mental images, even though both engage similar neural populations in the visual system (Ganis and Schendan 2008).

A study by Amedi et al. (Amedi, Malach, and Pascual-Leone 2005) in which the negative BOLD signal was considered and functional connectivity analyses were performed, adds supports to the view that a similar level of activation in the same visual areas during visual perception and visual imagery does not necessarily reflect identical processes. They demonstrated that if it is true that most brain areas that are activated during visual imagery are also activated by the visual perception of the same objects, the two conditions are significantly different in their brain-deactivation profile as measured by negative BOLD. In fact, in early auditory areas there was a minimal response to perception of visual objects whereas the authors observed a robust deactivation during visual imagery. Amedi et al. (Amedi, Malach, and Pascual-Leone 2005) explained these results by arguing that perception of the world is a multisensory experience in which seeing is inextricably associated with the processing of other sensory modalities that modify visual cortical activity and shape experience (for reviews see Stein, Meredith, and Wallace 1993; Pascual-Leone, Amedi et al. 2005). Conversely, when a purely visual image has to be generated and maintained, cortical areas processing sensory inputs that could potentially disrupt the image created by the mind's eye are deactivated. Hence, pure visual imagery corresponds to the isolated activation of visual cortical areas with concurrent deactivation of irrelevant sensory processing that could disrupt imagery processes.

Overall, these findings are extremely critical when thinking about imagery abilities in the blind. In fact, peripheral blindness only affects the eye (or the optic nerve), whereas visual cortical regions are virtually intact. Hence, if imagery is the result of a top-down process, in which fronto-parietal areas activate visual cortices, one may expect the same mechanisms to occur in blind subjects. What this implies for the imagery experience of blind subjects (e.g., do they experience visual imagery?) will be specifically discussed later in this book (see in particular chapters 4 and 8).

Neural Correlates of Visual and Spatial Imagery

Cognitive neuroscience studies (e.g., Farah, Hammond et al. 1988) have demonstrated that following brain lesions, patients can be extremely impaired in tasks tapping visual aspects of imagery while showing normal performance in tests of spatial imagery. The neural correlates of spatial imagery have been widely investigated, overall showing that bilateral fronto-parietal networks activated by perceptual visuo-spatial tasks also underlie the spatial analysis of mentally imagined objects (Kosslyn, LeSueur et al. 1993; Cohen, Kosslyn et al. 1996; Mellet, Tzourio et al. 1996; Kosslyn, DiGirolamo et al. 1998; Trojano, Grossi et al. 2000; Lamm, Windischberger et al. 2001). In particular, many studies have reported activity in the parietal cortex, and specifically in the intraparietal sulcus, during spatial imagery. For instance, in a task requiring subjects to imagine an analogical clock showing specific times on the basis of verbal instructions, and to judge which of two clocks had the larger angle between its hands, IPS was specifically active (Trojano, Grossi et al. 2002). In a meta-analysis carried out on thirty-two neuroimaging studies investigating the neural correlates of mental rotation, Zacks (2008) reported that mental rotation is usually accompanied by increased activity in IPS and adjacent regions, and that the amount of activation in these regions is consistently related to the amount of mental rotation required by each specific task. Interestingly, using effective brain connectivity analysis, it has been possible to identify the time-course of the involvement of the fronto-parietal network subtending spatial imagery (Sack, Jacobs et al. 2008). In Sack's study, participants were asked to "on-line" construct and spatially transform a visual mental object purely based on a sequence of six either acoustically or visually presented spatial instructions. Analyses showed that this task involved a series of sub-processes, starting with the convergence of information from modality-dependent sensory pathways to modality-independent fronto-parietal network, the online processing of sequentially presented modality-independent spatial instructions, the construction of a stepwise emerging final mental object and the spatial analysis of its content and, finally, the maintenance of the spatially rotated mental object in short-term memory and the preparation of motor response. Importantly, according to Sack et al. (Sack, Jacobs et al. 2008), the information upcoming from modality-specific sensory brain regions is first sent to the premotor cortex and then to the medial dorsal parietal cortex, indicating that the activation flow processes the construction and spatial transformation of visual mental images in a top-down manner from the motor to the perceptual pole of spatial imagery.

Interestingly, different patterns of cortical activation have been observed for *general* images and *specific* images (Gardini, Cornoldi et al. 2009). In particular, Gardini et al.

found that specific images took less time to be produced in response to word-stimuli if they had been preceded by the generation of a general image, suggesting that the process of mental image-generation proceeds in a sequential manner, starting from the retrieval of just enough basic knowledge to produce a blurred skeletal representation of a given object, which can be successively filled in with the required visual details to mentally visualize a specific exemplar (cf. Cornoldi, De Beni et al. 1989). Accordingly, different cortical activation patterns accompanied the generation of general and specific images: general images activated a set of bilaterally distributed regions involving the frontal, parietal and occipital areas (including the associative visual areas), whereas specific images activated the frontal cortex and the medial dorsal nucleus of the thalamus. Hence, the process of generating general mental images requires both the retrieval of conceptual knowledge mediated by the left temporo-frontal areas, and the retrieval of definite visual features through areas involved in processing visuo-spatial information, such as the precuneus (whose involvement in visuo-spatial imagery has been previously reported, see Maguire and Cipolotti 1998; Burgess, Maguire et al. 2001). In contrast, the generation of specific mental images is mediated by those brain regions which are responsible for attention to visual details, including the thalamus (cf. LaBerge 2000). Overall, these findings support previous behavioral data that the generation of different types of image relies on distinct cognitive mechanisms.

As we will see in the following chapters, the distinction between visual/specific and spatial/general images is a decisive aspect to consider when discussing the nature of mental images in blind individuals.

4 Imagery and Working Memory Processes in the Blind

For then my thoughts, from far where I abide,
Intend a zealous pilgrimage to thee,
And keep my drooping eyelids open wide,
Looking on darkness which the blind do see:
Save that my soul's imaginary sight
Presents thy shadow to my sightless view,
Which, like a jewel hung in ghastly night,
Makes black night beauteous, and her old face new.
—Shakespeare, *Midsummer Night's Dream*

4.1 Imagery Capacity in Blind Individuals

In chapter 3 we broadly discussed the relationship between visual perception and mental imagery, and the role played by imagery processes in many cognitive abilities. In this chapter we review studies that have investigated imagery abilities in blind individuals. Although mental images can be generated on the basis of multiple sensory inputs (e.g., Halpern and Zatorre 1999; Levy, Henkin et al. 1999), visual aspects are believed to play a major role in mediating cognitive processing in sighted individuals. Conversely, one may intuitively hypothesize that the mental world of blind individuals is purely "propositional," essentially based on abstract and semantic, language-mediated representations. According to this view, blind individuals would suffer of certain representational deficits that would make it harder for them to perform imagery tasks compared to sighted individuals (e.g., Zimler and Keenan 1983). Nevertheless, the assumption that the blind use abstract semantic representations in executing visuo-spatial tasks has not been supported by the evidence of blind individuals' performance of tasks that are widely held to involve *analogical* representations, such as mental rotation or mental scanning.

In fact, converging evidence suggests that congenitally blind individuals are able to generate and manipulate mental images in an analogical format, on the basis of haptic or verbal information or long-term memory (Kerr 1983; Arditi, Holtzman, and Kosslyn 1988; Klatzky, Loomis et al. 1990; Carreiras and Codina 1992; Vecchi, Monticellai, and Cornoldi 1995; Thinus-Blanc and Gaunet 1997; Vecchi 1998; Aleman, van Lee et al. 2001; Kaski 2002; Bertolo, Paiva et al. 2003; Vanlierde and Wanet-Defalque 2004; Vecchi, Tinti, and Cornoldi 2004; Tinti, Adenzato et al. 2006; Afonso, Blum et al. 2010; Cattaneo, Fantino et al 2010a). These findings sound less paradoxical if one regards mental images as the end product of a series of generation processes (e.g., Cornoldi, De Beni et al. 1998), rather than as mere perceptual traces. In fact, if some low-level images are the immediate result of a recent visual experience (visual traces) or of an automatic retrieval of a simple standard representation (possibly related to earlier generation processes), other high-level images involve complex cognitive processes and make use of different sources of information (haptic, auditory, semantic) (Cornoldi, De Beni et al. 1998; Eardley and Pring 2006). In this perspective, blind and sighted people's mental images would differ only in terms of the degree to which specific visual knowledge and processes are involved. Interestingly, some authors have also hypothesized that *visual* imagery is indeed possible in blind individuals, as the result of the activation of the visual cortex by non-visual inputs (cf. Bertolo, Paiva et al. 2003). Congenitally blind people cannot generate mental images on the basis of visual percepts; however, there are several "visual" characteristics—such as shape or texture—that can be easily perceived through touch and reproduced in an internal picture. The "visual" nature of mental images in the blind is still a matter of debate: on the one hand, visual and spatial features are highly interconnected and it has been suggested that blind individuals can even represent visual features such as colors in their mental representations (cf. Marmor 1978). On the other hand, the possible visual content of blind individuals' mental representations is hardly investigable, being extremely difficult to rule out the role played by semantic and linguistic processes.

Overall, blind individuals show some selective limitations in imagery tasks. These limitations have been interpreted both in terms of a "representational" deficit (see above, e.g., Zimler and Keenan 1983) and/or in terms of "operational/processing" deficits (e.g., Vecchi, Monticellai, and Cornoldi 1995; Vecchi 1998; Vecchi, Tinti, and Cornoldi 2004). According to the processing account, blind individuals' limitations in certain visuo-spatial tasks are likely to derive from deficits in their processes of generating, updating and manipulating a representation, and not from deficits in the very format of their representations. In the next paragraphs we will report results of studies that show how blind individuals are able to produce analog and vivid mental representations, although suffering from some representational and processing limitations. In particular, we will see how haptic perception, depending on sequential inputs from scanning movements, heavily affects the way information is mentally represented in blind individuals (see Cattaneo, Vecchi et al. 2008 for a review).

Imagery can be considered as a peculiar function of the working-memory system. According to the original model proposed by Baddeley (Baddeley 1986), WM refers to a multiple-component structure that can both temporarily retain and simultaneously process a limited amount of information, thus allowing the execution of a range of quotidian activities such as mental calculation, reading, decision making or comprehension (Baddeley 1986). In this chapter we will also discuss how blindness affects these different cognitive domains. In particular, the WM capacities of blind individuals will be considered, and evidence will be discussed showing that some WM processes develop normally even in the absence of vision, whereas others are critically affected by congenital blindness (see Cornoldi, Cortesi, and Preti 1991; Cornoldi, Bertuccelli et al. 1993; Vecchi, Monticellai, and Cornoldi 1995; Vecchi 1998; Cornoldi and Vecchi 2003; Vecchi, Tinti, and Cornoldi 2004).

4.2. Blind Individuals' Mental Images: Representational Format

Converging evidence suggests that blind individuals can experience mental images which are rich in sensory detail and that can be proficiently used to improve the recall of information from memory. Here we report evidence regarding the representational format of the mental images generated by blind individuals.

Images and Memory

In a study investigating autobiographical memories in sighted and blind individuals, Ogden and Barker (2001) observed that early blind participants reported only tactile, auditory and spatial features in their memories (with no reference to visual details), whereas sighted participants reported mainly visual details. Interestingly, late blind subjects reported predominantly visual features for childhood memories, and auditory, tactile and spatial features for more recent memories. Critically, when interviewed about the dominant imagery modality they were relying on currently and about the mental format of their dreams, the majority of the late blind as well as sighted subjects nominated visual imagery. In fact, consistent behavioral and neuropsychological evidence with normally sighted individuals suggests that visual imagery is critical to autobiographical memory functions (cf., Conway and Pleydell-Pearce 2000; Greenberg and Rubin 2003), whereas auditory, tactile, olfactory, gustatory or motor cues only play a minor role (see Williams, Healy, and Ellis 1999). Nonetheless, a series of experiments carried out by Linda Pring and colleagues suggests that blind and sighted individuals may use similar processes for autobiographical memory-generation. In fact, Pring and Goddard (2003) did not find any deficit in congenitally blind adults in memory specificity or retrieval time in either a cue-word task (in which positive emotional, negative emotional and neutral words were used as cues) or in semi-structured autobiographical memory interviews. In particular, high-imagery cue words generated significantly more memories than did low-imagery items in both sighted and blind participants (Eardley and Pring 2006). Interestingly, blind participants were found to generate an equal number of memories in response to visual, auditory and tactile cue-words, suggesting that visual words have cross-modal connections to other sensory or emotional encoding of self-related experiences that allow a privileged access to autobiographical memories in blind subjects.

Cesare Cornoldi and colleagues have carried out a series of experiments that clearly reveal that blind individuals can generate vivid mental images and make use of them in many situations. For instance, Cornoldi, Calore and Pra-Baldi (1979) required sighted and blind individuals to rate the vividness of imagery of nouns in each of three categories: high-imagery words whose referents could also be experience in the absence of visual experience (e.g., "cat"); high-imagery words referring to entities difficult to experience by touch, but with a high-imagery value (e.g., "palm tree"); and low-imagery or abstract words (e.g., "damage"). Blind and sighted subjects did not differ in their vividness rating for the first category of words; whereas words in the second category were rated higher by sighted subjects and words in the third category were rated slightly higher by the blind participants (see also Tinti, Galati et al. 1999). Zimler and Keenan (1983) found that when using a paired-associate task and a free-recall task for words varying for modality-specific attributes, such as color and sound (and hence being "high" in either visual imagery or auditory imagery), blind individuals performed as well as the sighted with "visual-related" words, and even outperformed the sighted for "auditorily related" words. Interestingly, Zimler and Keenan (1983) also measured the ability of blind and sighted subjects to create images of scenes in which target objects were described as either visible in the picture plane or concealed by another object and thus not visible. On an incidental recall test for the target objects, blind individuals, like the sighted, recalled more visible than concealed targets. These results indicate that the images generated by blind individuals on the basis of their available perceptual experience maintain occlusion just as the visual images of normally sighted individuals. The importance of "visualizing" information is extremely critical in education, where the use of graphs, pictures and figures have been found to significantly improve learning and memory in children. In light of this, Pring and Rusted (1985) studied whether presenting the to-be-remembered material in a pictorial format would also benefit individuals lacking visual experience. Blind children were required to haptically explore raised-line drawings of rare animals and to listen to a verbal description of these animals. It was found that blind children remembered more information about animals whose picture they had haptically explored, resembling the behavior of normally sighted individuals. Accordingly, Cornoldi and De Beni (1985; De Beni and Cornoldi 1988) found that blind individuals can use mnemonic strategies involving mental images similarly to sighted individuals.

How can these data be interpreted? Overall, they seem to suggest that blind individuals are able to generate mental representations containing accurate spatial relations and full of non-visual sensory details. In fact, as noted by Paivio (1986), the "visual" words used for instance by Zimler and Keenan (1983) referred to concrete objects ("apple," "blood," etc.) and thus could easily generate motor, tactile or olfactory imagery that could mediate memory performance in the blind. In fact, blind individuals might concretize even purely "visual" words like "shadow" through association with other modalities, such as temperature changes when one moves into the shade (Paivio 1971, 519–520). Of course, other explanations are possible. For instance, Zimler and Keenan (1983) argued that in the blind the advantage for high-imageability words reflected the operation of an effective non-imagery representation based upon propositional encoding of abstract semantic information. In contrast, others have suggested that the images of the blind may indeed contain *visual* details, thanks to the recruitment of the visual cortex by haptic or verbal processes (see for instance, Aleman, van Lee et al. 2001).

Dreams

The mental format of blind individuals' dreams have been the object of intense scientific interest. The widely accepted view is that congenitally or early blind individuals' dreams do not have visual content but contain sounds, touch-sensations and emotional experiences (Lavie 1996; Hurovitz, Dunn et al. 1999; Holzinger 2000). A person's age at the onset of blindness is critical on this regard: in fact, in an early study with blind children, Jastrow reported visual imagery only in those blind children that lost sight after five to seven years of age (Jastrow 1900), a result that has been confirmed by Kerr and colleagues (cf. Kerr, Foulkes, and Schmidt 1982; Kerr 2000). However, such evidence is mainly based on blind individuals' self-reports, thus suffering from the typical limitations of subjective measures. To obtain a more objective measure of such dreams' mental content, Bertolo and colleagues (Bertolo, Paiva et al. 2003) have investigated dreaming activity in blind individuals by using EEG recording. Bertolo et al. (Bertolo, Paiva et al. 2003) hypothesized that dreams with a visual content should be reflected by changes in the EEG alpha-rhythm. In fact, visual imagery is usually accompanied in normally sighted individuals by a decrease of alpha activity (8–12 Hz) recorded from the scalp (cf. Niedermeyer 1999). Participants were awakened every ninety minutes to be interviewed about their dreams, and a spectral analysis of the EEG preceding the moment of awakening was carried out. Bertolo et al. (Bertolo, Paiva et al. 2003) showed that the dream reports of blind subjects were vivid with tactile, auditory and kinesthetic references, but also contained visual elements. Accordingly, blind subjects were even able to graphically represent the dream-scenes they had previously described in words, and these reports and drawings contain visual detail to a similar extent as those produced by control sighted subjects. The most critical finding was the significant correlation between the reported visual content of the dreams and the decrease of the alpha-rhythm strength (see also Bertolo 2005) that, according to the authors, would prove that blind individuals were indeed experiencing *visual* images. Although intriguing, results by Bertolo and colleagues have been interpreted with caution. In fact, according to Lopes da Silva (2003), although Bertolo's study shows that the dreams of congenitally blind subjects involve the activation of areas of the cortex that are responsible for visual representations, this does not automatically imply that dreams also have a *visual* content (Lopes da Silva 2003). Rather, auditory and tactile inputs can create virtual images in the brain of congenitally blind subjects, but these images are not necessarily visual. We will go back to the issue of whether mental images of the blind can be visual later in this chapter.

"Chronometric" Functions: Mental Rotation and Mental Scanning

Studies with blind individuals have mainly employed the imagery paradigms (adapted to haptic or auditory presentations) traditionally used with normally sighted individuals, such as mental rotation and mental scanning (for a discussion of these paradigms, see chapter 3). Most behavioral findings suggest comparable chronometric functions (e.g., reaction times) in sighted and blind individuals in these types of task (but see Afonso, Blum et al. 2010). Using a haptic version of the mental-rotation task (Shepard and Metzler 1971), Marmor and Zaback (1976) observed that the time taken by blind participants to decide whether two figures differently oriented in the third dimension were identical or not depended upon their rotation angle, suggesting that blind individuals were "visualizing" the figures in their mind in order to rotate them, as is the case with sighted individuals (Shepard and Metzler 1971). Similar results were obtained by Carpenter and Eisenberg (1978) using verbal material such as single letters variously oriented (see also Dodds and Carter 1983; Hollins 1986; Barolo, Masini, and Antonietti 1990; Röder, Rösler et al. 1993). Accordingly, Kerr (1983) found that the time needed to mentally scan an image increased at the increase of the distance to be mentally computed, resembling the typical "distance effect" observed in mental-scanning tasks with sighted subjects (cf. Kosslyn, Ball, and Reiser 1978). (It should be noted though that in Kerr's experiment [Kerr 1983] six out of the ten blind subjects were not totally blind but could count on minimal light perception and on a spared capacity of perceiving contrast.) Similarly, Röder and Rösler (1998) used an image-scanning paradigm in which subjects were instructed to memorize the position of a series of landmarks on a tactile map, and to learn the association between each landmark and a specific sound tone. During the test, participants had to mentally move from one landmark to the other (on the basis of a given sequence of tones that had been previously associated to the different landmarks).

Image-scanning times were found to increase linearly with increasing distance in all participants, regardless of their visual status.

Nonetheless, a recent study by Afonso and colleagues (Afonso, Blum et al. 2010) suggests a partially different picture. In Afonso et al.'s study, congenitally blind, late blind, and blindfolded sighted subjects were required to learn a small-size spatial configuration, either by listening to a verbal description or by exploring the configuration haptically. After this learning process, they performed a mental scanning task. Their chronometric data revealed distinct patterns, namely, a significant positive correlation between scanning times and distances for the sighted and late blind participants, but not for the congenitally blind. This indicated that the congenitally blind participants did not generate the kind of metrically accurate mental representations that the other two groups formed, although they had reached the learning criterion just as their counterparts of the other two groups. However, a different pattern emerged in a second experiment (Afonso, Blum et al. 2010, experiment 2) in which the same groups of participants had to perform an image-scanning task after learning the position of a series of landmarks in a full-scale navigable space (created by an immersive audio virtual reality system) either by processing a verbal description or by direct locomotor exploration of the environment. In this second experiment, all three groups were able to transform the verbal descriptions into spatial representations that incorporated the metric distances between different locations in the navigable environment. However, sighted people were unable to generate a metrically valid representation of the environment by means of direct locomotion. Conversely, the congenitally blind participants performed particularly well after exploring the environment through direct locomotion, showing that metric information was validly represented in their mental representations (late blind participants were also able to generate valid spatial representation incorporating metric information, but they took longer compared to the congenitally blind). Hence, the capacity of congenitally blind individuals to generate analog spatial representations likely depends on how the information is acquired (haptically, through real locomotion, on the basis of a verbal description) and on whether the space to be represented is "near" (manipulatory space) or "far" (locomotor space). Notably, possible differences in the exploratory strategies—free exploration of the configuration with no time limits as in Röder and Rösler (1998) or more controlled exploration mode, as in Afonso et al. (Afonso, Blum et al. 2010)—may at least partially account for controversial results across studies.

Overall, these early findings indicate that blind individuals are able to represent sensory information in an analogical format, although this process may be more demanding when sight is lacking. In fact, blind individuals take longer overall than normally sighted subjects do, to rotate a stimulus or scan an image (Marmor and

Zaback 1976; Kerr 1983). In this regard, Marmor and Zaback argued that the limitations shown by the blind in mental rotation were not due to their use of a propositional rather than analogical representation, instead they concluded that overall "mental rotation is easier to perform upon visual representations than non-visual ones" (Marmor and Zaback 1976, 520). In fact, the limitations shown by the blind in these tasks have been interpreted—as we have already mentioned—both in terms of representational or/and operational deficits. According to the representational account, blind individuals may be initially troubled in coding the spatial form of the unfamiliar object of the type that is typically used in tactual mental rotation tasks. This would result in less accurate and slower performances in visuo-spatial tasks, particularly when objects irrelevant to the everyday experience of blind people are used as stimuli. Nevertheless, once the object is successfully recoded (with the additional time and loss of information that this might imply), the representation would be manipulated in a fashion similar to a sighted person's representation, and so comparable patterns of performance between sighted and blind participants would be observed. However, a purely representational account cannot explain why no differences are reported between blind and sighted performance at zero degrees of rotation (Heller 1989b). Alternatively, mental-rotation differences can be explained as depending on the increasing amounts of manipulation that are required at larger angles, which would slow down blind performance (i.e., a processing deficit). This is consistent with the hypothesis that the visuo-spatial processing capacity of congenitally blind participants is lower than that of sighted individuals. We will specifically discuss this issue later in the chapter, when considering the results of a series of studies we have carried out to investigate working memory capacity and processes in the blind (see Vecchi, Monticellai, and Cornoldi 1995; Vecchi 1998; Vecchi, Tinti, and Cornoldi 2004). Here it is worth reporting that the disadvantage of the blind compared to the sighted in chronometric tasks diminishes or disappears when more familiar stimuli are used. In fact, when Braille stimuli were used, blind individuals even outperformed sighted ones in mental rotation (Heller, Calcaterra et al. 1999), and no differences were reported between blind and sighted individuals when required to estimate the absolute distances between a series of objects in an indoor office environment with which they were familiar (Haber, Haber et al. 1993; see also Bliss, Kujala, and Hämäläinen 2004).

Images for Picture Recognition and Drawing by the Blind

In two-dimensional pictures, variations in depth are projected to a picture plane, from which the third dimension must be inferred. This is quite an automatic process in the visual modality, but less so in the haptic modality (Lederman, Klatzky et al. 1990). Usually, in tasks requiring that they recognize two-dimensional pictures by touch, individuals who have (or have had) visual experience attempt to generate a visual image of the object and recognize it by its visual mediation (Lederman, Klatzky et al. 1990). Accordingly, in sighted individuals measures of imagery positively correlate with performance in haptic recognition (Lederman and Klatzky 1987). But what is the case for individuals who cannot count on *visual* imagery processes? Are they able to recognize and produce 2D drawings? Blind individuals are of course less familiar than sighted individuals with the conventions governing the translation of 3D space into a 2D picture plane (Millar 1975, 1991). Nonetheless, the experiments carried out by Morton Heller, John M. Kennedy, Amedeo D'Angiulli and others have provided consistent evidence for the capacity of blind individuals to perceive and understand the rules subtending 2D representations of objects and to apply them (see for reviews, Kennedy 1993; Heller 2006; Kennedy and Jurevic 2006). Here we briefly report some of the most significant findings on this topic, which shed further light on the imagery capacity of blind individuals: in fact, in order to recognize a picture or draw an object, one has first to create a spatial mental representation of it.

In a picture-matching task (requiring that subjects match a target picture with an identical one to be chosen among a set of other pictures), Heller, Brackett and Scroggs (2002) found that congenitally blind individuals were as accurate and even significantly faster than blindfolded sighted individuals, suggesting that *visual* imagery and visual experience were not necessary for the perception of tangible pictures. However, in order to succeed in this task, one has to create a spatial mental representation of the target picture based on the tactile and kinesthetic inputs, maintain it in memory and match the newly experienced picture with the first one—but no identification of the picture is required, nor a matching between the real 3D object and the picture. Nevertheless, what is more interesting in haptic picture-recognition and reproduction is whether the blind are able to understand and apply some specific perceptual rules that apparently apply to visual perception only, such as perspective laws or viewpoint dependency. In fact, the shapes of objects are made of surfaces that can be experienced by both touch and vision (D'Angiulli, Kennedy, and Heller 1998), given that surfaces' edges are both visible and tangible. Hence, haptics and sight provide similar information about contours, directions and other spatial features of a scene (see Kennedy 1993; Kennedy and Jurevic 2006). According to this view, one may reasonably hypothesize that blind children may spontaneously implement, through outline, the basic principles of object-edges representation in much the same way as sighted children. However, tactile perception is not directly affected by *perspective* (contrarily to visual experience); similarly, when grasping an object, the agent usually gets all the possible planes of the object at the same time, as long as the object is small enough to be explored as a whole. Conversely, a visual observer can only ever *selectively* look at the frontal, lateral, upper or lower view of an object regardless of size. Hence, a blind person may not be so familiar with the notion of *vantage point* (see Heller, Brackett et al. 2002; Heller, Kennedy et al. 2006).

Vantage point Heller and Kennedy (1990) found that early blind individuals performed comparable to late blind and blindfolded sighted subjects in selectively drawing top or lateral sides of haptically perceived shapes, according to the received instructions (see also Heller, Brackett et al. 2002; D'Angiulli and Maggi 2003; Heller, Kennedy et al. 2006). Still, the early blind may experience more difficulties than late blind and sighted controls when required to "visualize" an object from a particular viewpoint in more complex situations (Heller, Kennedy, and Joyner 1995; Heller, Kennedy et al. 2006; Heller, Riddle et al., 2009). For instance, Heller and colleagues (Heller, Kennedy et al. 2006) compared blind and blindfolded sighted individuals in a series of tasks aimed to investigate the effect of viewpoint (3D-, top-, frontal-, side-view) and orientation in picture recognition. Briefly, a series of solid objects had to be haptically explored and then matched with one of four possible raised-line pictures depicting the object in the particular viewpoint previously indicated by the experimenter. In one condition (experiment 3), the solid object was rotated 45 degrees when compared to the tangible pictures. Participants were informed that the stimuli were turned counterclockwise, and that they needed to compensate for this when making their matches with the pictures (which were drawn while the objects were in their straight-ahead position). In these situations, the performance of early blind individuals was particularly impaired. Similarly, early blind participants may find it more difficult than late blind and blindfolded sighted subjects to match 3D haptically explored objects with 2D drawings, when objects have particularly complex forms (as in Heller, Riddle et al. 2009, experiment 1).

Perspective In an early study, Arditi, Holtzman, and Kosslyn (1988) required blind individuals to imagine familiar objects within "arm's reach." Subjects were then asked to point to the sides of objects of differing sizes at three distances. No evidence of alterations in arm angles as a function of distance was reported in the congenitally blind, suggesting that they were not following perspective rules. In a similar study by Vanlierde and Wanet-Defalque (2005), blindfolded sighted, late blind and early blind participants were asked to point to the left and right side of three objects, imagined at three increasing distances. The effects of perspective were present in the mental imagery of sighted and late blind subjects, whereas they were absent in the mental imagery of early blind participants. Nonetheless, others have reported different results: for instance, Kennedy (1993) found that when asked to point to the sides of an imagined wall at a near and far distance, blind participants bring their arms together when pointing to the wall at a greater distance. However, as noted by Heller (2006), interpreting perspective in drawings is likely to be a more difficult task than accounting for its effects in a pointing task. In this regard, Heller and colleagues (Heller, Calcaterra et al. 1996) observed that congenitally blind individuals did not spontaneously use foreshortening when required to produce raised-line drawings of a surface at different angles, whereas late blind and sighted individuals did. Moreover, an important factor to be considered is the experience that blind participants have with raised-line drawings: in fact, Dulin (Dulin, Hatwell et al. 2008) has recently demonstrated that prior experience in raised-line materials facilitated the performance of blind participants in a mental imagery task requiring that they estimate the length of a series of common objects (such as a credit card, a fork, a compact disk case). According to Dulin (Dulin, Hatwell et al. 2008), a high level of expertise with raised-line materials in the congenitally blind population may compensate for the impairment in spatial representation, often resulting from their lack of visual experience. Hence, different studies may lead to a different output because of the varying features of the participants involved or the particular paradigm used in constructing the tests. In fact, in a following study by Heller and colleagues which required subjects to explore two intersecting planes at different angles and select the correct perspective to match the object (drawing out of four choices), the congenitally blind performed as well as sighted subjects and late blind subjects, suggesting that performance on this perspective-task did not depend upon visual experience and visual imagery (Heller, Brackett et al. 2002).

Overall, these findings suggest that blind individuals do not spontaneously apply the rules of perspective in their mental representations, but they can learn from the reports of sighted individuals how to apply them successfully, if required. Even more importantly, these results indicate that blind individuals are able to "visualize" objects and to reveal their internal representations through highly detailed drawings that are unequivocally understandable by sighted individuals. Of course, this also depends on the drawing ability of the blind person involved, but this is a technical issue that doesn't have to do with the content of the representation; in fact, even a sighted person can find it very difficult to draw a horse though he/she has a clear image of a horse in mind. In this regard, a recent fMRI study by Amedi et al. (Amedi, Merabet et al. 2008) carried out to investigate the neural and behavioral correlates of drawing in EA, an early blind painter, is critical.

The case of EA is particularly important, because, given the talent of EA for painting (see figure 4.1), it is possible to study how mental images appear to the blind (without the limitations due to technical problems associated with paint). In particular, Amedi et al. (Amedi, Merabet et al. 2008) looked at the neural correlates associated with EA's ability to transform tactilely explored three-dimensional objects into drawings and contrasted these findings with meaningless scribbling conditions (i.e., sensory-motor control condition). Critically, this study reported significant activation during drawing (compared to scribbling) in cortical regions usually associated with vision (including primary and secondary visual cortical areas), along with frontal and parietal cortical regions. Some of these areas were also activated when EA mentally imagined the pictures he had to draw (although to a lesser anatomical extent and signal magnitude). Hence, Amedi et al.'s (Amedi, Merabet et al. 2008) results suggest that the occipital cortex plays

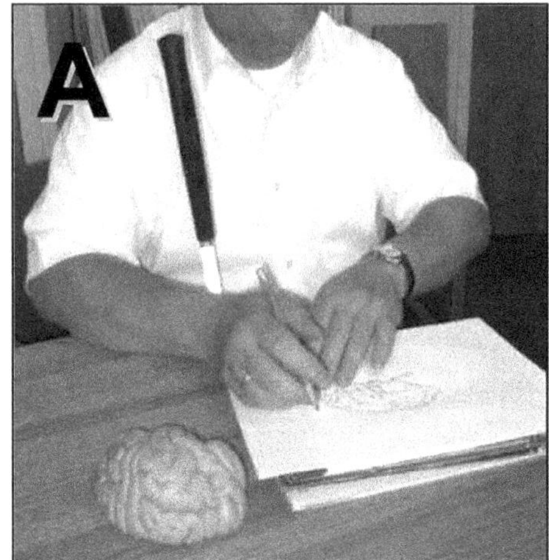

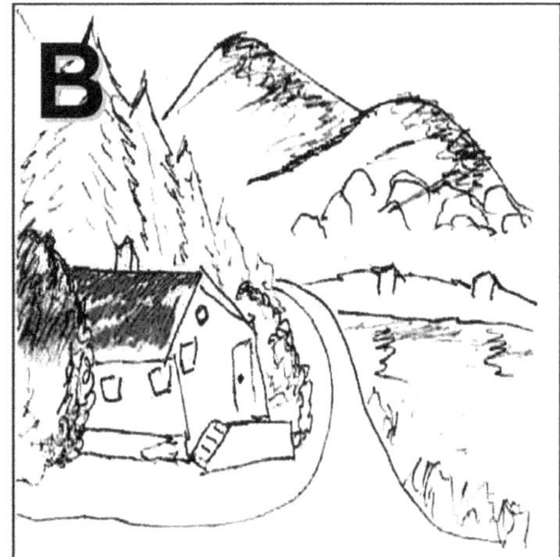

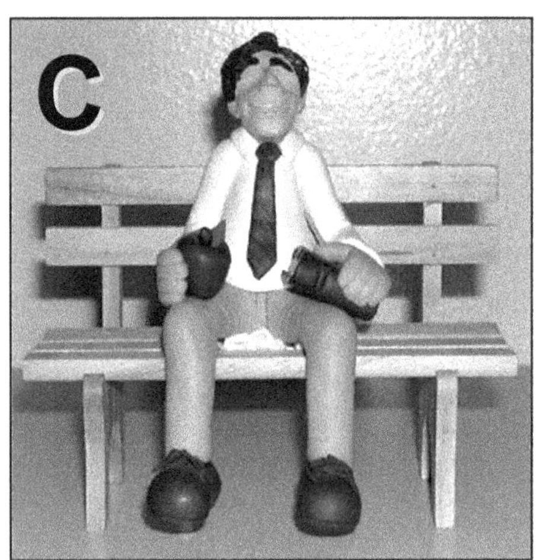

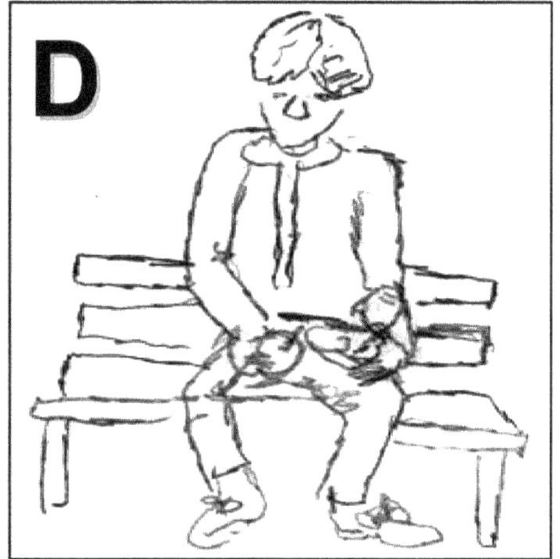

Figure 4.1

Examples of subject EA's drawing abilities. (A) EA drawing a novel object (a model of the brain) using a pencil and paper and a specially designed rubberized writing tablet (Sewell raised line drawing kit). This technique allows him to generate relief images that he can subsequently detect and explore tactilely. (B) The themes of his drawings and paintings vary and include both tactile and non-tactile subjects. The drawing shows a landscape scene. His paintings often contain vibrant color, and he uses shading, depth cues, and perspective akin to that employed by sighted artists. (C) Example of a complex and novel object which EA had never encountered. Once EA explored the object by touch for a few minutes, he was able to render a very accurate drawing of the object (D).

Reprinted from Amedi, Merabet et al., "Neural and behavioural correlates of drawing in an early blind painter: A case study," *Brain Research* 1242 (2008): 252–262. (© 2008. Reprinted by permission of Elsevier) a key role in supporting mental representations even without prior visual experience. Does this imply that blind individuals experience visual images? This is also the question raised by Bertolo's studies (see Bertolo, Paiva et al. 2003) on the dreaming content of the blind. We will go back to the format of the mental representations in blind individuals at the end of this chapter; in the following paragraphs we will discuss studies that have investigated visuo-spatial working memory processes in blind individuals.

4.3 Manipulating Mental Images in Working Memory

In the previous paragraphs we have mainly discussed evidence about the representational format of blind individuals' mental images, although also referring to possible difficulties of blind individuals in *processing* images once these have been properly generated. Here we discuss more specifically studies that have investigated the ability of blind individuals to manipulate and reorganize mental images in working memory; data from these studies are of course also indicative of the representational format of the generated images.

Passive and Active Visuo-Spatial Working Memory Processes

In the last decades, Cesare Cornoldi, Tomaso Vecchi and colleagues have carried out a series of experiments to investigate imagery and visuo-spatial WM abilities in blind individuals. In particular, Cornoldi and colleagues have adapted to a haptic presentation and modified (according to the specific cognitive processes under investigation) a series of tasks originally developed to study imagery processes and WM abilities in normally sighted individuals (cf. Attneave and Curlee 1983; Kerr 1987). In their studies, Cornoldi et al. were specifically interested in verifying whether blindness affects to a similar extent "passive" and "active" WM processes. Specifically, according to Cornoldi and Vecchi's view (see Cornoldi and Vecchi 2000, 2003), passive WM processes are involved when a variable amount of information has to be remembered. Conversely, when the original input has to be manipulated—as it is the case for instance in mental rotation or when different inputs have to be combined together—active processes are involved to a greater extent. In this regard, it is worth noting that the passive/active distinction is not indicative of a task's complexity: in fact, memorizing one hundred pictures (a passive process) is certainly harder than rotating a single picture (an active process) in the mind. Furthermore, this distinction between passive and active processes has been corroborated by neuroimaging findings (see Smith and Jonides 1999), showing a major role of amodal prefrontal areas for active processes, whereas the neural activation associated with passive storage was highly dependent upon the specific nature of the stimuli involved.

In the "active" imagery condition created by Cornoldi et al. in their experiments (Cornoldi, Cortesi, and Preti 1991; Cornoldi, Bertuccelli et al. 1993), blind and blindfolded sighted participants have to haptically explore a matrix composed of different wooden-made cubes (see figure 4.2 panel A). Hence, they are required to follow a pathway within that configuration on the basis of statements of direction (e.g., left/right, forward/backward) given by the experimenter: at the test, participants have to point to the cube corresponding to the last position of the pathway. In order to successfully carry out this task, participants need to generate and update a mental representation of the pathway on the basis of the sequential information (e.g., the number of statements of directions) that is progressively given. Levels of complexity can vary according to the size of the matrix (3 × 3, 5 × 5, etc.), the dimensionality of the matrix (two-dimensional or three-dimensional: 3 × 3 × 3, 5 × 5 × 5, etc.), the number of direction changes and the speed at which instructions are given (one every second, one every two seconds, etc.). Using this task, Cornoldi, Cortesi and Preti (1991) and Cornoldi, Bertuccelli, Rocchi, and Sbrana (1993) found that blind subjects were able to successfully generate a mental representation of the explored configuration, but experienced greater difficulty than the sighted when the complexity of the matrix was increased and—especially—when 3D matrices were used. It is possible that the difficulty in dealing with 3D mental images is a partial consequence of blind people's problems with the simultaneous treatment of the different spatial dimensions (vertical, horizontal and depth): in fact, although blind individuals experience the dimension of depth, it is very uncommon for them to simultaneously experience all the spatial planes together. Indeed, it is essentially through visual experience that an individual can get a simultaneous view of all the three spatial dimensions. However, blind individuals have certainly more experience with 3D objects than with 2D representations (Millar 1975, 1991) and other studies have questioned the hypothesis of a selective difficulty of blind individuals in manipulating 3D representations (cf. Eardley and Pring 2007).

In another version of the task proposed by Cornoldi and Vecchi, the surface of some of the matrices' cubes (targets) is covered by sandpaper in order to be highly recognizable by touch. Subjects are required to explore the matrices with the two hands (sighted controls perform the task blindfolded) and to memorize the location of the target cubes (see figure 4.2, panel B). Again, the task's complexity can be manipulated by increasing the number of targets to be remembered, the size and dimensionality of the matrix (two-dimensional: 3 × 3, etc.; or three-dimensional: 3 × 3 × 3, etc.), the number of matrices presented (one or two), or the time for exploration that is allotted. During the test, participants have to indicate on one/two corresponding blank matrix/matrices the location of the target cubes. In the simplest "single matrix" condition, only one matrix is used. In the so-called "multiple matrices" condition, targets are equally presented on two different matrices and have to be recalled on two corresponding blank matrices during the test. In the "integration" condition, again targets are presented on two different matrices, but have to be recalled

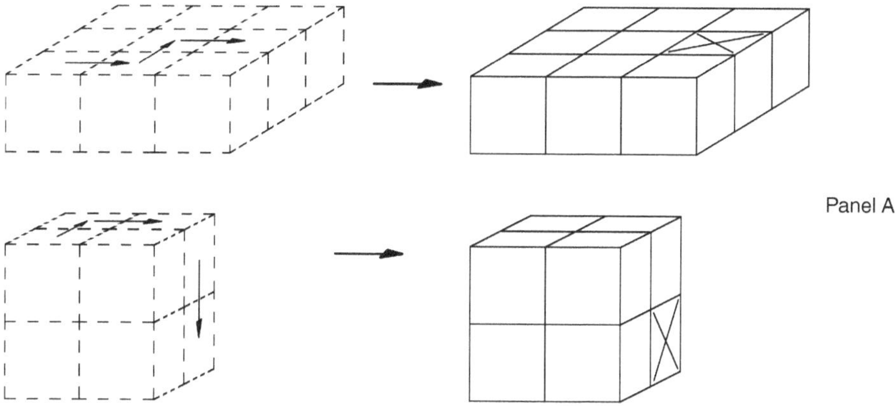

Figure 4.2

Examples of the "active" (panel A) and "passive" (panel B) matrix task used by Cornoldi and colleagues. In the active task, blind and blindfolded sighted participants have to haptically explore a matrix composed of different wooden-made cubes. Hence, they are required to follow a pathway within that configuration on the basis of statements of direction (e.g., left/right, forward/backward) given by the experimenter: at test, participants have to point to the cube corresponding to the last position of the pathway. (Adapted and modified from Cornoldi and Vecchi 2003: *Visuo-Spatial Working Memory and Individual Differences*, Hove: Psychology Press.) The passive task includes different conditions, requiring the memorization and recall of single (a) and multiple (b) matrices or an active manipulation involving the integration of the targets in a single response matrix (c). Target cells are covered with sandpaper so as to be easily recognizable at touch. The level of complexity in both tasks varies depending on the number of target cells (passive task) or directions (active task) to be retained, and on the matrices' size (3×3, 5×5, etc.) or dimensionality (2D or 3D).

Reprinted from Vecchi, Tinti, and Cornoldi, "Spatial memory and integration processes in congenital blindness," *NeuroReport* 15(18) (2004): 2787–2790. (Reprinted by permission of Wolters Kluwer Health)

on one single matrix (hence requiring an integrative—i.e., active process). Using this task, Vecchi, Monticellai, and Cornoldi (1995) found that blind and sighted participants' performance was similar in retrieving targets when one single matrix was used (even when the memory load was high—i.e., eight targets). However, when two matrices had to be distinctly retained in memory (multiple matrices conditions), blind subjects' performance was specifically affected, whereas the integration process was not (Vecchi, Tinti, and Cornoldi 2004). The authors hypothesized that blindness specifically affects the simultaneous maintenance of multiple images in memory, and that this may depend on the essentially sequential nature of the perceptual experience of the blind. In fact, haptic exploration only allows one to acquire information about

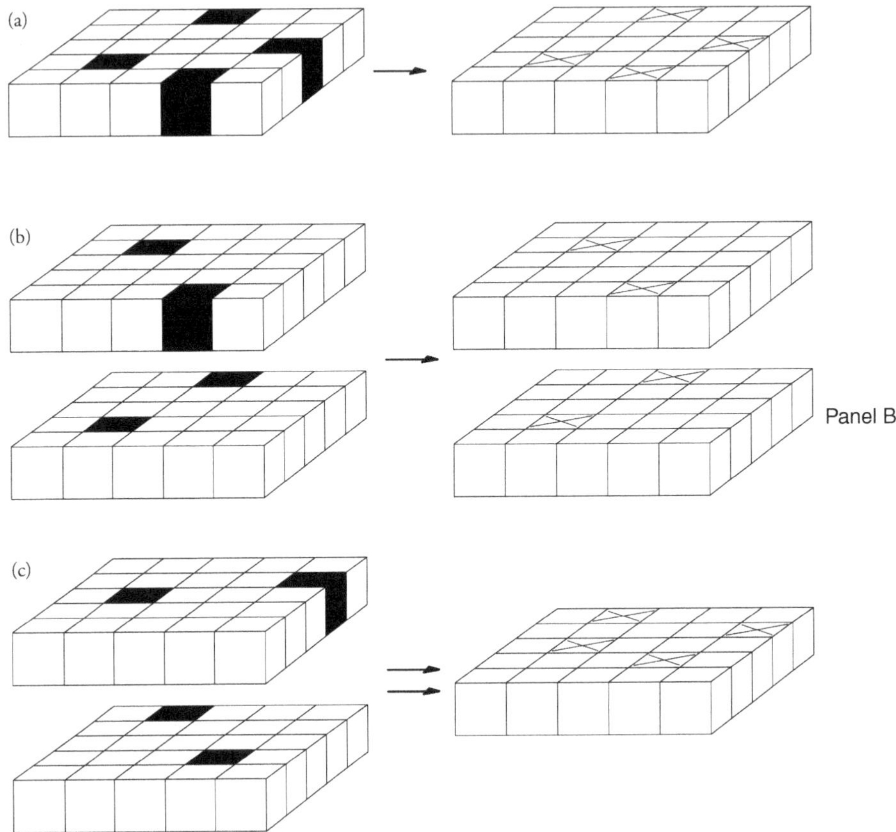

Figure 4.2
continued

the external environment piece-by-piece, whereas vision allows one to code with a single gaze complex scenes containing many different objects. Hence, Vecchi et al.'s findings (Vecchi, Tinti, and Cornoldi 2004) suggest that while the simultaneous maintenance of different spatial information is selectively affected by congenital blindness, cognitive processes that require a sequential manipulation are not.

In a recent study, Cattaneo and colleagues (Cattaneo, Fantino et al. 2010a) required early blind and blindfolded sighted subjects to haptically explore and memorize a series of target cells presented on a 2D 7 × 7 matrix. In some conditions, the overall configuration created by the target cells was symmetrical either along the vertical or the horizontal axis of the matrix. Subjects were not informed that in some trials configurations were symmetrical. Notably, both blindfolded sighted and congenitally blind subjects were better in recalling the location of the target cells when the configurations were symmetrical compared to when they were not (for the effect of symmetry in haptic perception see also Ballesteros and Reales 2004; Rossi-Arnaud, Pieroni, and Baddeley 2006). However, the performance of the blindfolded sighted participants was significantly higher with vertical symmetrical configurations than with horizontal symmetrical ones, whereas no difference depending on the orientation of the axis of symmetry was observed in the blind (Cattaneo, Fantino et al. 2010a). These findings suggest that symmetry efficiently works in the blind as a gestalt principle of perceptual organization (see Machilsen, Pauwels, and Wagemans 2009), although with specific limitations depending on the absence of the visual experience. In fact, visual perception inherently affects the way mental images are generated in the sighted: indeed, there is large evidence that the visual system detects vertical symmetry more easily than horizontal symmetry (e.g., Wagemans 1997), a preference that in the sighted participants is likely to be transferred to the haptic modality (possibly due to the generation of a visual image on the basis of the haptic input) (Cattaneo, Fantino et al. 2010a). Hence, although both blind and blindfolded sighted subjects represented the haptically acquired information in a spatial format, the mental images generated by the blind lacked of some specific characteristics that are typically associated to vision (e.g., the salience of vertical symmetry for the visual system) (Cattaneo, Fantino et al. 2010a).

An active visuo-spatial memory task was also used by Vanlierde and Wanet-Defalque to investigate imagery abilities of early blind and late blind individuals. Basically, the task required blind individuals to haptically explore a 6 × 6 2D matrix and then listen to a series of verbal instructions indicating which positions of the matrix were filled in. In the verbal instructions, the term "white" was used to indicate empty squares, whereas the term "black" was used to indicate filled-in squares (typical instructions being in this form "First line: white, white, white, black, white, white; second line: black, etc."). During the test, subjects had to indicate how many filled-in squares were mirrored in the matrix according to a given grid axis. Hence, in order to succeed in the task, participants had to (1) generate the mental representation of the 2D matrix, (2) integrate a large amount of sequential information in memory, and finally, (3) manipulate this information in order to give their response. Interestingly, blindfolded sighted, early blind and late blind participants were found to perform similarly in this task. However, when interviewed about the strategies they used in the task, late blind and sighted subjects reported having generated a visual mental representation, whereas the early blind mainly reported having relied on an "XY strategy," in which an (X,Y) coded grid representation was used to encode the location of each filled-in square in the grid. The number of filled-in cells that appear in corresponding positions according to a given grid axis was subsequently assessed by comparing one filled-in square (X,Y) location to another. Hence, with this strategy the early blind subjects did not use any visual representation.

The results by Vanlierde and Wanet-Defalque (2004) underline the importance of the strategy used to perform a particular task. In fact, even if the final output might be the same, the way early blind and sighted subjects cope with the task is likely to be different, at least in some situations. However, the use of a verbal strategy to perform imagery tasks by the early blind has not always been reported. Röder, Rösler, and Henighausen (1997) recorded slow event-related brain potentials in groups of sighted and blind individuals during a haptic mental-rotation task. Again, response times increased as a function of the rotation angle in both sighted and blind participants. Parietal areas—known to mediate spatial representation—were found to be activated in both groups, discouraging the hypothesis that spatial cognition is mediated by verbal processes in blind individuals (see Dodds and Carter 1983). Accordingly, blind subjects were not found to rely on a verbal rehearsal strategy more than sighted subjects in the mental-pathway task used by Cornoldi et al. (Cornoldi, Cortesi, and Preti 1991; Cornoldi, Bertuccelli et al. 1993), as demonstrated by the fact that a concomitant articulatory suppression task only produced a modest and generalized drop in performance in both sighted and blind individuals (Vecchi 1998). Cornoldi et al. (Cornoldi, Tinti et al. 2009) have re-used this paradigm, devoting particular attention to the role of individual strategies in determining performance. Notably, in Cornoldi et al. (Cornoldi, Tinti et al. 2009), half of the participants had to retrieve the entire pathway rather than the last position only; moreover, only 2D (5×5) matrices were used. On completion of all tasks, participants were required to indicate the strategy they adopted. Congenitally blind individuals were found to perform closely to the blindfolded sighted when only the last position of the matrices had to be retrieved, supporting the view that blindness does not necessarily prevent the use of efficient spatial imagery mechanisms. Nevertheless, when the entire pathway had to be retrieved, blind individuals were outperformed by the blindfolded sighted, probably reflecting an overload of their working-memory capacity. Three main strategies were identified: spatial (involving mental imagery), verbal and mixed (spatial and verbal). Critically, sighted participants who declared that they used a spatial strategy benefited from it, whereas this was not the case for blind participants. In fact, the blind participants who declared that they relied upon a spatial strategy performed poorer than both the blindfolded controls and the blind participants who adopted a verbal strategy. Accordingly, when analyzing the performance of subjects who used mixed or especially verbal strategies, Cornoldi et al. (Cornoldi, Tinti et al. 2009) found no difference between the performance of blind and blindfolded sighted participants. Once more, this study critically shows the importance of the strategies spontaneously used by individuals in affecting their performance. It is likely that when the task is relatively simple or quite suitable for being verbally mediated, blind individuals can reach a good level of performance—that is, comparable to that of sighted subjects (see for instance, Vanlierde and Wanet-Defalque 2004). However, when the task becomes more demanding, requiring an active mental manipulation of the material or the continuous updating of a spatial representation, then blind individuals tend to show specific deficits (e.g., Cornoldi, Tinti et al. 2009).

Imagery and Creativity

Eardley and Pring (2007) have investigated the ability of blind individuals to manipulate their mental images by means of the creative mental synthesis task (Finke and Slayton 1988). This task requires subjects to mentally manipulate shapes and generate new forms: in the traditional version of the task, subjects are given the verbal label of three shapes and they have to combine all three shapes into a recognizable form, which they are then required to verbally describe and draw. Previous research with the sighted has shown that this task has a mainly spatial component, whereas the role of visual processes is only marginal (Pearson, Logie, and Gilhooly 1999). Eardley and Pring (2007) created a haptic version of the task; in one condition 2D shapes were used, in another, 3D shapes were used. Overall, blind individuals were able to generate something novel using imagery, indicating that vision is not a requisite for active spatial processing. Nevertheless, sighted subjects produced more legitimate patterns than did the early blind, but only when the task involved 2D shapes. With 3D objects, no differences were reported between blind and sighted individuals. In fact, as also underlined by Heller (see Heller 2006), touch has a clear advantage over vision for the perception of 3D objects: in fact, it is possible to grasp the front and back of an object at once, whereas individuals cannot normally see multiple views of an object at the same time. As we will discuss further in this chapter, blind individuals are less familiar with the conventions of 2D representations (Millar 1975, 1991) and have less direct experience with this type of representation. Hence, as suggested by Eardley and Pring (2007), the greater difficulties blind participants experienced with 2D shapes are likely to reflect differences in experience and familiarity with the medium, rather than any underlying deficit in the capacity of their imagery system (see also Heller 2006). In fact, even studies with sighted individuals have demonstrated that haptic exploration is more effective at identifying objects in three dimensions than in two dimensions (Klatzky, Loomis et al. 1993; Ballesteros and Reales 2004). These findings appear in contrast to the greater difficulty with 3D matrices that is reported by Cornoldi et al. (Cornoldi, Cortesi, and Preti 1991; Vecchi 1998). In that case, it is possible that the unfamiliar nature of matrix-stimuli for blind individuals contributed to their disadvantage in comparison with the sighted.

Imagery and Reasoning

In chapter 3 we discussed the importance of visual imagery and spatial imagery in reasoning processes, particularly referring to the studies by Knauff and colleagues (Knauff and Johnson-Laird 2002; Knauff, Fangmeier et al. 2003; Knauff and May 2006).

According to Knauff and May (2006), relational terms that lead naturally to spatial representations (for instance, *above-below*) facilitate the process of reasoning. Conversely, visual relations, which are hard to envisage spatially (such as *cleaner-dirtier*), lead to a mental picture whose vivid details may impede the process of thinking, giving rise to the so-called *visual impedance effect* (Knauff and Johnson-Laird 2002). Knauff and May (2006) have carried out an experiment on blind individuals to further test this hypothesis. According to Knauff and May (2006), if it is true that relations that elicit visual images (containing details that are irrelevant to an inference) impede the process of reasoning in sighted individuals, this should not be the case for congenitally blind individuals, since the capacity to generate mental representations with visual details is impaired in this population. Three sets of verbal relations were presented to participants: (1) visuo-spatial relations (such as front-back, above-below); (2) visual relations (such as cleaner-dirtier, fatter-thinner); and (3) control relations (such as better-worse, smarter-dumber). Blind individuals performed less well and more slowly compared to the sighted, irrespective of the type of relations (visual vs. spatial), suggesting that visual experience may overall facilitate reasoning processes. However, if sighted participants were distracted by the visual details when the deductive reasoning involved visual relations, the blind were not. Hence, these data suggest that the blind were relying on another non-visual type of mental representations, as was confirmed by the blind participants themselves in post-test interviews, reporting that they tried to locate the objects of the inference on a spatial/degrees scale, representing the different concept (for instance, "dirtiness"). Moreover, further research on auditory-based reasoning carried out by the same group (Fangmeier and Knauff 2009) has emphasized the role of modality-independent spatial representations in reasoning processes, suggesting that visual imagery is not necessary in drawing inferences.

In an interesting study, Puche-Navarro and Millan (2007) have tested the ability of blind children to perform in a problem-solving situation in which information could be presented either in a "manipulative"/haptic format (i.e., models of houses, animals, or different types of food) or in a verbal format. The results showed that visually impaired children were able to solve the task of making proper inferences, although they did so better in the verbal than in the haptic version of the task. Overall, the performance of blind children was lower than that of age-matched sighted children in the manipulative/haptic version of the task, but slightly superior when the task was presented in a verbal format. According to the authors, the verbal problem-solving task allowed blind children to store a wider range of information than did the sighted (supporting previous findings on the superior verbal-memory capacity of the blind: e.g., Raz, Striem et al. 2007) and to use it to make the pertinent inferences. Conversely, in the haptic version of the task, irrelevant spatial elements inherent to the models used may have become salient so that the child needed to overcome this aspect, making the inference process more difficult (or slower): this would particularly be the case for the blind, who are more used to extracting spatial information from touch. Although this explanation is not completely convincing, the results by Puche-Navarro and Millan (2007) are important in suggesting that the format in which a task is presented can influence performance more than the child's degree of visual ability, and should then be considered in educational contexts.

4.4 Are *Visual* Images Possible in the Blind?

The format of the mental representations in the blind is still a highly controversial issue. In fact, while some researchers have used the term "visuo-spatial" to refer to the mental images of the blind, thus suggesting that those images may be somehow "visual," others have argued that the mental images of the blind only contain non visual-sensory information (auditory, tactile, olfactory) and abstract semantic content. Importantly, shared by both views is the idea that blind individuals can generate mental representations that contain spatial information (see also chapter 5, which deals with spatial cognition in the blind).

Behavioral Evidence

Aleman et al. (Aleman, van Lee et al. 2001) have carried out a study to disentangle pictorial imagery processes and spatial imagery processes in blind individuals. In the pictorial imagery task, blind and sighted individuals were asked to indicate the odd-one-out in terms of form characteristics of a triad of common objects. Specifically, three object-names were read to the participants and they had to decide which was the most deviant in terms of form characteristics. This has been considered as a pictorial task because it is indeed difficult to respond on the basis of semantic information only. A second spatial task was used (the matrix task), requiring subjects to explore two-dimensional or three-dimensional matrices and memorize a series of positions on the matrix or follow a mental pathway. In some trials of the pictorial and the spatial task, participants were also required to perform a tapping task, which is known to selectively interfere with spatial processing. Critically, it was found that blind individuals were able to accurately perform both when pictorial imagery was required and when more spatial capacities were tapped, although in both tasks they performed significantly lower than the sighted. However, the blind disadvantage was comparable in the pictorial and in the spatial task, and the blind were not more affected by the concurrent spatial task than were the sighted. The authors suggested that blind individuals were able to generate *visuo-spatial* representations of the stimuli.

Our view is that the mental images of congenitally blind individuals are not "visual" in a narrow sense, although we believe that objects are mentally represented by the blind in an analog format, enriched by all the semantic knowledge pertaining that specific object (in this sense, mental images of the blind may also be vivid). In other words, congenitally blind individuals might think about the sun as "a yellow circle," but although they can *visualize* the "circle" (spatial information), they cannot mentally *see* its being "yellow" (visual information): they know it is yellow, but they cannot see the color. We used the term "visualize" here intentionally. In fact, we are inclined to think that blind individuals do not necessarily represent information about objects' shapes in the form of kinesthetic/motor/tactile traces, nor as purely abstract (verbal-like) information. Rather, we argue that such information is maintained in an analog/spatial format that may contain sensory information to a different extent. Indeed, there is nothing as a *pure* spatial sense: that is to say, it is not possible to perceive a purely spatial input; rather, spatial information is always conveyed by sight, hearing, touch, or by proprioceptive and vestibular information. Hence, purely spatial mental images are unlikely to exist. Spatial information—when present—is embedded in mental representations that also present visual details, or tactile details, or auditory details, with the degree of each sensory-modality content depending on the dominant perceptual experience. Given this premise, the results we reported above on the performance of congenitally blind individuals in mental-scanning or mental-rotation tasks, and their capacity to produce drawings whose content is immediately understandable by a sighted person, suggest that blind individuals mentally *see* the shapes of objects. This is the most economical way to explain these results. The analogical images produced by the blind are likely to be very schematic, containing spatial information with no (strictly speaking) visual details, although visual information in the form of semantic knowledge or through association with other sensory experiences may also be present (see Knauff and May 2004). In this sense, the mental images generated by the blind are unlikely to exactly resemble those experienced by normally sighted individuals. Moreover, as we will discuss below, the way these images are mentally explored and manipulated by blind and sighted individuals is likely to be different: in fact, blind individuals seem to rely on sequential mental processes, due to the inherently sequential character of their dominant perceptual (tactile and auditory) experience; and they encounter specific limitations at the increasing of memory-load and operational processes.

Note that the visual cortex has been found to be recruited by other sensory modalities in the blind, as a result of cortical plasticity phenomena (see chapter 8). Hence, one may hypothesize that the activation of the visual cortex may indeed subtend some sort of visual imagery (Aleman, van Lee et al. 2001; Bertolo, Paiva et al. 2003), although this hypothesis is controversial and data are open to other interpretations (see Lopes da Silva 2003).

Neurophysiological Evidence

As we will discuss primarily in chapter 8, fMRI and PET studies have shown that the visual cortex of blind individuals may activate during tactile, auditory and verbal tasks (e.g., Sadato, Pascual-Leone et al. 1996; Sadato, Pascual-Leone et al. 1998; Burton, Snyder et al. 2002a). Though quite impressive, these findings indicate that visual areas may be recruited to process non-visual information, but they do not necessarily imply that such activation is associated to a *visual* internal experience. In a way, these findings are related to the results of research on rewired animals: in particular, a quite famous experiment (von Melchner, Pallas, and Sur 2000) showed that if retinal inputs from one eye are redirected to the auditory cortex at birth, the auditory cortex develops similarly to the visual cortex, and visual stimuli are indeed perceived as visual rather than auditory. Hence, it is the sensorial input that drives the activity of the various cortical regions, at least to a certain extent (for review, see Swindale 2000; Majewska and Sur 2006). In fact, there is also evidence that many forms of cortical organization develop without environmentally driven stimulation (such as orientation columns and ocular dominance columns). Hence, if the visual cortex retains part of its original structure and network properties, one can assume that although the visual cortex is usually recruited in blind individuals to process tactile and auditory stimuli, it would still be able to respond and process visual stimuli when perceived and could be used for pictorial representation in imagery.

Although visual stimuli cannot reach the occipital cortex due to the peripheral blindness, they can nonetheless be induced by directly stimulating the occipital cortex. In fact, if one assumes that the visual cortex retains a specific "predisposition" to processing visual stimuli even if it has never been reached by an external visual stimulus, it is possible that stimulating the cortex will induce a visual percept, in particular the experience of a flash of light (i.e., phosphene). Although this would not automatically imply that the blind experience visual images, it would support the idea that the visual cortex retains at least part of its original functions, and is not entirely re-routed to process tactile and auditory stimuli. Otherwise, if the activity in a given cortical area only reflects the characteristics of its novel sensory input source (tactile and auditory in case of the blind), then no visual sensations should be evoked in the blind. In one way, this question is related by the debate William James started when he wondered whether, if the eyes were forced to connect to the auditory centers of the brain, and the ears with the visual centers, we would "hear the lightning and see the thunder" (James [1890] 1950). This question voiced by James is more recently known as the cortical "dominance versus deference" debate (see Kupers, Fumal et al. 2006).

A few studies using transcranial magnetic stimulation have directly addressed this issue. In particular, the results of a TMS study by Kupers et al. (Kupers, Fumal et al. 2006) seem to suggest that the subjective character of the percept induced by TMS depends on the stimulated sensory channel (e.g., somesthesis) and not on the activated cortex (e.g., visual). In particular, Kupers et al. tested a group of blind and sighted controls that had been previously trained to use a sensory substitution device able to translate visual images into electrotactile tongue stimulation. Kupers et al. (Kupers, Fumal et al. 2006) found that when TMS was applied over the occipital cortex, the blind reported somato-topically organized tactile sensation on the tongue—while this was not the case with sighted subjects, who only reported TMS-induced phosphenes—although all subjects were trained to a high level in the use of the device. In a subsequent experiment, Ptito and colleagues (Ptito, Fumal et al. 2008) similarly reported that TMS over the occipital cortex induced tactile sensations in the fingers of a group of blind Braille readers. These data seem to support the "cortical deference" view, according to which the qualitative character of the subject's experience is not determined by the area of the cortex that is active (cortical dominance) but by the source of the input to it. Cowey and Walsh (2000) tried to induce visual phosphenes by applying TMS over the occipital cortex of a 61 year old totally retinal-blind subject, who had been completely blind (no light perception) for at least 8 years. Critically, this individual was found to experience TMS-induced phosphenes (see also Gothe, Brandt et al. 2002). However, to date, no cases have been reported of visual phosphenes induced in congenitally totally blind subjects.

The Molyneaux Question

Investigating whether the blind can experience some sort of visual imagery is directly connected to the famous philosophical "Molyneaux's query." In a letter to John Locke, after the publication of the first edition of Locke's *Essay Concerning Human Understanding* in 1690 (see Paterson 2006), William Molyneaux, an Irish politician, husband of a blind woman, interrogated the philosopher about the hypothetical case of a man born blind who could start to see: "Suppose a man born blind, and now adult, and taught by his touch to distinguish between a cube and a sphere of the same metal, and nighly of the same bigness, so as to tell, when he felt one and the other, which is the cube, which the sphere. Suppose then the cube and the sphere placed on a table, and the blind man be made to see: *quaere*, whether *by sight before he touched them*, he could now distinguish and tell which is the globe, which the cube" (Locke [1690] 1959).

Impressively, this question was posed before cataract operations were possible, and was indeed routed in the old debate about innate ideas and sensory experience. In fact, Locke gave a negative answer to the Molyneaux's question: according to Locke's empiricism, although a blind man following the restoration of vision could "see" the objects, he would be unable to name them, lacking any visual component in his previous ideas of "cube" or "sphere." Early experimental findings seemed to support Locke's theoretical expectations. In 1728, the surgeon William Cheselden removed the cataracts from a thirteen year old boy who had been blind since birth. The surgery restored the boy's vision but, although immediately after the surgery he was able to see and to visually differentiate between objects and even to make aesthetic judgments about them, he had no idea of distances, sizes, and space, was utterly bewildered by the appearance of shapes and distances, was not able to recognize objects with which he was familiar, and felt as though objects were touching his eyes. However, as noted by Gregory (2004), it would be wrong to answer the Molyneaux's question on the basis of the results of such "primitive" operations (as were those reviewed by Von Senden 1932, mainly involving patients with lens cataracts, with sight being restored by removal of the lens), since the available surgery did not allow a decent retinal image for weeks or months. This raises the problem of a possible confusion between low-level perceptual processes (i.e., being able to see) and higher-level processes mediating object recognition. In fact, one can be able to see objects, colors and faces but be completely unable to connect the visual percept to the semantic knowledge and the sensory experience based on non-visual modalities. Accordingly, as noted by Held (2009), some conditions should hold for an experiment to really address Molyneaux's issue. First of all, blindness must have been verifiably congenital and continuous. Moreover, standardized measures of pre- and post-surgery visual functions should be provided (and this is rarely the case for the earlier reports). In fact, if the patient is (or has been for a period) somehow able to see before the operation, a crossmodal transfer between touch and vision would be possible, thus making any inferences on the effects of vision-restoration uncertain. Moreover, the blind patient should demonstrate to possess a light perception, a condition for the normal functioning of the retina and of the optic nerve (accordingly, operable cases of blindness—or better, "near-blindness," since the retina has to be functional and eye tissues are never entirely opaque—are of two kinds: cataract of the lenses and opacity of the corneas; see Gregory and Wallace 1963). After surgery, the patient should have enough visual acuity to visually discriminate between objects, and testing should immediately follow surgery in order to prevent visual skills acquisition by experience (Held 2009).

Although a number of experiments have been carried out on blind individuals undergoing visual restoration (e.g., Gregory and Wallace 1963; Valvo 1971; Carlson, Hyvarinen, and Raninen 1986; Sacks 1993; Le Grand, Mondloch et al. 2001; Fine, Wade et al. 2003; Ostrovsky, Andalman, and Sinha 2006; Levin, Dumoulin et al. 2010), only a few are in line with the above mentioned recommendations. Moreover, a further *caveat* concerns the fact that a great part of the available data is based on subjective (or even anecdotal) observations. SB was a blind man that regained sight when he was 51 years old and who was studied by Gregory and Wallace (1963) a few weeks after his first operation. Although SB could "see" after the operation, pictures looked flat and meaningless to him, his responses to illusionary figures were far from normal (for instance, he did not experience the flipping ambiguity of the Necker Cube) and perspective did not make any sense to him. Still, he was able to estimate distances and sizes of objects that he was familiar with by touch, whereas he seemed completely lost with untouchable objects (such as the moon) or with pictures. Similar results have been obtained with patient MM by Fine et al. (Fine, Wade et al. 2003). MM lost his sight at 3.5 years and received a corneal and limbal stem-cell transplant at age 43. Before that age, MM had some light perception but no experience of contrast or form. Importantly, when first tested five months after surgery, he could perceive orientation changes and also easily recognize simple shapes and colors, but he was impaired in form tasks requiring integration of texture elements, or with subjective contours (e.g., Kanisza figures) (see figure 4.3). He was also impaired in interpreting 3D retinal images and perspective cues. Critically, MM's performance was particularly bad in object and face recognition; accordingly, fMRI data indicated that face and object recognition evoked little activation in MM's lingual and fusiform gyri (i.e., the cortical areas usually devoted to the recognition of objects and faces). Conversely, MM was successful at many motion tasks (as also confirmed by normal BOLD activation in the motion area MT). Notably, two years after the operation neither MM's form processing or neural resolution had improved, whereas interpreting motion and shading cues was better (see also Levin, Dumoulin et al. 2010).

Le Grand et al. (Le Grand, Mondloch et al. 2001) studied the effects of visual restoration in children: critically, deprivation of patterned vision due to a dense central cataract in each eye until 2–6 months of age was found to impair configuration face processing (specifically, differentiating faces that differed only in the spacing of their features) even after 9 years of restored vision, suggesting that normal visual experience during the first few months of life is necessary for the normal development of expert face processing. Recently, Project Prakash has provided the opportunity to work with restored-vision blind subjects. Project Prakash (see http://web.mit.edu/bcs/sinha/prakash.html; also see Mandavilli 2006) is a charitable and scientific initiative launched in 2003 that aims to locate congenitally blind children in India, treat those whose blindness is correctable, and study their subsequent visual development. Pawan Shina (who runs the project) and colleagues have reported the case of a 29-year-old man who has been blind for his entire life due to congenital aphakia (a rare condition in which the eyeball develops without a lens). His visual acuity was 20/900, far worse than the WHO definition of legal blindness. After wearing proper glasses for eighteen months (with glasses, SK's visual acuity was raised to 20/120), SK showed the ability to recognize objects with varying colors and brightness. Moreover, although at the beginning he had to rely on motion to integrate objects, over the next eighteen months he learned to recognize objects even when they were still. However, as noted by the authors, prior to this corrective intervention SK was able to visually perceive light and movement, which possibly allowed his visual cortex to develop normally. In a subsequent study, Ostrovosky, Andalman, and Sinha (2006) reported the case of SRD, a 34-year-old Indian woman born with dense cataract formation. For the first

FORM

a) Outlined form

What is the outlined shape?

MM = 100%; C = 100%, 100%, 100%; *P* = 1

b) Texture segmentation

What orientation is the rectangle of different contrast?

MM = 96%; C = 100%, 100%, 100%; *P* = 0

c) Line contour integration

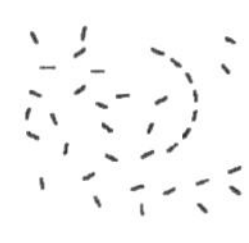

Is there a pathway of lines within the random lines?

MM = 80%; C = 100%, 90%, 95%; *P* = 0.02

d) Glass pattern

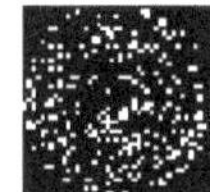

Is there a circular pattern within the random noise?

MM = 73%; C = 80%, 85%,100%; *P* = 0.06

e) Illusory contours

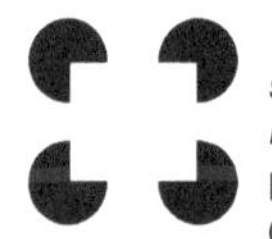

What is the 'hidden' shape outlined by the black apertures?

MM = no response; C = t

DEPTH

f) Occlusion

What is the color of the object in front?

MM = 100%; C = t

g) Texture segmentation

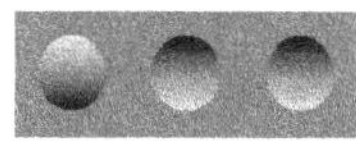

Which sphere bulges out?

MM = 100%; C = t

h) Transparency

How many objects are there, and which is in front?

MM = 0%; C = t

i) Perspective

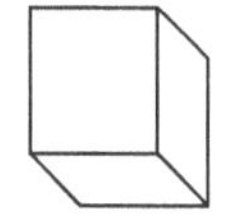

What is the shape of the object?

MM = no response; C = t

j) Shepard Tables

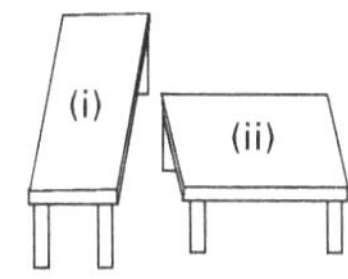

Which tables match in shape/use the same table-cloth?

width/height bias (100% veridical); MM= 100%; C = 63%, 63%, 47%; *P* = 0.009

MOTION

k) Simple/complex/barber pole motion

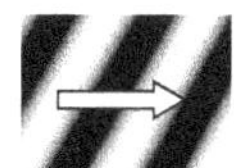

What direction is the pattern moving in?

MM = 100%; C = t

l) Form from motion

What is the orientation of the rectangle of different motion?

MM =1 00%; C = t

m) Motion Glass patterns

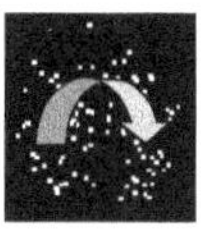

Is there a circular/swirling pattern within the random noise?

MM = 90%; C = 95%, 80%, 85%; *P* = 0.74

n) Kinetic depth effect

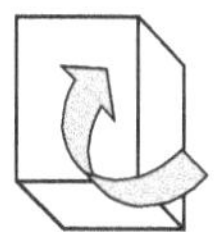

What is the shape of the object?

MM = 100%; C = t

o) Biological motion

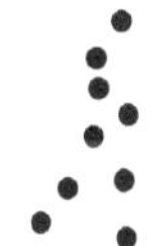

What do the moving dots represent?

MM correctly identified a moving walker.

Figure 4.3

Stimuli, tasks and performance for tests of MM's form, depth and motion processing. Stimuli shown to controls (C) were always blurred using a low-pass filter to match MM's spatial resolution losses. Some tasks were trivial (=t) for controls and were not formally tested. When *P*-values (one-tailed *t*-tests) are reported , MM worse than controls.

Reprinted from Fine, Wade et al., "Long-term deprivation affects visual perception and cortex," *Nature Neuroscience* 6(9) (2003): 915–916. (© 2003. Reprinted by permission of Macmillan Publishers Ltd.)

12 years of her childhood SRD did not experience any patterned visual stimulation. At the age of 12 years, she underwent cataract-removal surgery, but the operation succeeded only for the left eye. According to her mother's report, SRD learned to recognize her siblings and parents six months after surgery, and after one year could name objects around the house purely by sight. When tested at 34 years old she showed significant functional recovery, since she could successfully perform form-recognition and face-recognition tasks. On the basis of other experiments, Sinha and colleagues (Held, Ostrovsky et al. 2008) suggested a complete lack of transfer from normal tactile discrimination to vision immediately after sight onset; however, already one week after surgery, touch-to-vision transfer and crossmodal recognition are likely to occur. Accordingly, Ostrovsky and colleagues (Ostrovsky, Meyers et al. 2009) highlighted the importance of motion cues in improving object perception skills in three congenitally blind individuals whose vision had been restored, confirming that the human brain retains the ability to learn visual skills even after extended periods of visual deprivation. In summary, it is still difficult to draw any definitive conclusions regarding Molyneaux's question on the basis of the available findings. The results obtained so far—with all the methodological limitations of each case—seem to converge in suggesting that visual functions are not innately available but have to be acquired through learning. This conclusion (i.e., visual functions are not innately available) indicates that although spatial features can be acquired in a different sensory modality, and despite the existence of supramodal representations of objects (see the next section of this chapter), it takes time to translate a novel sensory experience into pre-existing categories built on the basis of other sensory modalities. This does not necessarily imply that blind individuals do not experience spatial mental images in an analogical format. Rather, it suggests that visual features—such as colors, brightness or the rules of perspective—may at the beginning make it hard to extract spatial features from the visual percept and match this percept with the mental image of a specific object that has been built up on the basis of tactile experience. In fact, the finding that blind individuals can learn to recognize visual objects after a few weeks following the restoration of vision, indicates that the visual cortex is able to retain its function even across several years of visual deprivation, and that a crossmodal matching between vision and touch remains possible even in adulthood. Although it may turn out to be impossible to verify empirically, Molyneaux's query still represents a fascinating "thought" experiment (cf. Jacomuzzi, Kobau, and Bruno 2003) that should continue to provoke discussion and inspire new experimental paradigms.

Finally, the practical implications of vision restoration after a long-term blindness should be seriously considered: in fact, regaining sight may induce depressive states in individuals who until that moment were perfectly at peace with living in a non-visual world (see Gregory and Wallace 1963).

4.5 Supramodal Mental Representations

In the previous section we have discussed whether blind individuals can experience visual mental images. As we have anticipated, regardless of the possibility that the mental images of the blind contain visual details, it is clear that blind individuals can represent spatial information and that their mental representations need to be built on the basis of a non-visual perceptual experience. Still, representations generated by the blind are similar to those generated by the sighted, at least to a certain extent, as is demonstrated by their similar patterns of performance in different visuo-spatial tasks: blind and sighted individuals can generate similar spatial representations on the basis of different perceptual experiences. Depending on the theoretical approach of different researchers, these representations have been regarded as "multimodal," "supramodal" or "amodal" (see Struiksma, Noordzij, and Postma 2009 for a review) (see figure 4.4).

Notably, the review by Struiksma and colleagues (Struiksma, Noordzij, and Postma 2009) is the first to clarify the difference between these terms that are often confused or used as interchangeable, although their theoretical assumptions are slightly different. In particular, the "multimodal" view assumes that spatial representations are related to the input-sensory modality and are subtended by modality-specific cortical regions. Accordingly, only modality-specific brain areas will activate to generate the image, without the involvement of other regions which are devoted to processing spatial information per se. Conversely, the "supramodal" account assumes that spatial representations, although maintaining modality-specific information, exceed the input from different modalities (Barsalou 1999; Pietrini, Furey et al. 2004). At the neural level, this should be reflected by the activation—during a spatial-imagery task—of both modality-specific regions and other "supramodal" areas devoted to processing spatial information per se, regardless the input-sensory modality. Finally, according to the "amodal" account, spatial imagery is an abstract process, independent from the input modality and not necessarily derived from multiple input sources. Hence, the same pattern of cortical activation would be observed regardless of the sensorial channel that conveyed the input. According to the amodal account, once the spatial image is generated, the modality-specific input can no longer be reactivated. Common to the supramodal and multimodal view is the idea that different input channels contribute in different measures to the generation of a spatial image, depending on the available perceptual experience. Moreover, the combined inputs from different modalities strengthen the spatial mental representation.

What do these models imply for congenitally blind individuals? As illustrated by Struiksma et al. (Struiksma, Noordzij, and Postma 2009), according to the multimodal view, the spatial representations generated by blind individuals would lack the con-

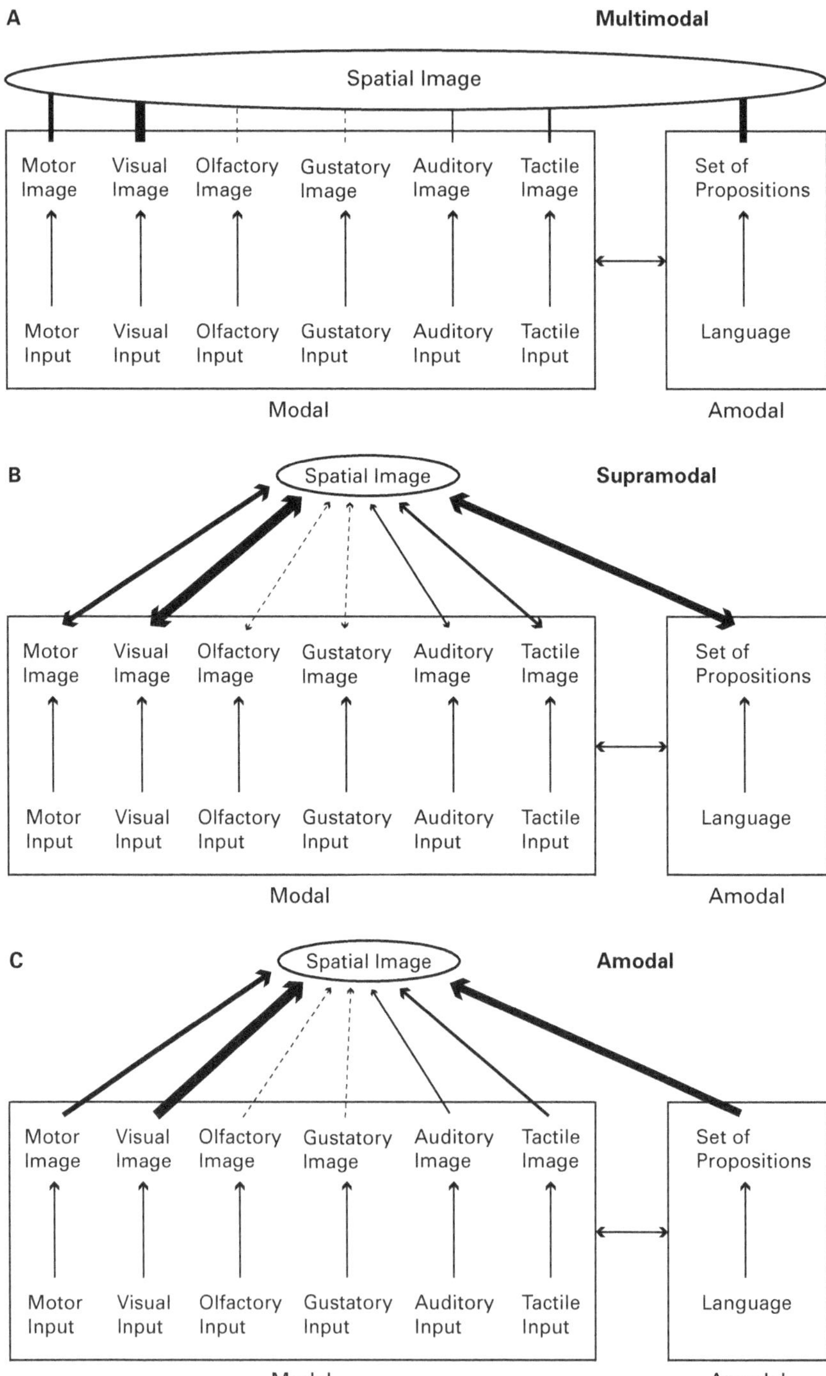
A
Multimodal
Spatial Image
Motor Image
Visual Image
Olfactory Image
Gustatory Image
Auditory Image
Tactile Image
Motor Input
Visual Input
Olfactory Input
Gustatory Input
Auditory Input
Tactile Input
Set of Propositions
Language
Modal
Amodal
B
Spatial Image
Supramodal
Motor Image
Visual Image
Olfactory Image
Gustatory Image
Auditory Image
Tactile Image
Motor Input
Visual Input
Olfactory Input
Gustatory Input
Auditory Input
Tactile Input
Set of Propositions
Language
Modal
Amodal
C
Spatial Image
Amodal
Motor Image
Visual Image
Olfactory Image
Gustatory Image
Auditory Image
Tactile Image
Motor Input
Visual Input
Olfactory Input
Gustatory Input
Auditory Input
Tactile Input
Set of Propositions
Language
Modal
Amodal

tribution of the visual input: therefore, behavioral differences are likely to emerge between sighted and blind subjects in spatial-imagery tasks. Nonetheless, blindness should not prevent the generation of a supramodal spatial representation, although the lack of visual input in the blind would change the distribution of the inputs from the other sensorial channels (i.e., sensory compensation), possibly resulting in behavioral differences between the sighted and the blind. Finally, according to the amodal account, no differences should be observed between sighted and blind individuals, since the spatial representations generated on the basis of a visual or a tactile input are supposed to be functionally identical. In light of the studies we reviewed above, it seems that spatial images are indeed "supramodal." For instance, in a study by Röder and Rösler (1998), blind and sighted subjects were required to perform a mental navigation task in which a series of landmarks haptically explored had to be memorized. Sighted subjects that explored the landmarks only visually performed similarly to the sighted and blind subjects that explored the scene only haptically, suggesting that a similar underlying supramodal spatial representation can be generated on the basis of either visual or haptic inputs. In fact, blind individuals have been found to perform similarly to sighted individuals in other spatial tasks, although also presenting certain specific limitations which depend on the dominant perceptual experience (see for instance the difficulty with simultaneous processing of multiple information in the blind: Vecchi, Tinti, and Cornoldi 2004). This has also been confirmed at the cortical level. For instance, in a study by Pascual-Leone et al. (Pascual-Leone, Theoret et al. 2006), blind and sighted subjects were required to imagine the shape of a letter presented auditorily and to answer about specific spatial features (such as whether the letter contained a specific vertical line, a diagonal line and so forth). Subjects were tested at baseline and after rTMS over sensorimotor and occipital cortex. Interestingly, blind subjects reported having imagined the feeling of the letters on their fingers as tracing each letter's outline in their imagination to cope with the task.

Figure 4.4
Three different models of how different sources of information can contribute to the generation of a spatial image as proposed by Struiksma, Noordzij, and Postma. The line width represents a schematic weighting of the contribution of the different sources. Panel A is a multimodal representation established in modality-specific brain areas. Together these form the multimodal representation. Panel B is a supramodal representation, which exceeds modality-specific input to generate a spatial image, but maintains a bi-directional link with modality-specific input. Panel C is an amodal representation in which a spatial image is extracted from the input and no backward connections remain.
Reprinted from Struiksma, Noordzij, and Postma, "What is the link between language and spatial images? Behavioral and neural findings in blind and sighted individuals," *Acta Psychologica* 132(2) (2009): 145–156. (© 2009. Reprinted by permission of Elsevier)

Conversely, sighted subjects reported visualizing the characters. Accordingly, rTMS over sensorimotor cortices significantly affected blind subjects' performance more than rTMS over occipital areas; whereas in the sighted, rTMS over occipital areas impaired performance more that rTMS over sensorimotor regions. If spatial representations were amodal, no differences should have been reported. Of course, a multimodal account might also be suitable, but neurofunctional findings mostly support the supramodal view. In fact, as we will see in more detail in a following chapter, neurofunctional evidence has showed that some regions (especially in the parietal lobe) mediate spatial mental processes, independently of the input modality. Critically, both the "dorsal" and the "ventral" pathways are likely to contain supramodal regions that allow us to encode the shape and location of objects regardless of the specific sensory modality that is in play (e.g., Pietrini, Furey et al. 2004; Ricciardi, Vanello et al. 2007; Bonino, Ricciardi et al. 2008; and for review, see Pietrini, Ptito, and Kupers 2009).

4.6 Blindness and the Mental Representation of Numerical Magnitude

Several studies indicate that individuals tend to mentally organize numerical magnitude along a left-to-right oriented horizontal mental number line, with the smaller numbers occupying leftward and larger numbers occupying rightward positions (see Dehaene, Bossini, and Giraux 1993). Critically, the correspondence between the ordinal sequence of numbers and their mental representation extends to a more general representation of space, with small numbers being internally associated with the left-side of the space and large numbers with the right-side of the space (Dehaene 1992; Dehaene, Bossini, and Giraux 1993). Accordingly, numbers have been found to directly modulate the allocation of attentional resources to particular portions of both egocentric and allocentric space; reaction times to smaller numbers (relative to larger numbers) are faster when responses are made with a left button-press, and the opposite pattern is found when responses are made with a right button-press (cf. The Spatial-Numerical Association of Response Codes = SNARC; e.g., Dehaene, Bossini, and Giraux 1993). Similarly, subjects are faster in detecting targets presented in the left hemifield if previously presented with a small-magnitude number and conversely, reaction times to right-hemifield targets are decreased by previous processing of a high-magnitude number (Fischer, Castel et al. 2003; Fischer, Warlop et al. 2004). Notably, the left-to-right orientation of the mental number line may be due to reading habits in Western culture, as suggested by the finding of a weaker or reversed SNARC-effect with Iranian subjects who read from right to left (Dehaene, Bossini, and Giraux 1993).

Whether early blind individuals also represent numbers in a spatial format, and, particularly, if they do so in the form of a left-to-right oriented linear analog mental representation, has been investigated only recently (Szucs and Csepe 2005; Castronovo and Seron 2007a,b; Salillas, Grana et al. 2009; Cattaneo, Fantino et al. 2010b). The issue is indeed of extreme interest both for research on the effects of blindness on representational processes and for research on the basis of numerical cognition development. In fact, on one side visual deprivation affects the way space is mentally represented (for review, see Thinus-Blanc and Gaunet 1997). On the other side, as noted by Castronovo and Seron (2007a,b), visual experience may be necessary for the proper development of numerical cognition (Trick and Pylyshyn 1994; Simon 1997, 1999; Newcombe 2002), especially in light of theories arguing that visual subitizing—the pre-attentive capacity of fast and precise quantification through vision of small sets of entities (up to three or four elements)—may be responsible for the numerosity discrimination abilities of preverbal infants, thus providing the basis for the development of numerical skills. According to this view, visual cortices and visuo-spatial information would play a major role in mediating the development of numerical cognition (Trick and Pylyshyn 1994; Simon 1997, 1999; Newcombe 2002). Although touch and hearing may also support numerical processing, they may not be as efficient as vision, especially when large numerosities are involved. In fact, in the sequential mode, hearing and touch put a heavy load on working memory and hence have a limited capacity, whereas in the simultaneous mode, hearing suffers from discrimination limitations and touch from exploration limitations. Conversely, vision allows for simultaneous perception of small and large sets of entities and is less affected by memory, discrimination and exploration limitations. Accordingly, there is evidence that children find numerical discrimination of sequential sets of objects more difficult than that of static sets (Mix 1999). Hence, by lacking experience with visual numerosities, blind individuals may represent numbers in a different way than do the sighted. Nevertheless, this may not be the case if one assumes that individuals possess an innate abstract and approximate sense of numbers that allows them to understand numerical quantities, regardless of their modality of presentation (Gallistel and Gelman 1992, 2000; Gelman and Gallistel 2004; Dehaene 1997). Similarly, visual experience may not be so critical for numerical cognition in light of the "undifferentiated amount hypothesis" (Mix, Huttenlocher, and Levine 2002), suggesting that the development of numerical abilities may be based on an analog mechanism that is suited for all types of continuous perceptual variables (such as brightness, density, weight, rhythm pattern, rate, duration) and not for numerosity per se (Clearfield and Mix 2001; Mix, Huttenlocher, and Levine 2002; Rousselle, Palmers, and Noël 2004).

The findings by Castronovo and Seron (2007a,b) have shed light on these issues. In a first study (Castronovo and Seron 2007a), a group of congenitally or early blind and sighted subjects were compared in classical numerical tasks on small numbers (comparison task to 5 and parity-judgment task with small numbers) and on large numbers (comparison task to 55). Blind and sighted subjects showed similar patterns of performance on numerical-comparison tasks in both ranges in the auditory modality, suggesting that the blind were representing numerical magnitude in the form of a numerical number line oriented from left to right (Dehaene, Bossini, and Giraux 1993; Fias, Brysbaert et al. 1996; Dehaene 1997; Dehaene, Dehaene-Lambertz, and Cohen 1998; Reynvoet, Brysbaert, and Fias 2002). In fact, the blind, as well as the sighted, were less accurate when the numerical distance between the compared numbers was small than when it was large, thus showing the so-called "distance effect"; and both groups were faster in responding to small numbers when they were responded to on the left side and to large numbers when they were responded to on the right side (SNARC effect). On the basis of these findings, Castronovo and Seron (2007a) concluded that vision is not indispensable for the development of numerical representation in the form of an analog mental number line, even for large numerosities. According to Castronovo and Seron (2007a), the similar left-to-right orientation of the mental number line in blind and in sighted individuals likely depends on the fact that Braille, like the Western alphabets, is "read" from left to right (all the blind subjects tested were Braille readers). Similar results were also obtained in a previous study by Szucs and Csepe (2005), who also reported a distance and a SNARC effect with congenitally blind people on a comparison task to 5. Critically, Szucs and Csepe also recorded electroencephalography data showing that blind participants activated a parietal network similar to that used by sighted subjects when representing small numerical magnitudes.

A following study by Castronovo and Seron (2007b) investigated the impact of blindness on the obedience to Weber's law in number processing: according to Weber's law, the larger the numbers and quantities are, the more their processing becomes approximate and imprecise. This effect has been consistently reported in sighted subjects, and likely depends on individuals' experience with numbers and quantities (e.g., Verguts and Van Opstal 2005; Booth and Siegler 2006). Castronovo and Seron (2007b) hypothesized that since blind individuals experience numbers in a different way than sighted subjects, they may also be affected by Weber's law to a different extent. In order to test this, a group of blind subjects and a group of sighted subjects were compared in two numerical-estimation tasks, a keypress estimation task and an auditory events estimation task. Specifically, in the first task, subjects had to press a key at rates that made vocal or subvocal counting impossible until they felt that they had approximately reached the given target number; in the second task they had to estimate the number of tones emitted in unique, non-periodic timed sequences. Both blind and sighted subjects' performance (Szucs and Csepe 2005) was found to obey Weber's law, but—critically—blind subjects demonstrated better numerical-estimation abilities than did sighted subjects, especially in contexts involving proprioception (i.e., keypress). Castronovo and Seron (2007b) interpreted these results as suggesting that blindness and its following experience with numbers might result in better accuracy in numerical processing, especially when the task is presented in the haptic modality. In fact, since they cannot count on vision, blind individuals are somehow "forced" to rely on number processing to carry out many everyday activities: for instance, in locomotion they often estimate distances in terms of number of steps, and have to rely on the numerical information provided by their own proprioception to continuously update their spatial position. Therefore, proprioception is likely to be the blind individuals' preferred modality to process numerosities. Accordingly, Szucs and Csepe (2005) also found remapping of number into somatosensory representations in their blind participants.

Recently, Cattaneo et al. (Cattaneo, Fantino et al. 2010b) have also investigated whether the mental number line can modulate the representation of external space crossmodally in a group of early blind individuals and sighted controls by using a line-bisection paradigm. Visual-line bisection is a widely used task for investigating the allocation of spatial attention (Jewell and McCourt 2000), and it has hence also been used to explore the influence of numerical magnitude on the allocation of spatial attention. For instance, a leftward spatial bias was observed when the bisected line consisted of series of small digits and a rightward bias was observed for lines consisting of series of large digits (Fischer 2001; see also de Hevia, Girelli, and Vallar 2006). Similarly, in left-neglect patients the bisection error was shifted contra-lesionally when the digit "1" was presented at each end of the to-be-bisected visual line, whereas it was shifted ipsi-lesionally when the digit "9" was presented (Bonato, Priftis et al. 2008). It has also been reported that priming by large numbers eliminates pseudo-neglect (i.e., the tendency to perceive stimulus midpoint to the left of its actual physical midpoint; cf. Bowers and Heilman 1980) in visual-line bisection (Cattaneo, Silvanto et al. 2009). In a recent study, Cattaneo et al. (Cattaneo, Fantino et al. 2010b) required blind and blindfolded sighted participants to haptically explore wooden rods of different lengths and indicate their midpoint. During each trial, a number from either the low ("2") or high ("8") end of the mental number line was presented in the auditory modality. In both the blind and sighted subjects, this bias was significantly increased by the presentation of the number "2" and significantly reduced by the presentation of the number "8." Hence, these results demonstrated that the mental number line can modulate the allocation of attention to external space crossmodally even in the absence of any visual experience. When no numbers were presented, both blind and blindfolded control subjects tended to bisect the rods to the left of the actual midpoint. This tendency of bisecting to the left of the veridical center is usually referred to as "pseudoneglect" (cf. Bowers and Heilman 1980), and it has been reported both in the visual and the haptic modality (for a review, see Jewell and McCourt 2000). Pseudoneglect is believed to reflect an attentional asymmetry which is biased in favor of the left side of space, resulting from the dominant role of the right hemisphere in the allocation and control of spatial attention (McCourt and Jewell 1999). In fact, the direction of this bias is the opposite to that displayed in neglect patients who typically suffer from a lesion to the right inferior parietal lobule or to the right temporo-parietal junction (cf. Vallar 2001). Cattaneo et al. (Cattaneo, Fantino et al. under revision a,b) have demonstrated that pseudoneglect is also evident in line and numerical bisection in early blind individuals, suggesting that it does not depend on prior visual experience.

Although blind individuals seem to represent numbers spatially, the processes underlying the mapping between numerical magnitude and space may be different in the blind and in the sighted. In this regard, a study by Salillas and colleagues (Salillas, Granà et al. 2009) has shown that the attentional shifts generated by numbers have different electrophysiological correlates in early blind and sighted individuals. In particular, the auditory presentation of numbers was found to shift attention to either the left or right auditory space according to numerical magnitude in both groups, but this effect was associated with the modulation of a sensory ERP component in the sighted (N100), and to the modulation of a more cognitive ERP component (P300) in the blind. The results by Salillas et al. (Salillas, Granà et al. 2009) suggest that blind individuals may have a spatial representation of numbers that is more dependent on working memory mechanisms as compared to that of the sighted: in other words, the absence of visual input and the use of the auditory modality (with less discriminative power and greater working-memory requirements), may force blind individuals to manipulate the mental number line in a more controlled way than do sighted people, relying on working memory processes to a greater extent while showing no effects at the sensory level.

4.7 Visual Deprivation and Semantic Knowledge

Research dealing with language functions in the blind has mainly focused on language acquisition, thus mostly considering the linguistic skills of blind children. On one side, their lack of vision has been found to interfere with specific aspects of language acquisition, but on the other side, language has been reported to play a crucial compensatory role in blind children's development. Indeed, language is—first of all—a *social* skill. In this book we have decided not to specifically deal with social implications of being blind. Accordingly, our aim in this section is to show how the lack of visual inputs can interfere with the way conceptual/semantic knowledge develops, and not to discuss the critical implications that blindness has for communicative/social abilities.

Blind children have been found to suffer delays and deviations in the acquisition of different aspects of language, showing semantic, syntactical and phonological deficits (for reviews, see Mills 1983; Perez-Pereira and Conti-Ramsden 1999). Nonetheless, the linguistic problems of blind children may rather reflect a more general deficit in the way their semantic knowledge is organized: specifically, the lack of vision may impair category formation (e.g., grouping objects according to similar visual features including motion, color and shape), thus for instance accounting for the lack of overgeneralization and the reduced number of word inventions often reported in blind children (Andersen, Dunlea, and Kekelis 1984, 1993). Linda Pring has extensively studied language acquisition in blind children. On the basis of the results of a series of experiments, Pring (1988; Pring, Freistone, and Katan 1990) hypothesized that the semantic network of blind children likely contains more abstract concepts. For instance, in one study memory for words that were either read or heard by sighted and blind children was tested; stimuli were either presented or had to be actively generated. Sighted children were found to recall better the words that they had generated compared to those that they had read or heard (showing the so called "generation effect"). Critically, blind children showed the reverse pattern. Since the generation effect is thought to be based on the "enhanced conceptual sensitivity" of self-produced items, the lack of generation in the blind was attributed to an impaired or less well-elaborated semantic network, depending on the fact that blind children had to acquire many concepts through language with less—or without any—direct sensory experience (Pring 1988; Pring, Freistone, and Katan 1990). For instance, as previously noted in this book, blind individuals usually have a good knowledge of colors, but this is entirely mediated by language, and is not accompanied by the *qualia* associated with the sensory experience. In this regard, by using an odd-man-out triad task to measure implicit pair-wise similarity judgments, Connolly et al. (Connolly, Gleitman, and Thompson-Schill 2007) have shown how the lack of first-hand experience with colors selectively affects implicit judgments about higher-order concepts, such as fruits and vegetables, but not about others, such as household objects. And this is because for fruits and vegetables color represents a "diagnostic" feature (a banana is—at least in normal conditions—yellow), whereas this is not the case for household items, for which color is not such a distinctive feature (a telephone may be black or red or yellow). Hence, whereas in sighted individuals color represents an immediate, possibly automatic form of knowledge (at least for certain categories of objects), in blind individuals color-knowledge is merely stipulated, with this knowledge not being spontaneously used in organizing similarity relations among concepts.

Although above we have underlined differences in the semantic organization of concepts in blind and sighted individuals, it should be noticed how equivalences are indeed more remarkable than differences between the two groups. This may depend on the ability of blind individuals to compensate for their lack of visual inputs by developing conceptual networks with more auditory and tactile nodes (see also Röder, Rösler, and Neville 2000; Röder, Demuth et al. 2002). For instance, Röder and Rösler

(2003) investigated whether blind adults can benefit from deep/semantic as opposed to physical/shallow encoding in a recognition task for environmental sounds, as sighted individuals usually do. All subjects (early, late and sighted) showed higher recognition rates after semantic encoding and, critically, blind participants outperformed the sighted under both physical and semantic encoding, thus contradicting the view that semantic networks in the blind are less elaborated and their concepts are more abstract.

5 Spatial Cognition in the Blind

Glaucus shouted her name. No answer came. They retraced their steps—in vain: they could not discover her—it was evident she had been swept along some opposite direction by the human current. Their friend, their preserver, was lost! And hitherto Nydia had been their guide. Her blindness rendered the scene familiar to her alone. Accustomed, through a perpetual night, to thread the windings of the city, she had led them unerringly towards the sea-shore, by which they had resolved to hazard an escape. Now, which way could they wend? all was rayless to them—a maze without a clue.

—Edward Bulwer-Lytton, *The Last Days of Pompeii*

5.1 *Visual* Spatial Cognition?

Spatial cognition is a general term we use to refer to a range of abilities that are of critical importance in our everyday life, such as representing the space that surrounds us and updating it whenever we move, localizing, grasping, or pointing to external objects, learning routes, understanding maps, orienting ourselves and so forth. Spatial cognition involves both dynamic aspects, such as navigation, and more static aspects, such as memory for object locations or topographic knowledge (e.g., Schacter and Nadel 1991; Janzen 2006).

Although we can obtain knowledge of our surroundings by seeing, hearing, touching and even smelling, vision is usually the primary sensory modality we rely on in spatial cognition (e.g., Pick, Warren, and Hay 1969; Eimer 2004). This is because our visual system allows the acquisition of highly detailed spatial information that cannot be obtained by other sensory modalities. In fact, through vision we can simultaneously perceive a large portion of spatial field; and even if the point of foveation is quite limited, objects falling in the periphery can still be detected as our attention moves around a particular scene. Conversely, when exploring a scene by way of touch, we can only attend to the objects that are currently touched and no cues are available to draw our attention in any particular direction. Moreover, tactile exploration is intrinsically limited to near objects, whereas distant objects cannot be explored. Vision is also more precise than audition in providing information about where objects are: in fact, hearing has often to deal with ambiguous and relatively imprecise cues (especially in case of distant object localization), and although it certainly contributes to sighted individuals' spatial cognition, usually the process of localizing sounds has the function of directing attention toward objects or events of interest, so that they can then be registered by vision. Furthermore, although objects always have visible features, they do not always emit sounds; and even when they do, the information that can be derived concerns where the object is but not the shape of the object itself. Moreover, although locomotion can rely upon proprioception and vestibular information as well, vision still plays the major role in supporting navigation (cf. the importance of peripheral optic flow in updating the relative positions of surrounding landmarks when one is moving: Gibson 1979).

Perceptual experience is normally so heavily vision-based that visual inputs affect the way spatial information is encoded by other sensory modalities (Pick, Warren, and Hay 1969; Kennett, Eimer et al. 2001; Röder, Rösler, and Spence 2004). Crossmodal perceptual illusions, such as the well-known "ventriloquism effect" (i.e., the mislocation of an auditory stimulus toward a simultaneous visual stimulus: Howard and Templeton 1966) or "visual capture" of touch phenomena (e.g., Singer and Day 1969; Pavani, Spence, and Driver 2000) are extreme examples of this. Notably, when the visual channel is temporarily impaired, the visual capture tends to disappear, as demonstrated for instance by the finding that blurred visual stimuli (which are difficult to locate) can be mislocalized toward clear auditory stimuli; an effect that immediately reverses as soon as visual stimuli are deblurred (Alais and Burr 2004). Beside the extreme case of crossmodal illusions, in normal conditions vision offers a sort of "reference frame" in which information coming from other sensory modalities is translated, thus providing "by default" the basis for multisensory integration and action control (e.g., Röder, Rösler, and Spence 2004; Röder, Kusmierek et al. 2007; Röder, Föcker et al. 2008; also see chapter 2 of this book). Therefore, even if we imagine (to refer to an example in Ungar 2000) walking in a dark room without any visual cues, still that experience cannot be truly compared to that of a blind person. In fact, although we might not be aware of it, in orienting ourselves we automatically rely on a series of spatial competences and skills that we have developed on the basis of our dominant visual experience. Indeed, "the very first time you, as an infant, watched your hand as you reached out for an object, you were already learning about space through vision" (Ungar 2000).

The privileged role of vision in spatial cognition suggests that individuals affected by visual impairment or blindness are likely to experience severe deficiencies in spatial abilities. Accordingly, consistent evidence indicates that visual experience is necessary for *efficient* spatial processing; nonetheless, good spatial skills and understanding can be acquired by blind people, thanks to compensatory task-related strategies, level of practice with spatial concepts, and cortical plasticity phenomena (see Thinus-Blanc and Gaunet 1997, for a review). Critically, in reviewing the published literature on spatial abilities in the blind, it is quite common to encounter apparently contrasting results. As we will specifically discuss later in this chapter (see section 5.5), the cognitive abilities exhibited by blind individuals depend on an interrelation between subjective and experimental characteristics, such as the specific ability being tested, the specific task used and the experimental context, so that differences in either the experimental setting or in individuals' characteristics may lead to a completely different behavioral output. In other words, on one hand "the blind" cannot be regarded as a homogeneous population, but must be considered according to individual variables such as age, onset-age of their visual deficit, duration and etiology of that deficit, mobility capacities, Braille-reading capacity and use of external devices, all of which are critical factors in predicting how well a blind individual will perform in a particular situation. On the other hand, the nature of the designated task (way-finding; object-location recall; real or virtual navigation; sequential vs. simultaneous spatial encoding; passive processing vs. active manipulation; auditory and/or haptic acquisition of information, etc.) and task-related strategies are also extremely critical in affecting the behavioral output.

5.2 Spatial Reference Frames

Whether a person wants to grasp an object, or moves toward a location or is simply aware of his/her surroundings, a spatial mental representation of the relevant scene has to be generated. Humans can rely on different *frames of reference* in locomotion and in representing the external environment and the locations of the various objects in it. Specifically, a reference frame can be defined as the particular perspective from which the observation of a spatial variable (position of an object, its velocity, etc.) is made. A well-established distinction is that between "egocentric" (or view-centered, viewpoint-dependent) and "allocentric" (or environmental, viewpoint-independent) spatial representations (e.g., Mou, McNamara et al. 2006; Mou, Li, and McNamara 2008; for recent reviews, see Burgess 2006, 2008).

In egocentric spatial representations, space is represented with reference to the observer's body; if the subject moves, the spatial representation needs to be updated accordingly. Conversely, an "allocentric" spatial representation is generated regardless of the individual's position, on the basis of coordinates which are external to the body, so that the absolute positions of the different objects in the scene and their relative spatial positions do not need to be updated every time the subject moves. Allocentric representations may be centered on a specific object or built with reference to a virtual point of view (cf. Grush 2000); similarly, egocentric representations may be either body-centered, eye-centered or hand-centered (Kappers 2007). The distinction between egocentric and allocentric spatial representations has also been confirmed at the neurophysiological level: in particular, the hippocampal complex is likely to be critical for allocentric spatial learning and recall, whereas other brain regions—such as the caudeate nucleus—may be specifically involved in the encoding of egocentric space (cf. Nadel and Hardt 2004; Burgess 2008 for review). Nonetheless, the distinction between egocentric and allocentric spatial representations is not always clearly defined: indeed, the two types of representation are likely to coexist in parallel, and to combine to support behavior according to a series of task-dependent factors such as the amount of required self-motion, the size and intrinsic spatial structure of the environment, or the extent of prior experience with it (see Burgess 2006). For instance, large spatial layouts that lie beyond reaching/peripersonal space may induce an allocentric mode of encoding, whereas small layouts are likely to be represented in a subject-centered perspective (e.g., Presson, DeLange, and Hazelrigg 1989; but see Roskos-Ewoldsen, McNamara et al. 1998).

Since blind individuals lack the capacity for embracing with a single glance all the objects in their surrounding environment, they have to rely mainly on an ego-centered (i.e., body-, hand- or arm-centered) perspective in representing external space. This mode of representing space might be quite efficient when limited to peripersonal/ "near" space (the "space of manipulation," in Thinus-Blanc and Gaunet's [1997] terminology); in fact, near objects can be easily touched and identified. Conversely, objects beyond the extension of the arm (or cane) cannot be identified and represented in the scene (unless of course they are identified by audition or olfaction: cf. Klatzky, Lippa et al. 2002, 2003; Porter, Anand et al. 2005). In fact, blind individuals can never experience a large place or number of objects within a short time: in the absence of vision, locomotion is required to explore larger-scale environments, forcing the blind to continuously re-code previously touched objects with reference to their moving body. This continuous *spatial updating* is likely to be very cognitively demanding when no visual feedback is available, and might indeed reduce spatial understanding.

As we will see in the next paragraphs, many different tasks have been used to assess the nature and reliability of blind individuals' spatial representations and the way in which these representations are updated, such as parallelity-setting tasks, pointing tasks, way-finding paradigms, memory/recognition of stable or rotated scenes and several others. An important factor to be considered in these studies is the extent to which the task requires participants to draw *inferences* on spatial relations that they have not directly experienced. In fact, the amount of inferential processes required by a specific task has been found to be of critical importance in determining the impact of blindness on that situation (see Thinus-Blanc and Gaunet 1997; see also Cornoldi and Vecchi 2003, for a discussion about the importance of distinguishing between "passive" and "active" processes in spatial cognition). Moreover, some of these studies have been conducted in small-scale (peripersonal/reachable) spaces, while others in larger environments that require locomotion. A majority of these studies have compared the ability of blindfolded sighted controls, congenitally blind and late blind individuals, thus helping to clarify the role of actual and/or prior visual experience in shaping an individual's spatial cognition.

5.3 Blind Individuals' Representation of *Near* Space

As we have already mentioned, different paradigms have been adopted to investigate the way blind individuals represent the location of objects in the near space. Here we present first the results of two paradigms—pointing and parallel-setting tasks—that tap directly into the type of mental representation generated by the blind, and that do not require (or only marginally require) inferential processes. Then we present the results from two other paradigms—object recognition for rotated configurations (or "perspective taking") and memory for pathways on 2D and 3D matrices—that indeed require a certain amount of "active," inferential manipulation.

Pointing Tasks

In pointing tasks, participants are usually required to indicate with a hand the position of a target-point that they have previously (proprioceptively or visually) memorized. The distribution (e.g., scatter) of the hand-pointing responses reflects the type of spatial representation (and the underlying cognitive mechanisms) an agent is relying upon (Paillard 1991): responses based on movement trajectory reveal a viewer-dependent/egocentric reference frame, while responses based on the spatial array of the targets indicate that the agent is encoding space in an allocentric fashion.

Yves Rossetti and colleagues have largely investigated pointing in *reachable* space, by asking sighted participants to indicate on a touch-screen the location of a visual target that had been briefly flashed at random locations (e.g., Rossetti 1998; Rossetti and Pisella 2002). Overall, their results showed that different frames of reference were used depending on whether the pointing test was immediate or *delayed* for a few seconds. In particular, they found that the orientation of the longer axis of the pointing distribution was mainly oriented along the movement direction of the pointing gesture when no delay was introduced between target presentation and pointing, indicating that an egocentric frame of reference was involved. Conversely, for longer delays (e.g., 8 seconds), the main axis of the pointing distribution was found to be oriented along the direction of the targets' array, reflecting the adoption of an allocentric representation and hence a dependency on the visual context provided by the experimental design. Similar results were obtained even when targets were proprioceptively (instead of visually) defined (Rossetti and Régnier 1995). In this version of the task, participants' left index finger was passively moved to touch the target on a sagittal plane: following a "go" signal, subjects had to point with their right index finger to the previously touched target. As in the visual version of the task, when a delay of a few seconds was introduced, responses indicated a shift from an egocentric reference frame to an allocentric one, revealing that—regardless of the sensory modality involved—individuals may initially rely on a precise but transient egocentric representation in encoding object locations, and hence shift to an enduring and more comprehensive representation of the array of objects (Waller and Hodgson 2006), that might be relatively imprecise in a novel environment but can gain in precision with experience (see also Burgess 2006).

Do the blind also shift from an egocentric to an allocentric spatial reference frame? Rossetti and colleagues (Gaunet and Rossetti 2006; see also Rossetti, Gaunet, and Thinus-Blanc 1996) have investigated this aspect by testing a group of early and late blind adults in the proprioceptive version of the pointing task (see figures 5.1 and 5.2). Overall, the mean absolute-distance error—defined as the unsigned mean distance between pointing and target—was significantly smaller in the two blind groups than in the sighted, possibly reflecting compensatory phenomena in the proprioceptive domain. In the no-delay condition, all participants were found to rely on an egocentric reference frame. However, in the delayed condition a clear group effect was found: blindfolded sighted subjects exhibited the typical shift from an egocentric to an allocentric reference frame, whereas the early blind individuals continued to rely on an egocentric reference frame and late blind individuals' responses were halfway between those of the blindfolded controls and those of the early blind. These findings suggest that the capacity of shifting from an egocentric to an allocentric reference frame critically depends on the previous available visual experience.

It is worth noting that Ittyerah and colleagues (Ittyerah, Gaunet, and Rossetti 2007) failed to replicate these results with congenitally blind children (range: 6–12 years) adopting a similar task. In fact, the pointing distribution observed in congenitally blind children in the delay condition was contingent upon the target array, similarly to that of the blindfolded sighted children. As suggested by the authors of the study themselves, this age-dependent difference in the use of reference frames might be related to the long-term memory experience adults have in space without vision for processes that rely on egocentric representations (such as a better trained capacity to avoid static and dynamic objects during locomotion: Ittyerah, Gaunet, and Rossetti 2007). Hence, it might be that the adoption of an egocentric frame of reference in spatial tasks by the early blind is strategic rather than predetermined by the absence of vision, despite the fact that the adoption of such an egocentric representation might even be—in some situations—detrimental to performance.

Parallel-Setting Tasks

In a typical haptic parallel-setting task, participants have to put two perceived bars into the same orientation. The parallel-setting task is another very sensitive tool to

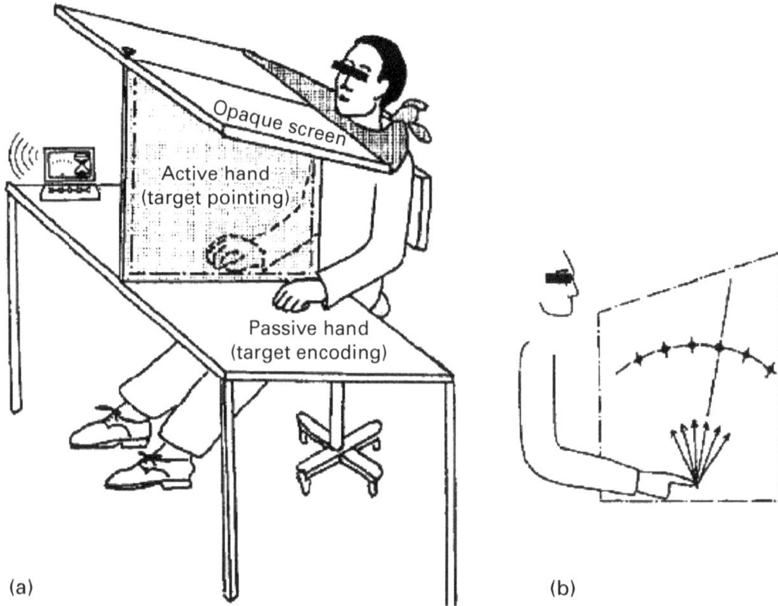

Figure 5.1
The experimental setting in Gaunet and Rossetti's (2006) study. (a) Apparatus: the left hand (passive hand) is placed on the table and the right hand (active hand) is placed on a tactile mark affixed to the bottom of the panel (starting position). The index finger of the left hand is put by the experimenter on the target and then back on the table; computer tones are triggered manually by the experimenter, to signal the moment when the participant has to point toward the memorized target. (b) Spatial configuration of the target array. Targets are arranged along an arc centered on the starting position of the finger.
Reprinted from Gaunet and Rossetti, "Effects of visual deprivation on space representation: Immediate and delayed pointing toward memorised proprioceptive targets," *Perception* 35/1 (2006): 107–124. (Reprinted by permission of Pion Ltd.)

reveal the way individuals represent space. In fact, if one relies on a purely allocentric representation, no systematic errors should be observed in consecutive performances. In contrast, if participants rely upon an egocentric reference frame, then systematic deviations should be reported.

Kappers and colleagues have carried out many experiments (e.g., Kappers 1999, 2002, 2003, 2004, 2007; Kappers and Koenderink 1999) to investigate the cognitive representational mechanisms subtending parallel-setting tasks in the haptic modality, with the bars placed either on the horizontal or fronto-parallel planes (cf. Zuidhoek, Kappers et al. 2003; Hermens, Kappers, and Gielen 2006; Volcic, Kappers, and Koenderink 2007), and in three-dimensional space (Volcic and Kappers 2008). Large

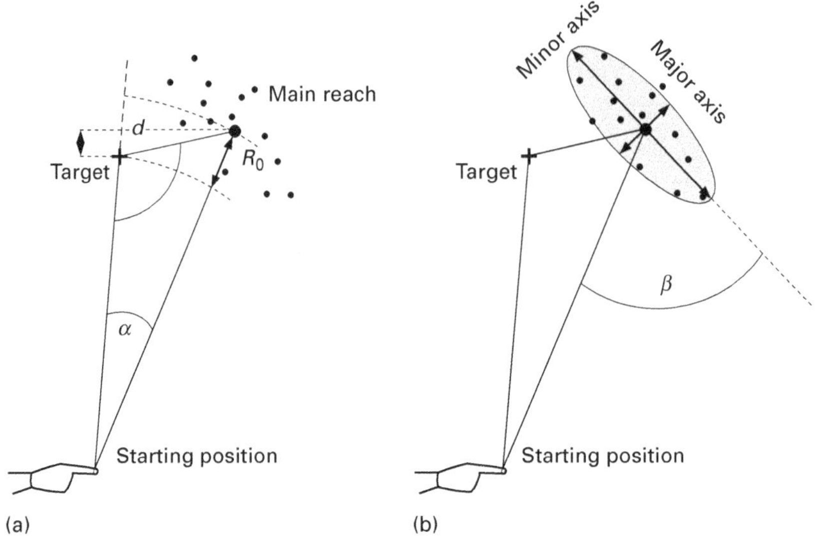

Figure 5.2
Computation of dependent variables in the study by Gaunet and Rossetti (2006). The larger black circle represents the target and the smaller black circles represent attempts to proprioceptively match the black cross target. (a): d, absolute-distance error between pointing distribution and target; a, movement-amplitude error of the pointing distribution; R0, movement-direction error of the pointing distribution. (b): Minor and major axes length of pointing distribution; b, orientation of the ellipse major axis.
Reprinted from Gaunet and Rossetti, "Effects of visual deprivation on space representation: Immediate and delayed pointing toward memorised proprioceptive targets," *Perception* 35(1) (2006): 107–124. (Reprinted by permission of Pion Ltd.)

systematic errors—clockwise with test bars to the right and counterclockwise with test bars to the left of the reference bar (Kappers 1999, 2003; Zuidhoek, Kappers et al. 2003; Zuidhoek, Visser et al. 2004)—have been reported, indicating the activation of an egocentric reference frame (systematic deviations have been reported in all the three main orthogonal planes). In fact, it is likely that parallel-setting tasks involve both an allocentric and an egocentric (mainly hand-centered, see Kappers and Viergever 2006; Kappers 2007; Volcic and Kappers 2008) reference frame: deviations vary largely across individuals depending on the extent to which the two reference frames combine with each other. Interestingly, as in the case of pointing tasks, the specific involvement of each representation seems to depend on the time between exploration and test: in fact, Zuidhoek et al. (Zuidhoek, Kappers et al. 2003) found that the retention of the reference-bar orientation for 10 seconds before rotating the test bar resulted in smaller deviations in parallel-setting performance than those found for non-delayed perfor-

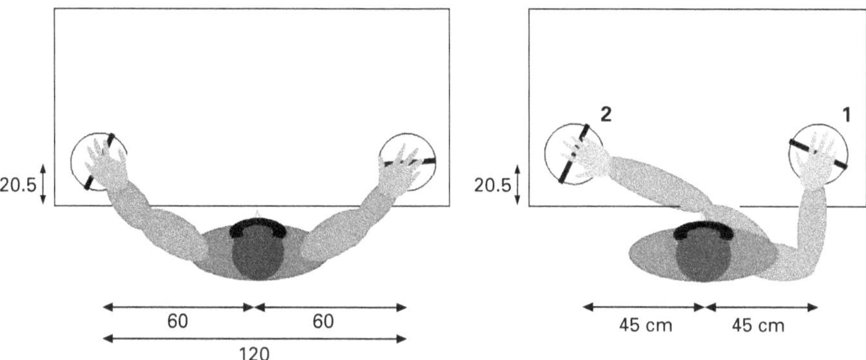

Figure 5.3
The experimental setup used by Postma, Zuidhoek et al. (2008). (A) Top view of the experimental setup used in the parallel-setting task. (B) Top view of the experimental setup used in the verbal judgment of an orientation task.
Reprinted from Postma, Zuidhoek et al., "Haptic orientation perception benefits from visual experience: Evidence from early-blind, late-blind, and sighted people," *Perception and Psychophysics* 70(7) (2008): 1197–1206. (Reprinted by permission of the Psychonomic Society)

mance, reflecting a shift from an egocentric to an allocentric spatial representation during the time delay.

The parallel-setting paradigm has been used to explore the nature of spatial mental representations in blind individuals (Postma, Zuidhoek et al. 2008) (see figure 5.3). Sighted, early blind, and late blind participants were required to rotate a test bar in order to put parallel to a previously touched reference-bar orientation, either with or without a 10-second delay. When the test was immediate, all groups made comparable errors with respect to size and direction, suggesting the use of a similar (predominantly egocentric) reference frame. However, in the delayed trials, the late blind and blindfolded sighted subjects became more accurate, suggesting that they shifted in this time to a more allocentric reference frame; in contrast, performance of the early blind was unaffected by the delay. Moreover, the delay-related improvement was higher for the blindfolded sighted than for the late blind group, indicating that the ability to generate allocentric representations benefit from being *continuously* exposed to a normal visual stimulation.

Spatial Updating for Rotated Configurations and "Perspective Taking"

As we have already mentioned, objects locations can be encoded either with reference to the observer or independently of the viewer's position. Previous research in the visual modality demonstrated that visual memory for scene is sensitive to the position of the observer (e.g., Simons and Wang 1998; Christou and Bulthoff 1999), indicating that objects relations may be preferentially encoded in an egocentric, orientation-dependent manner. Moreover, observers are likely to perform better in a new/old object-recognition task when view-changes are caused by active viewer movements rather than by object rotation (Simons and Wang 1998; Simons, Wang, and Roddenberry 2002). This is because proprioception or body movements can compensate for subsequent changes in the view of the object or of the scene by helping to update the spatial representation. In particular, body rotation would induce a specific egocentric recalibration, recruiting a short-term memory trace of the original forward-facing direction (Montello, Richardson et al. 1999). Interestingly, a series of experiments carried out by Fiona Newell and colleagues in normally sighted individuals have revealed that viewpoint-dependency also occurs when objects' configurations have to be haptically explored (in the absence of visual input) (e.g., Newell, Ernst et al. 2001; Newell, Woods et al. 2005; Pasqualotto, Finucane, and Newell 2005; Woods, Moore, and Newell 2008).

Moreover haptically based egocentric spatial mental representations can be updated according to agents' locomotion, whereas when the to-be-remembered configuration is rotated without any self-motion of the agent, scene-recognition is affected (Pasqualotto, Finucane, and Newell 2005). Although these experiments were carried out in the haptic modality, participants were all sighted individuals, and therefore, the role played by vision in determining the patterns of these results cannot be ignored. What is the case of blind individuals? Are the blind able to update the spatial representation of objects falling in their peripersonal space when the viewpoint from which objects are explored changes?

A study by Pasqualotto and Newell (2007) investigated this issue. A group of early blind, late blind and sighted individuals was required to memorize the relative position of a number of haptically explored novel/unfamiliar objects (see figure 5.4). After exploration, the location of one object was changed and participants had to report which object had changed position. In some trials, the configuration was rotated by 45 degrees, in other conditions participants had to walk to a new viewpoint position (resulting again in a 45-degree rotation compared to the study phase). Critically, rotation limits the use of previously stored movement memories and requires positional updating. Pasqualotto and Newell (2007) found an overall lower performance of the congenitally blind compared to the other two groups, and a cost in performance to a rotated scene relative to a stationary observer in all participants groups. However, the sighted and the late blind, but not the early blind participants, were able to compensate for the viewpoint-change when that was due to the observer's active locomotion.

Similar results were reported by Ungar, Blades, and Spencer (1995a) in a study with blind children. In this study, children had to haptically explore layouts of one, three or five shapes which they then attempted to reproduce. In some trials, children had

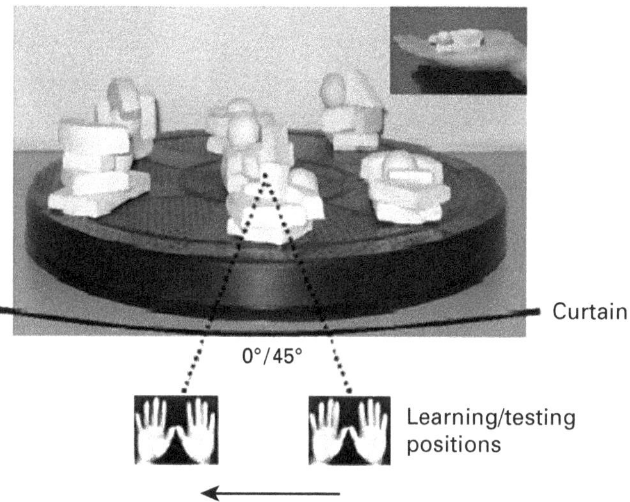

Figure 5.4
An illustration of Pasqualotto and Newell's experimental apparatus and novel stimuli used in the experiment. During the experiment, the circular platform could be rotated 45 degrees in a clockwise direction relative to the participant. Furthermore, in half of all trials, the participant was required to move in a clockwise direction from their original seating position to the new position.
Reprinted from Pasqualotto and Newell, "The role of visual experience in the representation and updating of novel haptic scenes," *Brain and Cognition* 65(2) (2007): 184–194. (© 2007. Reprinted by permission of Elsevier)

to move 90 degrees around the table between exploring and reproducing the layout: results showed that this manipulation critically affected the performance of blind participants (see also Hollins and Kelley 1988). Coluccia, Mammarella, and Cornoldi (2009) compared a group of congenitally blind individuals and blindfolded sighted subjects in an object-relocation task under different relocation conditions, in which again the position of the subject at relocation was different from that at learning, or the configuration itself was rotated by the experimenter between learning and test, or relocation took place from the same position as learning but started from a decentered point. Overall, the blind were found to perform lower than the sighted (experiment 2), and to be specifically affected when the object reference frame was rotated, supporting the view that the blind have difficulties in creating a mental representation of objects that is not related to their body (or hand). In this regard, Heller (1989b) has argued that blind individuals' spatial representations differ from sighted individuals' because the blind lack experience of an external reference frame or reference cues (e.g., knowledge of the horizontal and vertical) that normally aid in the construction of a more manipulable object-centered representation (Rock and DiVita 1987). This hypothesis was supported by the finding of less accurate recognition of rotated unfamiliar stimuli by the early blind and also by sighted groups who had frame of reference cues removed, compared to sighted participants who had frame of reference cues available (Heller 1989b).

Nonetheless, other findings suggest that blind individuals are able to efficiently update the position of objects falling in their peripersonal space. Postma, Zuidhoek, Noordzij, and Kappers (2007) have carried out a study in which they required early blind, late blind and blindfolded sighted participants to match ten haptically explored objects (shapes) to the cut-out in a board as fast as possible (see figure 5.5). In some conditions, performance was measured after a 90-degree rotation of the object configuration. Notably, the authors reported overall faster responses of the blind compared to the blindfolded sighted, even when the platform was rotated. In fact, although

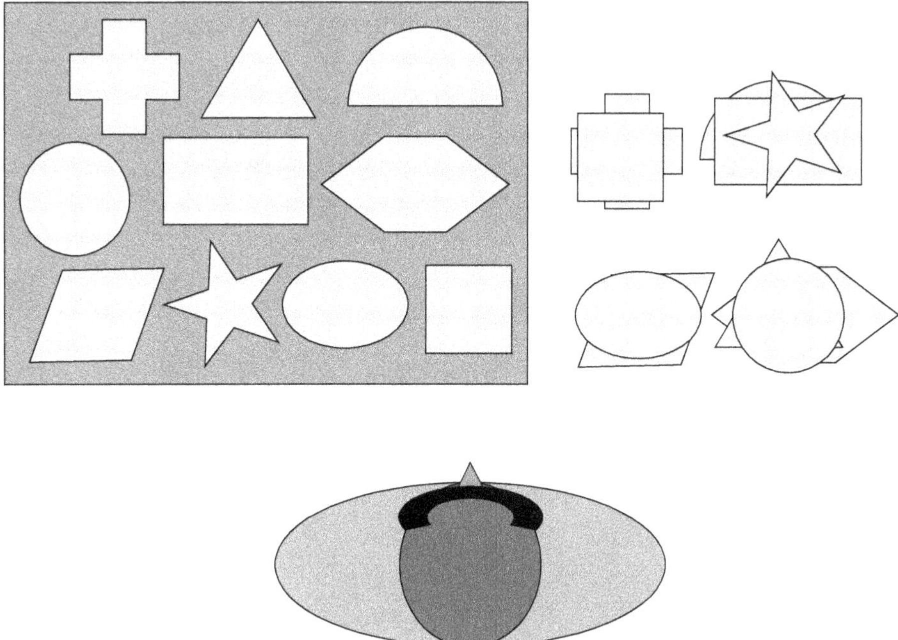

Figure 5.5

Top view of the board and objects of the portable Tactual Performance Test used by Postma, Zuidhoek, et al. (2007).

Reprinted from Postma, Zuidhoek, Noordzij, and Kappers, "Differences between early-blind, late-blind, and blindfolded-sighted people in haptic spatial-configuration learning and resulting memory traces," *Perception*, 36(8) (2007): 1253–1265. (Reprinted by permission of Pion Ltd.)

rotation caused an increase in completion time in all participants, this increase was the same for the congenitally blind, late blind and blindfolded sighted groups.

Hence, it seems that available literature is controversial regarding the ability of blind individuals to update the position of near objects. Once again, the origin of these inconsistencies among studies might be found in the specific nature of the task employed and in the individual characteristics of the participants. First of all, one should analyze the type of cognitive operation involved. In the studies described above, the viewpoint change essentially consisted of (different degrees of) a rotation. Mental rotation for haptically explored scenes was specifically investigated by Marmor and Zaback (1976) in one of the first studies on mental imagery processes in the blind (see also chapter 4 of this volume). Marmor and Zaback (1976) showed that congenitally blind individuals were able to mentally rotate an object that they had previously haptically explored, and suggested that they might have employed an *analog* representation in doing so, because of the linear increase in response times on increasing the angle of rotation. However, Marmor and Zaback (1976) also reported a blind visuospatial deficit, with the congenitally blind group being significantly slower and making more errors than both the late blind and sighted groups. This increased time indicates that the task is somehow more demanding for a blind person than for a sighted one. In fact, blind subjects have less everyday experience with tasks that involve the mental rotation of objects or patterns (Heller, Kennedy et al. 2006). Moreover, it has been suggested that the blind may encounter specific difficulties when an "active" operation is required or when the task becomes very complex (see Cornoldi, Cortesi, and Preti, 1991; Cornoldi and Vecchi 2000, 2003; Vecchi 1998; see also chapter 4 of this volume). Nonetheless, the specific nature of the task might be critical in determining whether rotation would affect scene recognition (see Postma, Zuidhoek et al. 2007): whether a task asks for an explicit relocation of objects or just for a shape/cut-off match, or whether updating is enforced by a whole-body movement of the observer relative to a fixed display, rather than by a rotation of the configuration relative to a stationary observer, are all important factors to be considered. Moreover, the degree of rotation may play a role as well. For instance, Millar (1976) used a rotated drawing task and found that that blind participants were worse than the sighted controls at oblique rotations but not at orthogonal ones (e.g., 90-degree and 180-degree rotations). This result is consistent with other reports by Heller and colleagues that found that early blind participants outperformed sighted controls when coping with Braille that was left-right reversed, but not with Braille rotated 45 degrees from the upright (Heller, Calcaterra et al. 1999).

Finally, the importance of individuals' strategies should not be underestimated. As pointed out by Ungar et al. (Ungar, Blades, and Spencer 1995b), it is likely that the use of strategies can account more for the pattern of obtained results than the visual status or the participants' age themselves.

5.4 Blind Individuals' Representation of Large-scale Environment (Locomotor Space)

When we move toward an object or toward the source of a sound (even when we can no longer perceive them), we are required to continuously update the representation of our intended destination while moving. Humans have been found to be able to efficiently cope with these situations (e.g., Ashmead, Davis, and Northington 1995; Farrell and Thomson 1999). Keeping track of self-to-objects relationships when we walk can be accomplished in different ways, some relying mainly on information from self-movement (such as proprioception or vestibular information), and some relying on the use of external reference frame information and landmarks.

"Route-like" and "Survey-like" Representations

According to Loomis, Klatzky et al. (1993) navigation requires five steps: (1) sensing, that is acquiring information about self-motion and landmarks; (2) creating a trace of the *route* (i.e., a sequence of contiguous segments and turns); (3) creating a *survey* representation; (4) computing the trajectories needed to reach the target; and (5) executing those trajectories. In route-like maps the environment is represented in a viewer-centered, egocentric frame of reference which reflects that individual's navigational experience, whereas in survey-like representations distant places are combined together into an integrated global overview of the entire environment (cf. Chown, Kaplan, and Kortenkamp 1995; Golledge 1999; Ungar 2000). Survey representations offer the advantage of allowing individuals to monitor their position within the entire environment during navigation, hence making it possible to plan new paths in advance. Nonetheless, to pass from a route-based representation to a survey-based representation some inferences have to be made. For instance, if reproduction of a previously explored pathway only requires a memory trace of the route, finding shortcuts requires building a survey representation and computing a completely new pathway.

It has been reported that blind individuals are able to generate survey-like representations, although they usually rely on route-like representations (Millar 1994). In fact, generating an integrated representation that simultaneously contains all the serially acquired bits of information places heavy demands on blind individuals' working memory system. Accordingly, Rieser et al. (Rieser, Lockman, and Pick 1980) reported that the blind found it difficult to estimate Euclidean distances between locations (a task that required generating a perspective structure of the layout), whereas they did not encounter specific problems in estimating "functional" distance (in units such as paces). Further support for the blind preference for relying on route representations can be found in a study by Noordzij and colleagues (Noordzij, Zuidhoek, and Postma 2006): in that study, early blind, late blind, and sighted individuals listened to a route-like and a survey-like verbal description of two environments before being presented with two different tests. The first task was an old/new recognition test, in which different prime-target pairs were used (i.e., close in text/close in space; far in text/close in space): if a spatial representation was generated following the descriptive text, then locations close in space should prime targets more than items far in space, independently of whether they were mentioned in the same or different sentences. In the second task, subjects were explicitly instructed to generate a spatial image of the verbal description: during the test, they had to perform a series of "bird-flight" distance comparisons, the hypothesis being that if participants formed a spatial mental model then their errors and response times should have increased when the metric distance increased. Interestingly, results from the first task indicated that both sighted and blind subjects represented the objects in a spatially organized mental model, and did not rely on the exact wording of the text. Nonetheless, results from the second experiment showed that overall, blind individuals were more efficient in forming a spatial mental model after listening to a route-like than a survey-like description, while the opposite pattern was found in the sighted controls. Interestingly, late blind participants' reaction times were not affected by increased distance after studying a survey-like description, while they always showed this effect after studying a route-like description.

In a recent study by Latini Corazzini and colleagues (Latini Corazzini, Tinti et al. 2010) the spatial exploration strategies of a group of congenitally blind individuals were examined using a modified version of the Morris Water Maze (Morris, Garrud et al. 1982). Congenitally blind individuals were again found to prefer an egocentric type of representation, even when allocentric cues were available (Latini Corazzini, Tinti et al. 2010).

The preference for route-like representations does not prevent blind individuals from generating survey-like representations. In this regard, tactile maps are particularly useful tools because they include only the essential spatial information (reducing the irrelevant noise), offering an almost simultaneous view of the to-be-represented space (e.g., Golledge 1991; Ungar, Blades, and Spencer 1994, 1995b, 1996, 1997a,b). In a study conducted to assess the effect of different instructions (direct experience vs. tactile map exploration vs. verbal description) on acquiring knowledge about a real unfamiliar space in a group of blind participants, it was found that even a brief exploration of a tactile map (but not a verbal description of the route) facilitated blind individuals' orientation and mobility in that environment (Espinosa, Ungar et al. 1998). Hence, tactile maps might be a more suitable tool in conveying survey-type knowledge among the blind than are verbal descriptions, probably because in tactile maps all the details are simultaneously available, whereas verbal descriptions put a higher load on the working memory system.

Spatial Updating in Navigation

In route-navigation, individuals do not refer to external landmarks but represent the route in terms of a "path structure" in which the information is coded like "go ahead three steps, then turn 90 degrees left" and so forth. In route-navigation tasks that simply require one to retrace a previously walked route, congenitally blind individuals have been found to perform similarly to sighted individuals (Loomis, Klatzky et al. 1993; Thinus-Blanc and Gaunet 1997). For instance, in one of the earliest studies on navigational abilities in the blind, Rieser, Guth and Hill (1986) guided blindfolded and blind participants to six different locations, always starting from the same position and returning after each visit to the same starting point. At test, participants had to point to the places they had previously explored while standing at the starting position. No differences were reported in this task between the blind and blindfolded sighted. However, when novel spatial relations have to be derived from previously experienced spatial measures, congenitally blind participants have been shown to encounter some limitations compared to sighted controls, although results are not always consistent (Loomis, Klatzky et al. 1993; Thinus-Blanc and Gaunet 1997). For instance, in Rieser et al.'s study (Rieser, Guth, and Hill 1986), when the task was made more complex by requiring subjects to stand in a new position and point to another location, blind individuals' performance was impaired. Hence, navigational tasks that cannot be solved by simply relying on a spatial memory trace but require drawing more complex inferences, may particularly benefit from survey-like representations and thus are potentially more difficult for a blind person.

Nevertheless, recent findings seem to suggest that even in some complex situations the blind are able to rely on survey-like representations. In particular, in a study by Tinti, Adenzato, Tamietto, and Cornoldi (2006), early blind, late blind and blindfolded sighted participants were first required to walk along predefined pathways of different complexity (e.g., with different numbers of turns) and then to perform a series of tasks that could be efficiently solved only by creating a survey-like representation of the pathways. During the pathway-walking, participants were required to count backward aloud, in order to prevent the generation of a linguistic representation of the pathway, and thus exclude the use of a verbal strategy. In a "find shortcuts" task, participants were required to walk through locations not linked by pathways directly experienced during the learning phase—for instance, once at the end of the pathway, they had to go back to the starting point taking the shortest way. In a second task, participants were taken to a random location on the explored pathway and then had to point to other places (such as the door, the starting and the end points of the pathway) and judge straight-line (Euclidean) distances from these points. In a further task, participants were asked to draw a map of the explored pathways. In contrast to previous evidence, Tinti et al. (Tinti, Adenzato et al. 2006) found that both congenital and late blind individuals performed well in these tasks (even outperforming the sighted group) (see also Loomis, Klatzky et al. 1993). Similar results indicating that blind individuals can update spatial locations while moving as efficiently as blindfolded sighted controls, have been reported by Loomis and colleagues (Loomis, Lippa et al. 2002). In particular, in Loomis et al.'s study (Loomis, Lippa et al. 2002), blind and blindfolded sighted observers were presented with auditory stimuli indicating a location in a grassy field; at test, they were required to walk to that location. Stimuli consisted of either a sound from a loudspeaker (positioned at the target location) or a series of verbal instructions indicating direction (in the form of the time on a clock) and distance to be walked (e.g., three o'clock, sixteen feet) to reach the target. In the "direct" walking condition, participants had to walk directly to the identified location. In the "indirect" walking condition, participants had to walk forward until the experimenter said "turn" (after 2.7 m), and hence attempted to walk the rest of the way to the identified location (spatial updating required). Blind individuals were able to spatial update their location according to both sound and verbal instructions, with similar deviations from their target as for the sighted.

Overall, these findings suggest that visual experience is not a necessary requisite for developing skills in spatial navigation and spatial updating. But why are blind subjects sometimes able to efficiently cope with tasks involving survey-like representations and sometimes not? It's possible that blind individuals who participated in more recent studies (Loomis, Lippa et al. 2002; Tinti, Adenzato et al. 2006) were more spatially skilled than participants in earlier studies, thanks to improved training programs for the blind. In fact, according to Ungar (2000), inefficient blind performance during inferential tasks may reflect higher inter-individual variability rather than a true deficit. As we will discuss later in this chapter, individual variables such as the degree of independent traveling, type of education and so forth may predict blind success in spatial tasks.

Vestibular Navigation

In navigation, normally sighted individuals usually rely upon vision (visual landmarks and optic flow), audition (auditory landmarks and acoustical flow), proprioception (information from muscles and joints about limb position) and vestibular information. Basically, proprioception is the sense that indicates whether the body is moving with required effort, as well as where the various parts of the body are located in relation to each other. The vestibular system—known as the balance organ of the inner ear—constitutes an inertial sensor which encodes the motion of the head relative to the outside world (see Angelaki and Cullen 2008 for review). As our movements consist of rotations and translations, the vestibular system comprises two components: the semicircular canal system, which indicates rotational movements; and the otoliths, which indicate linear accelerations. Notably, central vestibular processing is highly multimodal: in fact, signals from muscles, joints, skin, and eyes are continuously integrated with vestibular inflow. When sighted individuals walk in the dark, they can estimate their location through a process known as "path integration" (also defined as "dead reckoning" or "inertial navigation") in which the actual position is derived from inertial vestibular and proprioceptive signals (see Seemungal, Glasauer et al. 2007). Darwin (1873) noted a similar ability in animals that cannot be explained on the basis of external reference-frame information: in fact, early studies confirmed that animals could return directly to a starting point, such as a nest, in the absence of vision and having taken a circuitous outward journey. This process was referred to as "path integration" to stress the required continuous integration of movement cues over the journey.

For an individual who is totally blind, path integration is responsible for much of his or her knowledge about objects relationships. For instance, by first exploring object A and then object B, a blind individual gets to know—thanks to inferential rules—the spatial relationship between these two objects (what a sighted person would have immediately captured by sight). If haptic information is sufficient to allow a path-integration process during translational movements in the dark, only vestibular input updates position after walking turns (cf. Glasauer, Amorim et al. 2002; Seemungal, Glasauer et al. 2007). An fMRI study has indeed shown that blind subjects rely more heavily than sighted subjects on vestibular and somatosensory feedback for locomotion control, and that this is accompanied by enhanced voluntary motor control and enhanced motor-kinesthetic processing (see Deutschlander, Stephan et al. 2009). Related to this, Seemungal et al. (Seemungal, Glasauer et al. 2007) have investigated angular vestibular navigation for path reversal (route navigation) and path completion (inferential navigation) in sighted and congenitally blind subjects, in order to assess whether the difficulties experienced by the blind in many inferential navigational tasks (see Rieser, Guth, and Hill 1986) derive from a deficit in vestibular functions or in a suboptimal utilization of intact vestibular information. A first experiment was carried out in a dark room to investigate the impact of early visual loss on the perceptual velocity storage mechanism: sighted and blind subjects sat on a motorized but vibrationless wheel-chair that was passively rotated right or left in the vertical-axis: at test, subjects were required to indicate their perceived instantaneous angular velocity of the whole-body rotation. In two other experiments, subjects were again passively rotated and then instructed to return actively (by using a chair-mounted joystick) to the start position as accurately as possible: in one condition, the task could be performed through a reproduction of stimulus angle or kinetics (path reproduction, as in a route-navigation task), in another condition reorientation could only be performed with an accurate positional signal and required mental computation (path completion). Results suggested that in the congenitally blind velocity storage mechanisms are deficient—in agreement with previous animal (Harris and Cynader 1981; Tusa, Mustari et al. 2001) and infants' data (Weissman, DiScenna, and Leigh

1989)—indicating that vision continuously recalibrates the vestibular system. Interestingly though, blind and sighted individuals did not differ in path reproduction: therefore, some aspects of vestibular perception are entirely independent of visual mechanisms. Nonetheless, the blind participants showed worse performance in path completion (requiring inferences), in line with previous results (see Thinus-Blanc and Gaunet 1997). An analysis based on each single individual's performance showed that some of the blind participants performed comparably to the blindfolded sighted even when spatial inferences had to be drawn (these subjects also displayed ultra-short vestibular time constants, and they reported the higher scores in lifetime physical activity). Overall, Seemungal et al.'s data suggest that a deficit in the vestibular navigation component of locomotion (i.e., turning without vision) may—at least partially—account for the deficits in inferential locomotor navigation which are experienced by the blind (see Thinus-Blanc and Gaunet 1997). Notably, these findings also suggest that the promotion of physical activity in blind subjects may be a useful way to improve navigational skills and hence have implications for long-term orientation and mobility training for such subjects.

5.5 Role of Individual Variables in Determining Spatial Cognition Abilities of the Blind

In this chapter, we have often reported how different studies—although apparently investigating the same ability in comparable populations (e.g., congenitally/early blind or late blind)—have led to opposite conclusions, and we have explained these inconsistencies by stressing the role played by both experimental and individual variables (for an excellent review on this topic, see Thinus-Blanc and Gaunet 1997). In general, visual deprivation is more detrimental for tasks requiring that subjects draw spatial inferences or "actively" manipulate the original input, compared to situations that only require a "passive" retention of spatial information. This depends on specific limitations of the working memory system of blind individuals which mainly derive from the nature of their perceptual experience. In fact, the inherently sequential nature of tactile exploration puts a heavy demand on the working memory system, which needs to maintain a great amount of information in order to allow it to represent "as a whole" what the blind person has experienced "piece by piece." Although blind individuals develop specific (usually verbal) strategies to cope with spatial tasks, these strategies may become less efficient in case of increasing task demands (see Cornoldi, Tinti et al. 2009). In fact, when the task is relatively simple or quite suitable for verbal mediation, blind individuals can perform as well as blindfolded sighted individuals (see for instance, Vanlierde and Wanet-Defalque 2004). However, when the task becomes more demanding, requiring subjects to update a spatial representation by means of a mental rotation (e.g., Heller, Kennedy et al. 2006; Pasqualotto and

Newell 2007) or requiring them to draw high-level inferences (such as finding shortcuts), the lack of vision causes specific deficits, probably due to an overloading of the WM system. On this respect, according to Heller (Heller, Kennedy et al. 2006) the differences between sighted people and blind people in spatial tasks may be quantitative rather than qualitative.

Nonetheless, early blind individuals have been found to perform more poorly than the blindfolded sighted also in situations in which the WM system is not critically involved (as in the parallel-setting task, see Postma, Zuidhoek et al. 2008). In these cases, the difference between blind and sighted individuals seems to be qualitative rather than quantitative, depending on the adoption of a different spatial reference frame, such as a suboptimal egocentric representation when an allocentric one would have been more appropriate. In fact, blind individuals spontaneously rely on egocentric representations in representing the location of objects (Pasqualotto and Newell 2007). Therefore, if a task can be solved by relying on an egocentric representation, then blind individuals may perform similarly to the sighted; however, when the task requires them to generate an allocentric spatial representation, blind individuals are likely to be outperformed by the sighted. Notably, another factor that interacts with the generated type of mental representation is the existence of a delay between encoding and test: in fact, a delay of a few seconds facilitates a shift from an egocentric to an allocentric reference frame in late blind and sighted subjects, but not in early blind subjects (cf. Gaunet and Rossetti 2006; Postma, Zuidhoek et al. 2008). The specific response required at test also plays a role in determining how a blind person would perform in that particular situation. For instance, in memory for objects' configurations, different results have been obtained depending on whether that task implied an explicit recognition (Pasqualotto and Newell 2007) or just a shape/cut-off match (as in Postma, Zuidhoek et al. 2007): in fact, in the former case the capacity to generate an allocentric representation of the configuration may be more relevant (especially when the configuration is rotated), whereas in the second case good tactile skills of the blind may play a major role, possibly masking their representational deficit. The level of familiarity with the task or the task environment is also critical, so that it doesn't make too much sense to compare the results of studies that tested blind individuals' spatial abilities in familiar environments with those that tested their abilities in unknown environments. Ideally, an experiment comparing blind and sighted individuals' spatial capacities should be carried out in environments that are equally familiar to both sighted and blind groups, or unknown to both.

Critically, across studies, inter-individual variability appears more pronounced in blind than in sighted participants (Thinus-Blanc and Gaunet 1997); in other words, the blind groups appears more heterogeneous than the sighted ones. Accordingly, Ungar (2000) suggested that the usual worse performance of the blind compared to the sighted in spatial-inferential tasks reflects higher inter-individual performance variability rather than a true deficit, because some blind individuals are indeed able to attain sighted subjects' performance. This underlines the importance of a correct sampling procedure when carrying out research with blind individuals. In particular, some measurement of general cognitive ability should be provided (such as a verbal intelligence test or at least an evaluation of participants' sociocultural level), and factors such as gender, hand preference, Braille-reading ability and mobility skills should also be considered. Importantly, the etiology of their visual deficit also deserves to be taken into account, especially in case of late-blind individuals or low-vision individuals (who can rely on some residual vision), since different pathologies may affect visual acuity and visual field differently (and with a different temporal progression), thus also influencing the way in which a visually impaired person compensates—at the sensory and cognitive level—for his or her visual loss. The precise onset of visual deficit and the duration of visual deprivation are also extremely critical, as we will specifically discuss in chapter 7. Unfortunately, different studies have used different criteria to classify a blind person as either "early" or "late" blind, thus making it harder to compare their results. The age of subjects at testing is also important: in fact, results obtained with children are often markedly different from those obtained with adults, possibly depending on blind individuals' being able to adopt better spatial strategies which they learn to use over years of visual deprivation (see Ittyerah, Gaunet, and Rossetti 2007).

The personal history of each individual, specifically in terms of his or her experience with orientation and mobility (O&M) training and familiarity with the task (Loomis, Klatzky et al. 1993; Ochaíta and Huertas 1993), affects the choice of strategies that are used. In fact, physical training can improve performance in tandem with the use of a more allocentric-based navigation (Ungar, Blades, and Spencer 1997b; Ungar 2000; Seemungal, Glasauer et al. 2007). In this regard, Fiehler et al. (Fiehler, Reuschel, and Rösler 2009) found that the proprioceptive-spatial acuity of congenitally blind participants significantly co-varied with the age at which they attended O&M training. Specifically, the earlier that congenitally blind participants started O&M training the more accurate and less variable were their spatial judgments: in fact, those who received an O&M training after the age of 12 years showed poorer acuity than sighted controls, whereas those with an earlier O&M training performed similarly to sighted controls. The results by Fiehler et al. (Fiehler, Reuschel, and Rösler 2009) suggest that proprioceptive-spatial acuity in adulthood depends on the developmental experience of space irrespective of the sensory modality by which spatial information becomes available.

Finally, when considering individual variables, "affective" aspects should also be taken into account. In fact, blindness—especially late blindness following a sudden onset—is often associated with depression, and blind individuals are more likely to develop autism and stereotyped behavior patterns than sighted individuals are (Janson 1993; Pring 2005).

In summary, blind individuals' spatial deficits as reported in some studies may not directly depend on blindness, but on a number of idiosyncratic factors and on their interaction with the specific nature of the task that is used.

5.6 Rehabilitation and Sensory Substitution Devices

The results discussed in the previous sections are of critical importance for the design of navigational devices for the visually impaired. In fact, although blind individuals are usually able to move and navigate in familiar environments, they may be impaired in larger or unfamiliar environments that often present unexpected obstacles or deviations. During the last decades, several substitution devices have been developed and tested in order to help visually impaired people navigate in urban space (see discussion by Bach-y-Rita and Kercel 2003). The main rationale shared by the various types of navigational devices is that the information that cannot be acquired visually can be replaced by information that is provided in another modality, usually touch or—more frequently—audition. In this regard, a recent review by Auvray and Myin (2009) offers a clear summary of the available sensory substitution devices (SSDs) and their use in visual impairments. Briefly, SSDs for blindness assistance can be divided into two main categories: devices translating visual inputs in tactual stimulation and devices transforming visual information into verbal, auditory strings.

Tactile stimulators are mainly confined to simple object- or form-recognition and to reading, being of less "practical" utility in spatial navigation (Bach-y-Rita and Kercel 2003). Numerous SSDs are instead available which are capable of converting visual information into language or sounds. The findings by Loomis et al. (Loomis, Lippa et al. 2002) suggest that valid navigational aids might make use both of sounds to indicate objects of interest but also of spatial language descriptions—in terms of street and cardinal directions and information about the location of off-route landmarks and other points of interest—given by a speech synthesizer. Overall, the adoption of a visual-to-auditory converter offers many advantages and greater applications compared to a visual-to-tactile converter. In fact, the human auditory system has fine discrimination for sound intensity and frequency and is capable of dealing with complex materials even in difficult contexts (Hirsh 1988; Auvray and Myin 2009). Vision-to-auditory SSD are mainly based upon two different principles. The first one uses sonar characteristics in order to calculate the distance between the subject and objects in the surrounding space. This technique is often referred as "echolocation" (see chapter 2), and can be used for locomotion and for guiding visually impaired people (Heyes 1984; Kay 1985), as well as for conveying information about spatial layouts (Hughes 2001). The alternative system is based upon video-camera signals that are converted into auditory instructions. Different sound pitches, temporal intervals, frequencies and amplitudes are associated with the positions of the objects in space and to their luminosity (see Auvray and Myin 2009 for a review). In recent years, GPS-based wayfinding systems for the blind that provide a steady narrative on instantaneous location, travel directions and points of interest have also been successfully employed (see Loomis, Klatzky, and Golledge 2001).

Besides SSDs, visually impaired individuals usually participate in orientation and mobility (O&M) programs that aim to increase blind people's spatial competencies (cf. Blasch, Wiener, and Welsh 1997). O&M training began after World War II when different techniques were developed to help veterans who had been blinded during the war. In the 1960s, universities started training programs for O&M specialists who worked with adults and school-aged children; later, the importance of also providing services to preschool-aged children became clear. Nowadays, O&M specialists have developed strategies and approaches for supporting increasingly younger populations so that O&M training may begin even in infancy.

Basically, O&M training helps blind individuals first to know where they are in space and where they want to go (orientation), and then helps them be able to carry out a plan to get there (mobility). The training usually consists of a multi-stage education program in which motor and orientation skills are trained by teaching the visually impaired how to orient in small and large environments, how to be effectively guided by other individuals and how to protect their own body. Part of the training is specifically devoted to the use of the long cane that is critical for walking in and systematically exploring unfamiliar places. Moreover, different spatial-orientation strategies and abstract spatial concepts are also described and ingrained, such as the use of tangible street maps (Ungar, Blades, and Spencer 1995b; Blasch, Wiener, and Welsh 1997). In many cases, rehabilitation programs are also based on specific cognitive and motivational training in which a given spatial ability is associated with sport, art, or workplace activities.

6 Low Vision

"I have examined Bogota," he said, "and the case is clearer to me. I think very probably he might be cured." "That is what I have always hoped," said old Yacob. "His brain is affected," said the blind doctor. The elders murmured assent. "Now, what affects it?" "Ah!" said old Yacob. "This," said the doctor, answering his own question. "Those queer things that are called the eyes, and which exist to make an agreeable soft depression in the face, are diseased, in the case of Bogota, in such a way as to affect his brain. They are greatly distended, he has eyelashes, and his eyelids move, and consequently his brain is in a state of constant irritation and distraction." "Yes?" said old Yacob. "Yes?" "And I think I may say with reasonable certainty that, in order to cure him completely, all that we need do is a simple and easy surgical operation—namely, to remove those irritant bodies." "And then he will be sane?" "Then he will be perfectly sane, and a quite admirable citizen." "Thank heaven for science!" said old Yacob.

—H. G. Wells, *The Country of the Blind*

6.1 Beyond a Monolithic View of the Visual Experience

If the totally blind cannot count on any form of visual experience, many individuals are affected by less severe forms of visual impairment in which some residual visual experience is possible. In fact, visual impairment takes many forms and can be present to varying degrees, with scientific publications partially differing in the criterion used to define a person as being affected by blindness rather than having low vision (see chapter 1 of this volume). In this chapter we will see that "blindness" and "visual impairment" cannot be considered as homogeneous when analyzing their effects on cognition. Critically, if studies with congenitally totally blind individuals can only offer an "all-or-nothing" perspective on the effects of visual deprivation on cognitive abilities, in case of low vision the etiology of the visual impairment, the available visual field (central vs. peripheral visual-field loss), residual visual acuity, level of contrast sensitivity, possible imbalance between the two eyes, and the temporal onset and duration of the visual deficit are all factors that play a role in influencing cognitive performance and ultimately in impacting rehabilitative outcomes (cf. Merabet, Rizzo et al. 2005).

This chapter specifically considers the effect of different types of low vision (due to different pathologies) on perceptual, attentional and higher-order cognitive abilities in the haptic, visual and auditory modalities. The last section is entirely devoted to the case of individuals who are affected by monocular blindness.

6.2 Blurred Vision

We use the term "visually impaired" (VI) to refer to low-vision individuals, who—after treatment or refractive correction—can rely to some extent on vision to plan and/or carry out a task. Visually impaired individuals are unable to read the newspaper from a normal viewing distance, even with the aid of eyeglasses or contact lenses, and they usually rely on a combination of vision (although often requiring adaptations in lighting or size of print) and other senses to learn. If the ability of totally blind individuals to perform a spatial imagery task has been investigated in many studies, only a few studies have directly examined the effect of less severe forms of visual impairment on cognitive abilities. An important question regards whether increases in acuity in intact systems (e.g., hearing, touch) occur not only when the visual system undergoes total deprivation but also in case of only partial deficits.

Sensory Compensation

In France, the group of Dufour et al. (cf. Dufour and Gérard 2000; Déspres, Candas, and Dufour 2005b,c) has carried out a series of experiments to investigate intramodal compensation—specifically, enhanced hearing sensitivity—in individuals affected by partial visual impairment, such as myopia. In a first study, Dufour and Gérard (2000) found that a group of 9 myopic individuals, affected by severe myopia for at least 10 years (myopia ranged from 21.25 to 26.75 diopters), performed better and faster than sighted controls in a sound-localization task when sounds were emitted from both the frontal and the posterior hemifields. These results indicate that even a partial visual deficit like myopia can lead to an improved spatial auditory sensitivity (i.e., intramodal compensation). In fact, although myopia can be corrected to normal vision, the vision of myopic individuals remains altered in the periphery, as is suggested by different ophthalmic studies (cf. Ito, Kawabata et al. 2001; Koller, Haas et al. 2001), with such altered peripheral vision likely forcing myopic individuals to rely on auditory information more than normally sighted subjects do in everyday situations (Dufour and Gérard 2000).

In a follow-up study, Dufour and colleagues (Déspres, Candas, and Dufour 2005c) investigated whether auditory compensation in myopic individuals involves all, or only specific, sound-localization mechanisms of the auditory system. In fact, as we discussed in chapter 2, sound localization depends on the neuronal processing of implicit auditory cues that are encoded by independent binaural and monaural neural

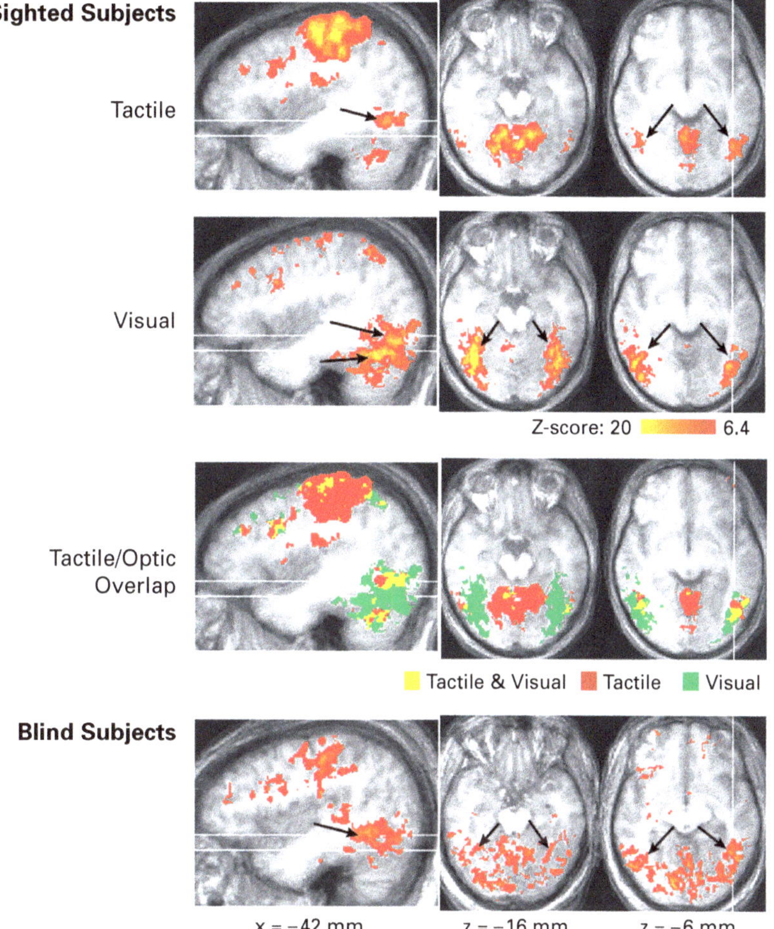

Plate 1

Brain areas that responded during tactile and/or visual object-perception in sighted subjects and during tactile perception in blind subjects in the study by Pietrini et al. (Pietrini, Furey et al. 2004). Sagittal and axial images from group Z-score maps of activated areas are shown for the sighted and blind subjects. The inferior temporal (IT) and ventral temporal (VT) regions activated by tactile and visual object-perception are indicated. The tactile/visual overlap map shows the areas activated by both tactile and visual perception (shown in yellow), as well as the areas activated only by tactile (red) and visual (green) perception. The white lines in the sagittal images correspond to the locations of the axial slices and, similarly, the white line in the axial slice indicates the location of the sagittal section.

Reprinted from Pietrini, Furey et al., "Beyond sensory images: Object-based representation in the human ventral pathway," *Proceedings of the National Academy of Sciences of the United States of America* 101(15) (2004): 5658–5663. (© 2004. Reprinted by permission of the National Academy of Sciences of the United States of America)

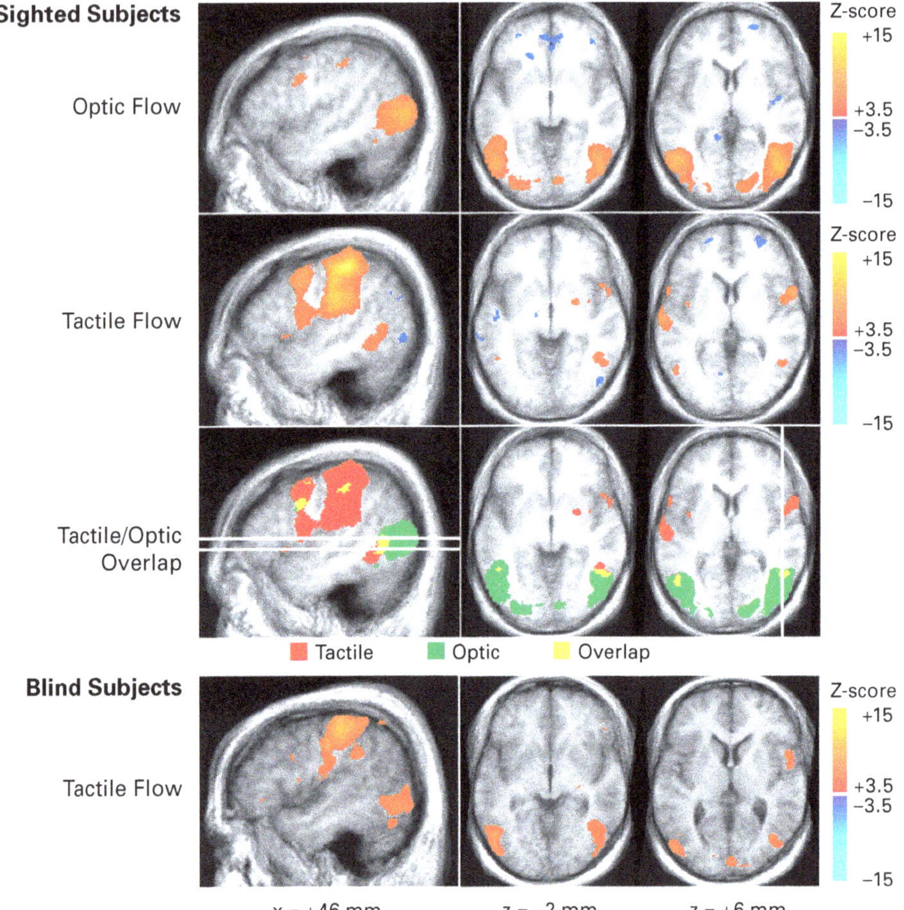

Plate 2

Brain areas that responded during tactile or optic flow perception in sighted subjects and during tactile flow-perception in blind subjects in the study by Ricciardi et al. (Ricciardi, Vanello et al. 2007). Sagittal and axial images from group Z-score maps of activated areas are shown for the sighted and blind subjects. The tactile/visual overlap map shows the areas activated by both tactile and optic flow perception (shown in yellow), as well as the areas activated only by tactile (red) and optic (green) perception. The white lines in the sagittal image correspond to the locations of the axial slices, and similarly, the white line in the axial slice indicates the location of the sagittal section.

Reprinted from Ricciardi, Vanello et al., "The effect of visual experience on the development of functional architecture in hMT+," *Cerebral Cortex* 17(12) (2007): 2933–2939. (Reprinted by permission of Oxford University Press)

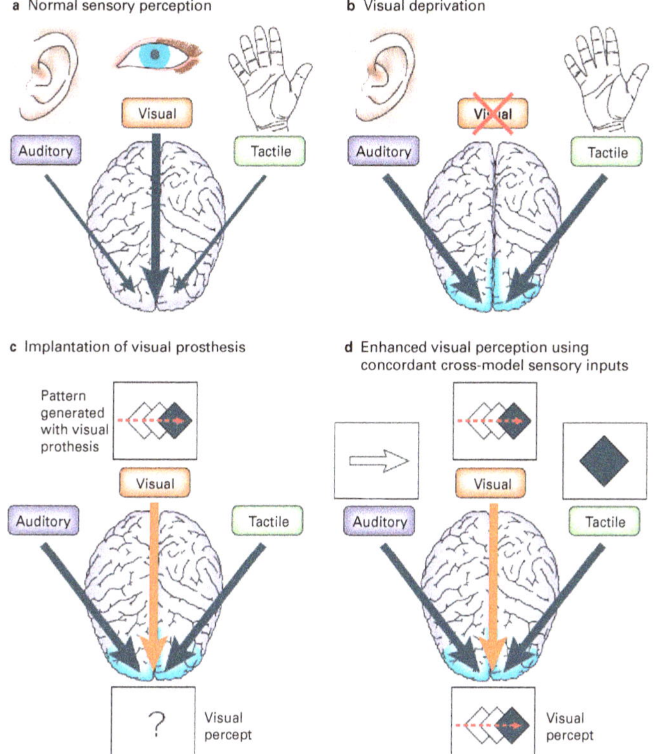

Plate 3

The multimodal nature of our sensory world and its implications for implementing a visual prosthesis to restore vision as discussed by Merabet et al. (Merabet, Rizzo et al. 2005). (A) Under normal conditions, the occipital cortex receives predominantly visual inputs but perception is also highly influenced by crossmodal sensory information obtained from other sources (for example, touch and hearing). (B) Following visual deprivation, neuroplastic changes occur such that the visual cortex is recruited to process sensory information from other senses (illustrated by larger arrows for touch and hearing). This might be through the potential "unmasking" or enhancement of connections that are already present. (C) After neuroplastic changes associated with vision loss have occurred, the visual cortex is fundamentally altered in terms of its sensory processing, so that simple reintroduction of visual input (by a visual prosthesis) is not sufficient to create meaningful vision (in this example: a pattern encoding a moving diamond figure is generated with the prosthesis). (D) To create meaningful visual percepts, a patient who has received an implanted visual prosthesis can incorporate concordant information from remaining sensory sources. In this case, the directionality of a moving visual stimulus can be presented with an appropriately timed directional auditory input and the shape of the object can be determined by simultaneous haptic exploration. In summary, modification of visual input by a visual neuroprosthesis in conjunction with appropriate auditory and tactile stimulation could potentially maximize the functional significance of restored light-perceptions and allow blind individuals to regain behaviorally relevant vision.

Reprinted from Merabet, Rizzo et al., "What blindness can tell us about seeing again: Merging neuroplasticity and neuroprostheses," *Nature Reviews. Neuroscience*, 6(1) (2005): 71–77. (© 2005. Reprinted by permission of Macmillan Publishers Ltd.)

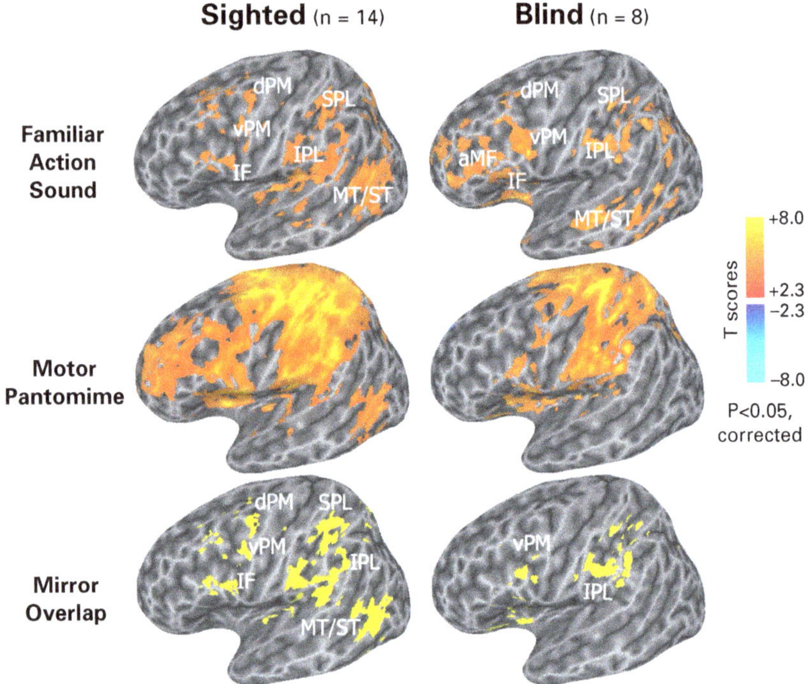

Plate 4

Statistical maps reported by Ricciardi et al. (Ricciardi, Bonino et al. 2009) showing activated brain regions during listening to *familiar* actions as compared to environmental sounds, and during the motor pantomime of action as compared to rest (corrected $p < 0.05$). In both sighted and congenitally blind individuals, aural presentation of familiar actions as compared to the environmental sounds elicited similar patterns of activation involving a left-lateralized premotor, temporal and parietal cortical network. Hand-motor pantomimes evoked bilateral activations in premotor and sensorimotor areas. Auditory mirror voxels are shown in yellow as overlap between the two task conditions in the bottom row. Spatially normalized activations are projected onto a single-subject left-hemisphere template in Talairach space. aMF = anterior middle frontal gyrus; IF = inferior frontal gyrus; vPM = ventral premotor cortex; dPM = dorsal premotor cortex; MT/ST = middle temporal and superior temporal cortex; IPL = inferior parietal lobule; SPL = superior parietal lobule.

Reprinted from Ricciardi, Bonino et al., "Do we really need vision? How blind people 'see' the actions of others," *Journal of Neuroscience* 29(31) (2009): 9719–9724. (Reprinted by permission of Society for Neuroscience) pathways (cf. Hofman, Van Riswick, and Van Opstal 1998). Previous research has shown that blind individuals can compensate for their visual loss by a general sharpening of spatial hearing (cf. Ashmead, Wall et al. 1998b; Lessard, Paré et al. 1998; Röder, Teder-Salejarvi et al. 1999), but also through developing echolocation skills (cf. Rice, Feinstein, and Schusterman 1965; Strelow and Brabyn 1982). In fact, sound waves are usually reflected from nearby surfaces, so each ear is reached by multiple echoes, and the auditory system has the ability to distinguish between the first sound (direct sound) and its reflections (echoes). Are the same compensatory mechanisms also at play in the case of visually impaired individuals? To address this issue, Déspres, Candas, and Dufour (2005c) compared sensitivity to binaural, monaural and echo cues in normally sighted and 15 myopic subjects. The group of myopic adults was affected by this visual deficit for at least 10 years, with myopia ranging from –6 to –1 diopters. Déspres et al. (Déspres, Candas, and Dufour 2005c) found that myopic individuals outperformed the sighted in the use of echo cues only, suggesting that the auditory compensation previously reported in myopic participants (Dufour and Gérard 2000) selectively depended on an increased use of echo information, and not on an enhanced sensitivity to either binaural or monaural cues. Moreover, according to Déspres et al. (Déspres, Candas, and Dufour 2005c), auditory compensation is achieved by different mechanisms in the blind and in the visually impaired: in partially sighted subjects compensation is likely to rely on visual inputs, while in the case of blindness other sensory feedback systems (e.g., proprioception, kinesthesis) may take over (Zwiers, Van Opstal, and Cruysberg 2001b). Interestingly, no significant correlation was found between myopic subjects' performance and their degree of myopia.

In a further experiment, Déspres, Candas, and Dufour (2005b) tested 20 blindfolded sighted, 24 myopic (who reported having had a visual deficit for at least 10 years; myopia ranged from –9 to –1 diopters), 5 amblyopic (i.e., suffering from a strong imbalance in the visual acuity of the two eyes), 11 adventitiously blind (with a visual deficit that had been manifest for at least 10 years) and 9 congenitally blind persons in a self-positioning task during which they were stimulated only by auditory cues. Results showed that visually deprived subjects used auditory cues to position themselves in their environment with a greater accuracy than normally sighted subjects. In addition, this time the magnitude of auditory spatial compensation was found to be strongly related to the extent of the visual deficit: in particular, if different degrees of myopia likely induce similar auditory compensation mechanisms (see Déspres, Candas, and Dufour 2005c), the presence of a residual visual capacity compared to total blindness has a significantly different impact on auditory compensation. In fact, analysis revealed that early blind subjects made smaller positioning errors than normally sighted controls, myopic, amblyopic and late blind subjects. Myopic, amblyopic, and late blind subjects performed to a similar level and were overall significantly better at self-positioning than normally sighted subjects. These findings confirm that even a small visual deficit such as myopia can give rise to auditory compensation, although the extent of such compensation is smaller compared to what accompanies a complete visual deprivation.

In fact, there is converging evidence that intersensory compensatory mechanisms are likely to be less robust in case of a partial visual loss compared to a total visual deprivation. For instance, Lessard et al. (Lessard, Paré et al. 1998) showed that VI participants performed worse than completely blind individuals in generating a spatial map of the environment on the basis of an auditory stimulation (Lessard, Paré et al. 1998). In particular, Lessard et al. (Lessard, Paré et al. 1998) compared 8 early totally blind subjects, 3 VI subjects with residual vision in the peripheral field, 7 normally sighted but blindfolded controls, and 29 sighted controls. Although VI subjects were expected to exhibit a normal localization behavior in peripheral fields (where vision was present), and a performance similar to that of the early blind subjects in the central visual field (where vision was lacking), the results were different: in fact, VI subjects were less accurate than all other subjects, particularly in the pericentral field. Lessard et al. (Lessard, Paré et al. 1998) hypothesized that the disadvantage of the VI participants tested in their study may have depended on three different factors: (1) VI subjects might have developed an auditory map of space in part supported by vision (peripheral field) and in part independent of vision (central field), which could have caused some confusion; (2) in general, cortical reorganization is less robust in case of partial visual loss than with complete blindness: in fact, if in blindness plasticity is mediated by the recruitment of the deafferented visual areas, the occipital cortex is still stimulated in VI subjects, albeit at a reduced rate, by its normal afferences; (3) a central visual loss determines abnormal orienting behaviors (such as fixating the source of the sound by turning the head, so that the sound-source falls in the peripheral/spared visual field), which might interfere with correct localization. Other evidence supports the view that having some residual vision compared to total blindness might be detrimental in auditory localization tasks: for instance, Lewald (2002b) reported that two VI subjects performed worse than blind participants in a vertical sound-localization task, possibly reflecting a sensory conflict between visual and nonvisual cues for recalibration of the auditory input.

Evidence for sensory compensation in tactile capacity in individuals with some residual vision has also been reported. In a grating-orientation discrimination task aimed at measuring passive tactile acuity, Goldreich and Kanics (2003) tested a heterogeneous group of blind individuals who differed as to degrees of blindness (residual light perception vs. none), light vision and prior visual experience (late blind vs. early blind). It was found that tactile acuity enhancement was not restricted to individuals who completely lacked light perception: in fact, 19 VI subjects with residual light perception—as stated by the authors, these subjects were unable to read print, even with magnification devices, but maintained an ability to distinguish light from dark, and in some cases, to discern vague shapes—significantly outperformed the sighted subjects. In a following study using a grating-detection task (requiring subjects to distinguish grooved from smooth surfaces pressed against the tip of their stationary index finger), Goldreich and Kanics (2006) found that the same severely visually impaired subjects performed similarly to totally blind subjects and better than sighted subjects. In a haptic angle-discrimination task in proximal space, Alary et al. (Alary, Goldstein et al. 2008) reported that three individuals with residual light perception performed similarly to the totally blind subjects and better than the sighted control group.

Overall, these findings suggest that even a severe but not complete visual deprivation may itself result in auditory and tactile acuity gains. However, in some specific situations (as in auditory spatial-localization tasks) the tendency of the brain to preferentially rely on the visual input over other sensory modalities may impair performance when the residual vision provides very distorted, or virtually no, spatial information. Finally, there is evidence for compensatory phenomena occurring within the visual system itself. For instance, Wolffe (1995) reported the case of a group of youngsters who were able to paint actual scenes or still-lifes as accurately as normally sighted people, despite a severe central-field loss. Thus, in the wake of a central vision loss the peripheral retina could convey fine details that are normally detected by the macula and fovea, allowing the visual cortex to generate a clearly detailed representation of the visual external scenes. That is, the visual cortex can develop the ability to optimize and integrate the information received from all the receptors over the whole retina (see also Trauzettel-Klosinski, MacKeben et al. 2002). Accordingly, Baker and colleagues (Baker, Peli et al. 2005) found that areas of the visual cortex usually devoted to process foveal stimuli were activated by inputs in the peripheral vision in individuals who were affected by macular degeneration (diagnosed nearly 20 years earlier), indicating a large-scale reorganization of visual processing associated with this deficit. However, the extent of cortical compensation within the visual system likely depends on the duration of the visual deficit: in fact, Sunness and colleagues (Sunness, Liu, and Yantis 2004) did not observe any significant plasticity in an individual affected by a partial macular lesion diagnosed two years before the test. An fMRI study conducted by Smirnakis and colleagues (Smirnakis, Brewer et al. 2005) showed that the topography of adult macaques' primary visual cortex did not change after several months of an induced binocular retinal lesion (resulting in a binaular scotoma). Taken together, these studies suggest that in visually impaired participants, large-scale cortical reorganization might not occur until at least several years after sensory deprivation.

Mental Representations

In previous chapters we have discussed how blindness affects imagery and working memory processes. Here we present a review of the few studies that have investigated VSWM processes in VI individuals.

Vecchi and colleagues (Vecchi, Cattaneo et al. 2006) compared a group of 10 congenitally severe VI individuals and a control group of 20 blindfolded sighted subjects in the "matrix task" (see chapter 4), requiring them to haptically explore for 10 seconds either one or two wooden-made 5×5 matrices, in which a number of target cells (covered with sand-paper and thus easily recognizable by touch) had to be memorized. When two matrices were presented, target positions at test either had to be retrieved on two corresponding empty matrices or be combined and retrieved onto a single matrix, thus allowing to measure both the ability to maintain multiple distinct spatial data in memory and the ability to integrate two spatial representations into a single one. All participants (VI participants included) were blindfolded during the exploration of the matrices and remained blindfolded at test, when they were required to haptically indicate the memorized locations on corresponding empty matrices. According to the Italian classification of severe visual impairment, all the VI participants had a visual acuity between 1/20 and 1/10, so that they could experience only blurred images. In a previous experiment (Vecchi, Tinti, and Cornoldi 2004; also see chapter 4), congenitally blind individuals performed significantly less accurately than age-matched sighted participants in this task, being particularly impaired (relative to controls) at simultaneously remembering and reproducing two separate spatially defined patterns. However, Vecchi et al. (Vecchi, Cattaneo et al. 2006) found that VI individuals did not differ from sighted controls in the different experimental conditions; specifically, VI were not selectively impaired in memorizing multiple images, as was the case for blind people. These results suggest that even highly degraded visual information is sufficient to allow the development of normal imagery and VSWM processes.

The ability of VI individuals to perform haptic tasks requiring them to draw spatial inferences has been specifically investigated by Morton Heller and colleagues (Heller, Brackett et al. 2001; Heller, Wilson et al. 2003; Heller, Riddle, et al. 2009). In a first study, a group of 9 congenitally blind, 9 late blind (mean onset-age of blindness was 20.8 years), 9 VI individuals (mean onset-age of visual deficit was 8.1 years) and 9 blindfolded sighted controls were tested in a haptic version of the Piaget water-level task (Heller, Brackett et al. 2001). In order to succeed in this task, one has to understand that the water stays horizontal despite possible tilts of the container. Is visual experience necessary for the development of such understanding? Interestingly, VI individuals outperformed both totally (early and late) blind and blindfolded sighted in this task. The overall advantage reported by the VI group was not obvious, especially considering that most of the VI subjects tested by Heller et al. (Heller, Brackett et al. 2001) defined themselves as "blind," were Braille readers and used a long cane for mobility. However, they could count on some residual light perception, and they could use it to maintain an upright posture: this—according to Heller et al. (Heller, Brackett et al. 2001)—might have played a critical role in coping with the task, because maintaining a postural stability aids in the interpretation of one's spatial surround by facilitating the use of a body-centered framework to guide haptic exploration (see Millar 1994). Furthermore, the fact that VI subjects overall lost their sight at an earlier age than late blind subjects further facilitated their performance: in fact, according to Heller et al. (Heller, Brackett et al. 2001), although VI individuals had more time to forget visual impressions, they could count on earlier exposure to education in the use of touch for pattern-perception and mobility, thus combining the benefits of early experience in education of touch with the advantages deriving from prior visual experience and from their remaining residual vision.

Similar results were obtained in a subsequent study, in which Heller et al. (Heller, Wilson et al. 2003) tested 9 VI individuals (all having light-perception, although participants considered themselves to be "blind" and were all Braille readers), 10 blindfolded sighted, 8 congenitally blind, and 9 late totally blind individuals in a haptic modified version of the embedded-figures test. In short, participants had to haptically explore a number of target raised-line drawings; at test, they had to explore four complex raised-line drawings and to indicate which one contained the target. Late blind and VI subjects were found to perform significantly better than the early blind and blindfolded sighted, again thanks to the combined effects of prior experience with pictures and increased haptic skills. In a further study carried out by Heller and colleagues (Heller, Riddle et al. 2009) 10 early-blind, 12 late blind, 10 very low-vision individuals (with light perception and able to locate strong lights), and 10 blindfolded-sighted were tested on the capacity to match haptically perceived complex objects with corresponding 2D drawings (depicting the 3D objects in different views). Low-vision individuals resulted to be more accurate in this task compared to the early blind and the blindfolded sighted (the performance of the late blind individuals was overall the highest; see chapter 7).

Unfortunately, in most of the studies carried out with VI individuals, the etiology inducing the visual deficit and age at onset are very heterogeneous. For instance, in Heller et al.'s study (Heller, Brackett et al. 2001) low vision was due to many different causes (retinopathy of prematurity—in one elderly subject associated with other diseases as macular degeneration—blood clots in the brain, retinal degeneration, chronic uveitis, hydrocephalus and retinitis pygmentosa). Moreover, the ages of participants ranged from 21 to 68 years old, and—critically—the age of onset of visual impairment was heterogeneous, ranging from congenital to 23 years of age. The majority of VI participants had no residual pattern-perception, and could not see hand motion or lines on paper, although some could see shadows, and two subjects could read large print very slowly with the help of specific visual aids. In Heller et al. (Heller, Wilson et al. 2003), VI participants' ages ranged from 19 to 71; the etiology included retinitis pygmentosa, microphtalamus, retinal degeneration, hydrocephalus and glaucoma, and retinopathy of prematurity; and the age of onset of the visual deficit ranged from congenital to a maximum of 34 years of prior normal vision. In Vecchi et al. (Vecchi,

Cattaneo et al. 2006), although all VI participants were congenitally so, they differed with regard to etiology, being affected by either profound bilateral myopia, bilateral cataract, retinitis pygmentosa and glaucoma; VI participants' ages at test ranged from 21 to 55.

This heterogeneity is somehow intrinsic to research considering VI to date, but must be taken into account when extending the results to a larger population.

Spatial Cognition

Available evidence on spatial cognition abilities in VI individuals is quite limited, but converges in indicating that low vision does not prevent the capacity to generate appropriate visual representations of familiar environments or to visually represent spatial information acquired from haptic maps. For instance, in an early study, Bigelow (1996) examined the development of spatial knowledge of the home environment in 20 normally sighted, two visually impaired, and two totally blind children. The two visually impaired children suffered from optic disc hypoplasia (damage to the nerves of the optic disc) and aniridia with nystagmus (absence of the iris, reduced central vision, and exaggeration of the natural involuntary movements of the eye) respectively, and they could only read print with high magnification or at very close range (unfortunately, visual acuity and visual field were not reported). VI and sighted children performed similarly, whereas totally blind children showed critical difficulties in performing the task, especially when they had to rely on a straight-line distance criterion: these data indicate that a reduced visual experience does not prevent the generation of an appropriate visual layout to be used to establish distances (Bigelow 1996). Similarly, Blanco and Travieso (2003) found that 7 VI participants performed closer to 7 blindfolded sighted than to 7 totally blind subjects in a task requiring haptic exploration and mental scanning of a map. All the VI participants had visual fields of less than 10 degrees and visual acuities of less than 1/10 on the Becker scale. The subjective reports of the participants indicated that the sighted and low vision individuals overall tended to generate a mental image of the island to cope with the task; whereas the totally blind group tended to project the haptic information onto representational devices that were frequent in their training as blind people (for example, three participants reported the use of the map of Spain, and two participants used geometric figures that fit the shape of the island).

Onset of Visual Impairment and Visuo-Spatial Working Memory Abilities

Research with totally blind individuals has shown that, on one hand, cortical and sensory compensatory mechanisms are more robust in case of a congenital deficit than in case of a deficit acquired later in life (Hubel and Wiesel 1977; Arno, De Volder et al. 2001; De Volder, Toyama et al. 2001), and, on the other hand, that prior visual experience may facilitate performance in spatial tasks (e.g., Gaunet, Martinez, and

Thinus-Blanc 1997; Vanlierde and Wanet-Defalque 2004; Gaunet and Rossetti 2006). However, VI individuals still have some residual vision and one might hypothesize that a normal visual experience prior to the deficit is less critical in case of low vision than in case of total blindness. In this section, we discuss results obtained in the studies that have directly compared congenitally/early VI individuals and late VI individuals in tasks that tap into spatial abilities.

In a series of studies, Cattaneo and colleagues examined whether a late emergence of a partial visual handicap weakens spatial memory or whether it has no effects whatsoever. In particular, Cattaneo et al. (Cattaneo, Vecchi et al. 2007) compared a group of 12 late VI participants and a group of sighted subjects in the haptic matrix task used by Vecchi et al. (Vecchi, Cattaneo et al. 2006: stimuli presented in haptic modality). In the VI group, the best-corrected visual acuity in the better eye ranged from 20/1000 to 60/200. Mean onset-age of the visual impairment was 27.7 years, and visual impairment had prevailed for at least 6 years. The majority of the VI participants were affected by retinitis pygmentosa (two participants were affected by Stargardt disease). Critically, late VI participants were found to be significantly impaired compared to the sighted controls in performing the task (Cattaneo, Vecchi et al. 2007), whereas this was not the case for congenitally VI subjects (Vecchi, Cattaneo et al. 2006). It is likely that in case of a late onset of visual deficit, the visuo-spatial working memory system tends to function by relying on the dominant perceptual experience on whose basis it originally developed—i.e., normally functioning vision. However, the visuo-spatial working memory system may not readapt perfectly to the impaired sensorial stimulation (Vecchi, Cattaneo et al. 2006), thus explaining the apparently paradoxical result that late VI individuals failed in a task where congenitally visually impaired individuals had succeeded as well as sighted individuals (cf. Vecchi, Cattaneo et al. 2006).

This hypothesis received support in a further experiment (Monegato, Cattaneo et al. 2007) that directly compared 16 early VI individuals and 16 late VI individuals (in the late VI group, low vision had prevailed for at least 15 years, and the age of onset of the visual impairment ranged from 15 to 38 years). Visual acuity was comparable in the two groups, with best-corrected visual acuity in the better eye ranging from 0.5 to 1.6 logMAR. The majority of participants in the late VI group suffered of retinitis pygmentosa. In the early VI group, the etiology was more various, including profound myopia, albinism, glaucoma, retinitis pygmentosa, cataract, and optic nerve atrophy. The experimental paradigm was similar to that used by Vecchi et al. (Vecchi, Cattaneo et al. 2006), but this time the same task was performed in the visual modality. In fact, the presence of a residual visual experience offers the opportunity to test participants with both visual and tactile stimuli, allowing a direct comparison between mental representations generated on the basis of different sensorial stimulation. All participants performed better in the visual than in the haptic modality, confirming that they were still able to make efficient use of their residual visual ability to carry out the task.

Critically, congenitally VI participants performed better than late ones when required to remember a number of locations presented on tactile or visual matrices, although their general pattern of performance was identical (i.e., relative level of performance in the different conditions requiring subjects to memorize targets on one single matrix, or on two matrices or an integration process). Hence, differences induced by the onset time of a partial visual loss are likely to be "quantitative" rather than "qualitative." One might hypothesize that other factors beyond the visual deficit onset have played a role in determining the pattern of results, such as different residual visual acuity and visual field, differences in mobility skills, and so forth. In fact, the two groups differed both in terms of deficit-onset and in terms of residual visual field: retinitis pygmentosa was the main cause of visual deficit in the late VI group, while the congenitally VI group was more affected by nerve atrophy, glaucoma and myopia. Retinitis pygmentosa is usually accompanied by a loss of the peripheral visual field while the central visual field can be relatively preserved; conversely, the congenitally VI participants overall presented a decrease in sensitivity in both the peripheral and central visual field. However, the different performances in this spatial task could not be caused by the differences in the remaining visual field: a preserved central visual field is more critical for this type of task (whereas the peripheral field is more important in navigational tasks), and hence, given that the majority of late VI subjects had a preserved central vision, they should have outperformed congenitally VI subjects.

Moreover, peripheral and tunnel vision led to comparable performances in a study assessing the role of concomitant vision in improving haptic performance (Millar and Al-Attar 2005). The task required subjects to memorize locations presented on a tactile map either without vision, with concomitant full vision, with peripheral vision, with tunnel vision or in a condition of residual diffuse light perception (by using particular spectacles). Millar and Al-Attar (2005) noticed that in the peripheral vision condition—thanks to appropriate head movements—participants could count on an adequate (although blurred) vision of the relevant stimuli. Similarly, in the tunnel vision condition, participants were able to obtain a clear view of any area of the map, by moving their head appropriately. In fact, peripheral and tunnel vision do not determine differences in perception as long as participants are free to move their heads. In Monegato, Cattaneo et al.'s (2007) study, participants were free to move their heads, and none of them reported difficulties in visualizing the matrices. Hence, data suggest a quite marginal role for the residual field of view in static spatial memory tasks (Millar and Al-Attar 2005).

To summarize, these studies suggest that a partial visual deficit might induce the development of functional compensatory mechanisms that are likely to be quantitatively and qualitatively different from those occurring in case of total blindness and to depend—as in case of blindness—on the time of onset of the visual deprivation (cf. Cattaneo, Vecchi et al. 2007; Monegato, Cattaneo et al. 2007). At a cortical level, changes are likely to occur also in case of a partial visual deficit, and these changes appear to be modulated by the duration and age of onset of the visual deficit (Sunness, Liu, and Yantis 2004; Baker, Peli et al. 2005; Smirnakis, Brewer et al. 2005).

6.3 Monocular Vision

Monocular blindness is a particular case of low vision that deserves attention since it allows us to specifically investigate whether and how binocularity affects visual perception and cognitive development. In fact, monocular deprivation has been extensively studied in animals as a model for cortical plasticity, allowing researchers to establish how visual information is normally represented in the visual system and how alterations at the perceptual stage result in cortical plastic changes (for a recent review, see Berardi, Pizzorusso, and Maffei 2000). In the visual system, information coming from the two eyes is kept separate through the early stages of visual processing. Retinal ganglion cell axons from the two eyes project to separate eye-specific layers in the lateral geniculate nucleus (LGN). Similarly, in the primary visual cortex (V1), LGN afferents of the two eyes are segregated into eye-specific stripes in cortical layer IV, thus forming the anatomical basis for ocular dominance columns, radial columns of cells throughout the depth of the cortex that tend to respond better to visual stimuli presented to one or the other eye. Following monocular deprivation, physiological and anatomical changes have been reported in both the LGN and V1. In the LGN axonal projections from the remaining eye tend to occupy nearly the entire LGN (cf. Chalupa and Williams 1984). Similar changes occur in V1, as firstly reported by Hubel and Wiesel, who showed that raising a kitten with one eye sutured interferes with the normal development of its primary visual cortex, so that cells can no longer respond to visual stimuli through the closed eye and are driven exclusively by the eye that remained open (Wiesel and Hubel 1963; LeVay, Wiesel, and Hubel 1980). These physiological changes are followed by anatomical rearrangements: the thalamo-cortical arbors from the closed eye shrink their arborizations and then the axonal arbors driven by the open eye expand; moreover, changes in horizontal connections between neurons in layer II/III have been reported (cf. Beaver, Ji, and Daw 2001; Trachtenberg and Stryker 2001). Similarly, in experimentally induced strabismic animals, in which the misalignment of the eyes causes the animals to see double, neurons in the primary visual cortex become almost exclusively monocular, driven by the one or the other eye but not by both (Hubel and Wiesel 1965; Van Sluyters and Levitt 1980). A reduction in horizontal connections for binocular vision in V1 has been observed in naturally strabismic monkeys (Tychsen, Wong, and Burkhalter 2004). According to the seminal work of Hubel and Wiesel, these cortical rearrangements in response to monocular deprivation occur during a relatively short time window in development that they referred to as the *critical period* (Wiesel and Hubel 1965).

In more recent years, advanced postmortem neurophysiological techniques have allowed us to investigate the effects of monocular deprivation on the human brain: as with animal monocular blindness, early monocular deprivation causes shrinkage of ocular dominance columns of the deprived eye in the primary human visual cortex with a corresponding expansion of the columns of the functioning eye (Horton and Hocking 1998; Adams, Sincich, and Horton 2007). In cases of severe unilateral visual deficit with no enucleation (such as in unilateral amblyopia) there are associated cortical changes in the primary visual cortex resulting in an overall loss of cortical binocularly and a shift in cortical eye dominance toward the unaffected eye (for a review, see Barrett, Bradley, and McGraw 2004).

Monocular Vision and Visual Perception

Steeves, González, and Steinbach (2008) have reviewed behavioral studies on visual performance in individuals who underwent unilateral enucleation to assess whether the remaining eye compensates for the loss of binocularity. Overall, the review shows that monocular blindness is associated with both enhanced and reduced visual functions depending upon the visual capacity that is being measured: specifically, some aspects of visual spatial ability—such as contrast sensitivity and Vernier visual acuity—benefit from the loss of binocularity; whereas motion processing and oculomotor behavior are impaired (Steeves, González, and Steinbach 2008). The type of monocular deficit is an important factor to be considered: specifically, unilateral enucleation likely represents a peculiar case that has different effects on the remaining eye's visual functions compared to other forms of monocular visual deprivation such as cataract, strabismus, ptosis (i.e., drooping of the upper eyelid) and anisometropia (e.g., McKee, Levi, and Movshon 2003; Mansouri and Hess 2006). In fact, unilateral enucleation results in the most complete form of deprivation because the brain loses any possible visual input from the enucleated eye, whereas other forms of monocular visual deprivation leave some, usually abnormal, visual input. Another important factor to be considered is age at onset of the monocular visual deficit (or of the enucleation). In fact, at the anatomical level, there is evidence that the reorganization of the ocular dominance columns varies with the onset-age of the deficit, being for instance less robust when enucleation occurred at the age of 4 months (Adams, Sincich, and Horton 2007) than at the age of one week (Horton and Hocking 1998). However, experience-dependent plasticity is also possible in adulthood, as is for instance demonstrated by the improvements in visual function in the amblyopic eye after a reduction of visual function in the non-amblyopic eye in adults, which is consistent with the animal data (Smith, Holdefer, and Reeves 1982; Harwerth, Smith et al. 1986; Horton and Hocking 1998; Prusky, Alam, and Douglas 2006). Overall though, plasticity phenomena following monocular deprivation in adulthood appear reduced, slower and—importantly—

qualitatively different from those occurring in the critical period (cf. Sato and Stryker 2008).

Different studies have shown that unilateral enucleated individuals can count on an enhanced luminance-defined form processing (such as perceiving *low contrast* letters or discriminating radial frequency patterns) as compared to monocular viewing (i.e., patched) controls, resembling the level of performance of binocular viewing controls (Reed, Steeves et al. 1996; Reed, Steeves, and Steinbach 1997; González, Steeves et al. 2002; Steeves, Wilkinson et al. 2004). Notably, improvements in contrast sensitivity likely depends on the onset-age of the monocular deprivation (i.e., during postnatal visual development or later in life): for instance, Nicholas, Heywood, and Cowey (1996) found that the earlier the enucleation occurred, the larger tended to be the improvement for specific spatial frequencies. Monocularly enucleated individuals have also been reported to possess enhanced foveal Vernier acuity (Freeman and Bradley 1980), but these results have been later questioned (González, Steinbach et al. 1992).

According to Steeves et al. (Steeves, González et al. 2008), the enhanced spatial-visual ability reported in one-eye observers might depend on different factors, such as the absence of inhibitory binocular interactions, the recruitment by the remaining eye of the resources normally assigned to the missing eye, and the level of monocular practice. Critically, superior visual functions compared to monocularly viewing sighted controls have not been reported in the fellow eye of strabismic individuals (Reed, Steeves et al. 1996; González, Steeves et al. 2002), suggesting that the absence of binocularly inhibitory interactions plays a major role in leading to superior performance in certain visual tasks. Nonetheless, level of practice is also an important factor. In a task that measures depth-perception, González et al. (González, Steinbach et al. 1989) found that enucleated young children were not superior to controls in the use of monocular cues for depth, as one might expect considering that depth from stereopsis is not available to them. However, after a short training in which González and colleagues instructed the children to move the head from side to side, depth-perception in the younger one-eye observers became comparable to that of an older control group viewing binocularly. In fact, individuals that have been affected by monocular blindness for years tend to rely on compensatory practices, such as the use of larger and faster head movements (cf. Marotta, Perrot et al. 1995; see also Goltz, Steinbach, and Gallie 1997). In particular, they tend to turn the head to bring the remaining eye closer to the midline of the body, thus reducing the occlusion of the visual field by the nose. If soon after the enucleation these compensatory practices may not be evident, they become frequent with the years, since one-eye observers learn to use as many optical variables as possible to compensate for the lack of binocular information. For instance, in a task requiring subjects to estimate the "time to contact" of an object,

Steeves et al. (Steeves, Gray et al. 2000) found that most one-eye individuals made use of variables that were irrelevant to the specific task—such as the stimulus' starting size—but that are useful in the real world where objects have familiar sizes. In this regard, it is worth noting that the superior visual functions of monocularly enucleated individuals might depend on the age at enucleation, more than on the number of years since enucleation (Nicholas, Heywood, and Cowey 1996; González, Steeves, and Steinbach 1998).

If some aspects of spatial vision are likely to be enhanced in the monocular blind, motion perception and processing have been found to be impaired (Steeves, Gray et al. 2000; Steeves, González et al. 2002), with age at enucleation again playing a critical role. For instance, Steeves et al. (Steeves, González et al. 2002) reported a nose-ward bias in horizontal motion direction discrimination in subjects who were enucleated before 36 months of age but not in those who had undergone enucleation at an older age (43 months), suggesting that normal binocular competitive interactions during a critical postnatal sensitive period are necessary for the establishment of symmetrical motion perception (Steeves, González et al. 2008; cf. also Reed, Steinbach et al. 1991; Day 1995). Additionally, it has been demonstrated that in early enucleated children (up to four years of age) the origin of visual direction or egocenter (that is, the spatial egocentric reference from which individuals judge direction, also called the "cyclopean" eye: see Barbeito 1983; Steinbach, Howard, and Ono 1985) shifts from the midline toward the functioning eye. Conversely, no change in the egocenter location was reported in either children with one eye patched (Moidell, Steinbach, and Ono 1988), in children with strabismus (Dengis, Simpson et al. 1998) or in normal binocular adults wearing a monocular patch for one month (Dengis, Steinbach, and Kraft 1992).

The data described here highlight the problems in studying the effects of binocular deprivation on basic visual functions and the difficulties in selecting appropriate control groups for one-eye observers. On the one hand, while strabismic amblyopia, anisometropia and unilateral cataracts all involve monocular deprivation, they also involve abnormal binocular interactions which result in inferior performance in many visual functions when compared to monocular enucleation. On the other hand, in normally sighted subjects, patching or closing one eye does not produce a "real" monocular vision but rather a condition of temporarily weak binocular rivalry with completely different effects at the cortical level (Dengis, Steinbach, and Kraft 1992; González, Weinstock, and Steinbach 2007).

Monocular Vision and Higher Cognitive Functions

Little research has been carried out on the effects of early monocular blindness on higher cognitive functions. A few studies have assessed the effect of eye-patching in normally sighted subjects on crossmodal sensory interactions and attentional tasks.

For instance, patching one eye in normally sighted individuals has been found to bias sound localization toward the viewing eye (Abel and Tikuisis 2005). Moreover, using a radial line bisection task, Roth et al. (Roth, Lora, and Heilman 2002) reported that eye-patching causes preferential activation of attentional systems in the controlateral hemisphere. Accordingly, eye-patching has been used as a treatment for visuo-spatial neglect sometimes resulting in improved performance in different spatial tasks, although data are not always consistent (cf. Butter and Kirsch 1992; Walker, Young, and Lincoln 1996; Beis, Andre et al. 1999; Barrett and Burkholder 2006). Overall, available findings suggest that unilateral eye-patching in normally sighted individuals might influence performance in spatial tasks.

In a study investigating cognitive and visual outcomes in children treated for retinoblastoma, both children with a unilateral tumor (all of which underwent enucleation) and children with bilateral tumors (only some of which were enucleated) were tested (Ek, Seregard et al. 2002). Despite the fact that children with bilateral tumors were severely visually impaired, while children affected by unilateral retinoblastoma could see almost normally from their remaining eye, the former scored higher in a series of tests measuring verbal development, short-term memory, understanding of concepts, and visuomotor and nonverbal reasoning ability (Ek, Seregard et al. 2002). These findings corroborate earlier evidence in favor of higher cognitive abilities in children bilaterally affected by retinoblastoma associated with blindness, that are probably due to the development of verbal and cognitive functions involving attention, memory and concentration to compensate for the visual deficit (e.g., Thurrell and Josephson 1966; Williams 1968; Eldridge, O'Meara, and Kitchin 1972). Such compensatory mechanisms would not develop in case of unilateral retinoblastoma, since these patients can normally see from their functioning eye.

The effects of congenital monocular blindness on cognitive abilities have been systematically investigated in a series of experiments (Vecchi, Cattaneo et al. 2006; Cattaneo, Merabet et al. 2008). In a first experiment (Vecchi, Cattaneo et al. 2006), blindfolded congenitally monocular individuals, visually impaired individuals, and blindfolded sighted controls were required to memorize a series of target locations presented on two-dimensional tactile matrices in different experimental conditions. In a similar experiment, congenitally totally blind individuals were found to be particularly impaired when required to memorize and retrieve target locations on two distinct matrices (Vecchi, Tinti, and Cornoldi 2004). Interestingly, Vecchi and colleagues (Vecchi, Cattaneo et al. 2006) found a similar pattern of performance in VI and sighted participants (for a discussion on the VI subjects' performance in this task, see earlier in this chapter), whereas the pattern of performance shown by monocular individuals was significantly lower in the condition requiring maintenance of multiple matrices in memory, thus resembling what had been found with congenitally totally blind individuals. Hence, surprisingly, the performance of monocular participants was closer to that of totally blind individuals than to normally sighted controls, despite the fact that monocular individuals could see perfectly with their single eye. Overall, the pattern of performance of monocular, visually impaired, congenitally blind and sighted individuals indicated that the critical variable influencing performance was not vision per se but rather the presence/absence of binocular vision (congenitally blind and monocular individuals showed the same pattern of performance). The absence of binocular vision and of simultaneous visual processes in monocularity may result, at a higher cognitive level, in a different development of the imagery cognitive system in turn determining a specific difficulty in simultaneously maintaining different representations in memory (Vecchi, Cattaneo et al. 2006).

In a follow-up study, the same experiment was presented in the visual modality (Cattaneo, Merabet et al. 2008). This time, the task required participants to memorize and retrieve a number of spatial cells (either 4 or 6) within 5×5 matrices that were *visually* presented for 10 seconds. A group of individuals affected by monocular blindness since birth due to different pathologies (including optic atrophy, choroidal hemangioma, toxoplasmosis and microphthalmos) and totally blind in the affected eye (no light-perception) was compared with a group of sighted individuals viewing binocularly and with a group of sighted individuals wearing a one-eye blindfold. The one-eye blindfolded control group was introduced to verify whether possible limitations experienced by the monocularly blind could be due to perceptual limitations (this comparison was pointless in the haptic modality since all participants performed the task blindfolded). Overall, congenitally monocular individuals performed worse than both monocular- and binocular-viewing normally sighted controls, whereas performance was similar for the monocular- and binocular-viewing controls. The fact that eye-patched controls were not impaired in the task, although temporarily viewing from just one eye, indicated that the limitations experienced by the congenitally monocular participants in the visual version of the task were not due to an impaired perception of the stimuli at a peripheral level, but were rather related to a higher central level of processing. Moreover, the hypothesis of a peripheral deficit experienced by monocular individuals would not be compatible with previous evidence indicating that visual-acuity and contrast-sensitivity performance in unilateral enucleated individuals is superior to that of monocular-viewing controls or at least comparable to binocular-viewing controls (for a review, see Steeves, González, and Steinbach 2008).

Available neurophysiological and neuroimaging evidence supports the hypothesis that the deficit observed in monocular individuals in the matrix task was likely to be inherently "cognitive": in fact, monocular early enucleation induces changes in the cortical organization in primary visual cortex (Horton and Hocking 1998; Adams and Horton 2002), and it is well known that the primary visual cortex is involved both in visual perception and visual imagery (cf. Kosslyn, Thompson et al. 1995; Kosslyn,

Thompson, and Alpert 1997; Kosslyn, Pascual-Leone et al. 1999). Similarly, it has been reported that in case of a severe unilateral visual deficit with no enucleation (such as in unilateral amblyopia) there are associated cortical changes in the primary visual cortex resulting in an overall loss of cortical binocularity and a shift in cortical eye-dominance toward the unaffected eye (for a review, see Barrett, Bradley, and McGraw 2004). The general deficit reported in the monocular blind group might also depend on an atypical engagement of the two hemispheres in the spatial task. In fact, monocular eye-patching has been found to affect the extent to which each hemisphere contributes to the allocation of visuo-spatial attentive resources (Roth, Lora, and Heilman 2002) and it has been successfully used as a treatment to reduce neglect symptoms (cf. Butter and Kirsch 1992). If temporary monocular patching is sufficient to modulate hemispheric competition, early monocular blindness is likely to critically interfere with the specific involvement of the two hemispheres in visual, attentive and visuo-spatial imagery processes. Notably, the deficit showed by the monocular individuals emerged in all the experimental conditions, but was significantly more evident when participants were required to maintain distinct representations in memory. Hence, although monocular blindness may generally affect the capacity to deal with spatial mental representations, a specific difficulty seems to be associated with the simultaneous maintenance in memory of distinct spatial representations. The fact that a similar specific deficit was reported in the haptic version of the task (cf. Vecchi, Cattaneo et al. 2006) might be explained by assuming the existence of supramodal representations depending on specific task-requirements, and indeed only marginally sensitive to the sensorial format of the entering input (cf. Pietrini, Furey et al. 2004; Ricciardi, Bonino et al. 2006; and see chapter 8).

7 The Importance of Blindness-Onset

Blindness has not been for me a total misfortune; it should not be seen in a pathetic way. It should be seen as a way of life: one of the styles of living.

—Jorge Luis Borges, *Seven Nights*

7.1 Distinguishing between "Early" and "Late"

In previous chapters we have mentioned the importance of a person's age at the onset of blindness, when considering the perceptual, attentional and cognitive capacities of the blind. This chapter focuses on the effects that blindness-onset exerts on sensory compensation phenomena, imagery abilities, working memory capacities and cortical plasticity phenomena. Although some of the findings discussed here have also been considered in other parts of this book, a chapter devoted wholly to this topic offers a more exhaustive view of the effects that the timing of blindness-onset plays at the functional and cortical levels.

Different studies have adopted heterogeneous criteria to classify early and late blind individuals (see table 7.1): in some cases, individuals who lost their sight after two to three years of life have been considered as "early" blind (e.g., Voss, Lassonde et al. 2004), in other cases as "late" blind (e.g., Gougoux, Belin et al. 2009). This is problematic when trying to compare the available experimental outputs, because of course the perceptual and cognitive consequences associated with sight-loss when individuals turn blind in their thirties or later are likely to be different from those at play when individuals lose visual capacity after a few months or years of life. Moreover, it is likely that blindness-induced changes in perceptual and cognitive capacity and cortical plasticity phenomena depend both on individuals' age at blindness-onset and on the duration of the visual deprivation, with effects that are often difficult to disentangle. Indeed, the visual system in humans seems to be highly plastic until 14–16 years of age (see Cohen, Weeks et al. 1999; Sadato, Okada et al. 2002), although the exact duration of the "critical period" in humans has not been clearly defined. The "critical period" should not be regarded as a single entity, since it varies for each particular

Table 7.1

Table summarizing the characteristics of blind (B=blind; EB=early blind; LB=late blind) and sighted (S) subjects participating in some of the experiments discussed in chapter 7 (M=mean; SD=standard deviation).

Study	Number of subjects [mean age [SD] and/or age-range in years]	Mean age and/or range of ages at blindness-onset	Mean deficit duration and/ or years range
Afonso, Blum, et al. (2010)	24 congenitally blind 24 LB 24 S All 72 subjects' age range 21–63	LB range 6–30	LB > 15 years
Alary, Goldstein, et al. (2008)	16 B [M=36.3, range 19–53] 17 S [M=28.4, range 22–50]	7 congenitally blind, 2 became blind at 2–3months, 3 became blind at 3 years, 4 became blind at 7, 8, 11, and 14 years	
Alary, Duquette, et al. (2009)	16 B [M=36.3, range 19–53] 2 groups of sighted: 17 S [M=28.4, range 22–50]; 30 S [range 21–58]	7 congenitally blind, 2 became blind at 2–3 months, 3 became blind at 3 years, 4 became blind at 7, 8, 11, and 14 years	
Buchel, Price, et al. (1998)	6 congenitally blind [M=49.2, SD=12] 3 LB [M=45, SD=7.6] 6 S [M=26.8, SD=4]	LB 18.3 (±3.8)	
Burton, Snyder, et al. (2002a)	9 EB [M=44.78, range 34–67] 7 LB [M=49.14, range 36–66]	EB range 0–5 LB 12.7, range 10–25	
Burton, Snyder, et al. (2002b)	8 EB [M=41.25, SD=10.5] 6 LB [M=50.5, SD=12] 8 S	EB range 0–3 LB 19.2 (SD=10.9), range 7–36	LB 31.3 (SD=15), range 11–51
Burton, Diamond, and McDermott (2003)	9 EB [M=45.8, SD=16.4] 7 LB [M=51.4, SD=11.2] 8 S [M=42.5, SD=14.9]	EB 0.9 (SD=1.83), range 0–5 LB 17.7 (SD=10.7), range 7–36	LB 33.7 (SD=14.2), range 12–52
Burton, Sinclair, and McLaren (2004)	9 EB [M=48.8, SD=16.7] 9 LB [M=46.2, SD=13.8] 8 S [M=45.5, SD=12.7]	EB 0.9 (SD=1.7), range 0–5 LB 20.6 (SD=11.9), range 6–41	LB 25.7 (SD=15.1), range 0–36

Table 7.1
(continued)

Study	Number of subjects [mean age [SD] and/or age-range in years]	Mean age and/or range of ages at blindness-onset	Mean deficit duration and/ or years range
Burton, McLaren, and Sinclair (2006)	9 EB [M=49, SD=16.7] 9 LB [M=43.8, SD=14.4] 10 S [M=43.2, SD=15.6]	EB 0.9 (SD=1.8), range 0–5 LB 16.3 (SD=11.4), range 7–41	LB 27.5 (SD=14.2), range 1–51
Cohen, Weeks, et al. (1999)	8 LB [M=48.25, SD=12.68]	LB 30.37 (SD=15.25), range 15–58	LB 17.9 yrs (SD 17.03), range 3–47
Collignon, Charbonneau, et al. (2009)	10 EB [M=40, SD=10, range 26–56] 11 LB [M=44, SD=9, range 24–60] 12 S [M=43, SD=10, range 28–56]	EB 0–2 months LB 17 (SD=5.1), range 8–27	LB 25, range 13–46
Cowey and Walsh (2000)	1 LB=61 6 S	53	8
Déspres, Candas and Dufour (2005b)	9 congenitally blind [M=35.9, SD=14.6] 11 LB [M=40.4, SD=14.3] 20 S [M=38, range 18–55]	LB 21.3 (SD=13.4), range 6–50	LB 19.1 (SD=7.8), range 10–30
Dufour, Déspres, and Candas (2005)	6 congenitally blind [M=27.5, SD=8.2] 6 LB [M=45, SD=7] 20 S [M=32, range 20–51]	LB 22.3 (SD=9.8), range 13–40	LB 22.7 (SD=6.3), range 15–30
Gaunet and Rossetti (2006)	13 EB [M=32.6, SD=8.8] 9 LB[M=33.3, SD=7.98] 7 S [M=30.85, SD=8.41]	EB range 0–1 LB > 4	LB 21, range 7–35
Goldreich and Kanics (2003)	47 S [median age=44 years 2 months, range 20 years 7 months–71 years 7 months] 43 B [median age=48 years 5 months, range 21 years 7 months –71 years] Authors did not categorize blind subjects according to their age at onset of blindness because this was indeterminate in a large number of subjects, who lost vision progressively over the course of many years.	Birth to 12 years	

Table 7.1
(continued)

Study	Number of subjects [mean age [SD] and/or age-range in years]	Mean age and/or range of ages at blindness-onset	Mean deficit duration and/ or years range
Goldreich and Kanics (2006)	47 S [median age=44 years 2 months, range 20 years 7 months–71 years 7 months] 37 B [median 49 years; range 19 years 8 months–71 years] Authors did not categorize blind subjects according to their age-at-onset of blindness.	Birth to 12 years	
Gougoux, Lepore, et al. (2004)	7 EB [range 21–40 yrs] 7 LB [range 24–26 yrs] 12 S [range 21–37 yrs]	EB range 0–2 LB range 5–45	
Gougoux, Belin, et al. (2009)	5 congenitally blind [M=30.4 yrs, SD=8.2] 10 LB [M=34.2 yrs, SD=8]	LB 18.5 (SD=16), range 1–45	LB 15.7 (SD=11.2), range 1–36
Goyal, Hansen and Blakemore (2006)	3 congenitally blind [M=21] 3 LB [M=62] 3 S [M=25]	LB 11	
Grant, Thiagarajah and Sathian (2000)	15 EB [M=39.2,SD=13.7] 9 LB [M=42.6, SD=7.36] 39 S [M=39, range 19–75]	EB range 0 (14 subjects)–5 (1 subject), range 23–67 LB > 10, range 12–37	
Heller, Wilson et al. (2003)	8 congenitally blind [M=41.9, SD=8.9] 10 LB [M=47.9, SD=11.6] 9 Low-vision [M=37, range 19–54] 10 S [M=35.1, range n.a.]	LB 12.6 (SD=12.4), range 2–43	LB 35.3 (SD=17.4), range 12–58
Heller, Riddle, et al. (2009)	12 EB [M=52, SD=12.78] 12 LB [M= 45.4, SD=11.97] 12 Low-vision: [M=38.5, SD=16.32] 20 S M= 41.2 [range 21–68]	EB 10 congenitally blind, 2 lost sight when 2 years old LB 19.3 (SD=11.57), range 4–42 Low vision: 6 congenitally low vision, 4 became low vision at a mean age of 19.8 (SD=11.20), range 8–37	LB 26.1 (SD=17.58)

Table 7.1
(continued)

Study	Number of subjects [mean age [SD] and/or age-range in years]	Mean age and/or range of ages at blindness-onset	Mean deficit duration and/ or years range
Kupers, Fumal, et al. (2006)	8 EB [M=36.5, SD=4.7] 5 LB [M=37, SD=7.6] 8 S [M=34.5, SD=11]	EB 1.75 (SD=3.24), range 0–7 LB 20.8 (SD=11.5), range 9–40	LB 16.2 (SD=9.45), range 7–29
Noordzij, Zuidhoek and Postma (2006)	13 EB [M=45, SD=9.75] 17 LB [M=53.5, SD=7.95] 16 S [M=49.3, SD=11.4]	EB 0.61 (SD=0.96), range 0–3 LB 23 (SD=13.2), range 4–49	LB 30.53 (SD=14.3), range 4–57
Occelli, Spence and Zampini (2008)	8 EB [M=34.2, SD=6.6] 9 LB [M=39.6, SD=11.5] 20 S [M=33, range 20–55]	EB range 0–3 months LB range 6–37	LB 15.1 (SD=4.1), range 11–22
Ogden and Barker (2001)	8 EB [M=35.6, SD=10.7, range 25–56] 8 LB [M=48, SD=13.2, range 32–70] 8 S [M=41.1, SD=13.7, range 23–65]	EB range 0–2 LB 24 (SD=12.9), range 12–45	LB 24 (SD=15.5), range 12–45
Pasqualotto and Newell (2007)	10 congenitally blind [M=37.3, SD=15.6] 12 LB [M=35.4, SD=14.6]	LB 12.3 (SD=8), range 2–21	LB 23.1 (SD=16.6), range 2–50
Postma, Zuidhoek, et al. (2008)	13 EB [M=44.9, SD=10.1] 17 LB [M=53.5, SD=7.9] 16 S	EB 0.6 (SD=1), range 0–2/3 LB 23 (SD=13.2), range 4–49	LB 30.5 (SD=14.3), range 4–57
Rao, Nobre, et al. (2007)	1 LB: 64	52	12
Röder and Rösler (2003)	20 congenitally blind [M=21.4, range 18–32] 20 LB [M=35.3, range 21–53] 24 S [M=21.5, range 19–25]		LB 14.5, range 5–32
Röder, Rösler, and Spence (2004)	10 congenitally blind [M=22.3, SD=4.4] 5 LB [M=26.2, SD=3.6] 12 S1 [M=22, range 20–26] 12 S2 [M=22, range 19–26]	LB 18.6 (SD=3.7), range 13–23	LB 7.6 (SD=3.2), range 5–12

Table 7.1
(continued)

Study	Number of subjects [mean age [SD] and/or age-range in years]	Mean age and/or range of ages at blindness-onset	Mean deficit duration and/or years range
Röder, Kusmierek, et al. (2007)	11 congenitally blind [M=35.7, SD=9.2] 7 LB [M=55.9, SD=15.5] 11 S1 (control group for the EB) [M=35.2, range 23–51] 7 S2 (control group for the LB) [M=56.6, range 38–72]	LB 34.1 (SD=16.2), range 15–58	LB 21.7 (SD=14.9), range 10–50
Sadato, Okada, et al. (2002)	9 EB [M=43.6, SD=13.5] 6 LB [M=44.5, SD=11.5] 8 S [M=29.0, SD=4.5]	EB 5.8 (SD=5.7), range 0–15 LB 33.2 (SD=11.6), range 20–51	EB 37.7 (SD=18.3), range 9–57 LB 11.3 (SD=5.2), range 2–17
Steven and Blakemore (2004)	6 LB [M=61.5, SD=10.9, range 10–35]		LB range 10–35 (2 subjects could still perceive colors)
Stevens and Weaver (2009)	7 congenitally blind [M=46.9, SD=11.13] 5 LB [M=52, SD=10.1] 6 S [M= 45.4, range 36–54]	LB 25.4 (SD=18.46), range 6–53	LB 26.6 (SD=16.9), range 13–52
Sukemiya, Nakamizo, and Ono (2008)	4 congenitally blind [M=32.5, SD=18.7] 12 LB [M=43.6, SD=15.1] 7 S [M=22.4, range 20–27]	LB 20.5, range 2–45	LB 22.9 (SD=12.4), range 2–42
Tinti, Adenzato, et al. (2006) (Experiment 2)	13 congenitally blind [M=44.2, SD=13.7, range 26–68] 13 LB [M=53.2, SD=15.3, range 19–77] 20 S [M=52.8, SD=17.3, range 21–78]	LB >12	
Vanlierde and Wanet-Defalque (2004)	10 EB [M=39.6, SD=13.4] 9 LB [M=52.2, SD=8.7] 27 S [M=43, SD=15.07]	EB 0.9 (SD=1), range 0–3 LB 26 (SD=11), range 9–40	LB 26.2 (SD=12), range 15–48

Table 7.1
(continued)

Study	Number of subjects [mean age [SD] and/or age-range in years]	Mean age and/or range of ages at blindness-onset	Mean deficit duration and/ or years range
Vanlierde and Wanet-Defalque (2005)	10 EB [M=40, SD=13.01, range 20–62] 9 LB [M=52, SD=8.42, range 37–61] 27 S [M=43, SD=15.07, range 22–68]	EB 0.9 (SD=1), range 0–3 LB 26 (SD=11), range 9–40	LB 26.22 (SD=12), range 15–48
Voss, Lassonde et al. (2004)	14 EB [M=36.6, range 21–54] 9 LB [M=41.6, range 23–55] 10 S [M=21.2, range 18–24]	EB <11 LB >16	EB 36.6 LB 20.2
Voss, Gougoux, et al. (2006)	6 LB [M=41.5, range 33–54] 7 S [M=27.9, range 22–48]	LB 26.3, range 18–37	LB 15.8, range 4–36
Voss, Gougoux, et al. (2008)	12 EB [M=31.3, range 21–41] 6 LB [M=41.5, range 33–54] 7 S [M=27.9, range 22–48]	EB 2.6, range 0–14 LB 15.8, range 18–37	EB 28.7, range 16–40 LB 15.8, range 4–36
Wan, Wood, et al. (2010a, 2010b)	11 congenitally blind [M=33, SD=14] 11 EB [M=42, SD=9] 11 LB [M=46, SD=7]	congenitally blind: 0.1 (SD=0.1), range 0–0.3 EB 7.9 (SD=4.8), range 1.4–13 LB 27.0 (SD=10.9), range 14.5–54	EB 34 (SD=8), range 17–47 LB 19 (SD=8), range 5–29

function and is modulated by the particular history of visual exposure with a particular kind of visual deprivation (see Daw 1995).

In fact, to have seen even for a short period means to have experienced shapes of objects in a visual format, and hence to have been familiar with notions such as perspective or visual occlusion, to have been exposed to two-dimensional pictures, to the faces of people, and the colors of various objects. Importantly, it means to have experienced the combination of a visual percept and a tactual experience, for instance, when holding a cup or a toy in one hand. Of course, these visual memories may fade after years of visual deprivation. Still, a visually based reference frame, which is useful for multisensory integration processes (Putzar, Goerendt et al. 2007; Röder, Kusmierek et al. 2007; Röder, Föcker et al. 2008), may remain available.

7.2 Behavioral Findings: Sensory Compensation and Blindness-Onset

Individuals blinded later in life may develop some super-normal auditory or tactile capacities, although the extent of such compensation is likely to be limited compared to that occurring in the congenitally blind (see chapter 2) and to be restricted to some specific contexts. Although cortical plasticity reorganization phenomena have often been observed in the late blind, they are not always reflected at the behavioral level.

Frequency Discrimination and Temporal Auditory Sensitivity

Gougoux and colleagues (Gougoux, Lepore et al. 2004) compared the performance of a group of early blind, late blind and sighted subjects at judging the direction of pitch-change between sounds. Early blind subjects outperformed both late blind and sighted subjects in this task, whereas no differences were reported between the late blind and the sighted participants. Notably, the level of performance inversely correlated with the age of blindness-onset (i.e., the earlier the onset of blindness, the better the performance), a correlation that remained significant even when controlling for blindness duration. In an earlier study, Bross and Borenstein (1982) compared the temporal auditory sensitivity in five adventitiously blind and five normally sighted subjects in a signal-detection paradigm, without finding any significant difference between the two groups. Wan and colleagues (Wan, Wood et al. 2010a) compared a group of congenitally blind, early blind, and late blind subjects with sighted controls matched for age, gender, musical experience and pitch-naming on tasks tapping into different aspects of auditory processing. Late blind subjects were found to perform similarly to the sighted controls in pitch-discrimination (i.e., deciding which of a pair of tones was higher) and pitch-timbre categorization (i.e., making judgments on both pitch and timbre), whereas the congenitally and early blind outperformed other participants in these tasks (Wan, Wood et al. 2010a).

Overall, these data suggest that the late blind do not compensate for their visual deficit by improving sensitivity in basic auditory functions. However, one may argue that these capacities are not so critical in coping with everyday situations; rather, what seems to be more critical is the capacity to localize external objects on the basis of auditory stimulation (safety in crossing the street, etc.). Accordingly, as we will see in the next paragraph, late blind individuals have been found to perform better than sighted subjects in localizing auditory stimuli.

Auditory Localization

Voss and colleagues have carried out a series of behavioral and PET studies to investigate the ability of late blind individuals to compensate for their acquired visual deprivation in auditory-localization tasks (Voss, Lassonde et al. 2004; Voss, Gougoux et al.

2006; Voss, Gougoux et al. 2008). It emerged that both early blind and late blind subjects are better than sighted controls in properly localizing auditory stimuli when these are presented in lateral positions in the rear hemifield, whereas no differences across groups seem to exist for auditory stimuli presented in the central hemifield (possibly due to overall ceiling effects) (Voss, Lassonde et al. 2004). Déspres et al. (Déspres, Candas, and Dufour 2005b) reported that late blind subjects performed better than the sighted in a self-localization task on the basis of auditory cues (although the advantage of the early blind was even greater). Moreover, the late blind, similarly to the early blind, are likely to possess a higher sensitivity to echo-cues compared to sighted individuals (Dufour, Déspres, and Candas 2005). Nonetheless, the auditory egocenter of late blind individuals is likely close to the midpoint of the interocular axis of visual egocenter as it is in sighted subjects, and not shifted to the midpoint of the interaural axis or the center of head-rotation as it is in the congenitally blind (Sukemiya, Nakamizo, and Ono 2008). In a temporal-order judgment task in which pairs of auditory and tactile stimuli were presented and subjects were required to indicate which sensory modality had been presented first in each trial, early and late blind subjects showed a similar pattern of performance: specifically, they were both affected by the relative spatial position of the auditory and tactile inputs (being more accurate when the two stimuli were not presented at the same spatial location), whereas the sighted subjects were not (Occelli, Spence, and Zampini 2008). The authors interpreted these results as depending on an improved ability of both late and early blind subjects to process spatial cues within the residual tactile and auditory modalities.

Overall, these findings suggest that even a late visual deprivation may induce some compensatory phenomena at the perceptual level, although these appear more limited compared to those associated to early blindness.

Tactile Discrimination

Using a grating-detection and a grating-orientation task (see chapter 2), Goldreich and Kanics (Goldreich and Kanics 2003, 2006) found superior performance of both late and early blind over the sighted, regardless of members of the former group having had normal childhood vision. Similarly, Alary et al. (Alary, Duquette et al. 2009) showed that both late and early blind subjects performed better than sighted controls in a texture-discrimination task, with no difference due to the time of blindness onset (early vs. late). These data, together with the findings that even a short visual deprivation can induce reversible passive-tactile acuity gains (e.g., Kauffman, Théoret, and Pascual-Leone 2002; Facchini and Aglioti 2003), seem to suggest that blindness at any age may result in enhanced tactile acuity, providing no evidence for a developmental critical period for the blindness-induced tactile acuity improvement. However, the enhancement in tactile discrimination of the late blind is not robust enough to be consistently detected across different tasks. For instance, Heller (1989a) failed to find any differences between sighted subjects and late (and congenitally) blind subjects in discriminating the texture of sandpaper. Similarly, Grant et al. (Grant, Thiagarajah, and Sathian 2000) reported that although the late blind performed better (in terms of mean accuracy) than the sighted in a dot-pattern discrimination task, this difference was not significant (whereas congenitally blind subjects clearly outperformed the sighted); moreover, no differences were observed between performances of late blind, early blind, and sighted subjects in a grating-discrimination task. Accordingly, Alary et al. (Alary, Goldstein et al. 2008) found that blind individuals performed significantly better than sighted individuals in a task requiring (proximal) exploration of haptic angles, but such advantage was mostly due to the congenitally blind subjects: in fact, discrimination threshold was found to covary with the age at onset of blindness. Furthermore, Wan and colleagues (Wan, Wood et al. 2010b) compared the performance of congenitally, early, and late blind individuals on a vibrotactile task and reported no differences between late blind and sighted control subjects. On the contrary, both the early blind and the congenitally blind participants performed better than the sighted in this task, with the congenitally blind even outperforming the early blind.

7.3 Late Blindness and Compensatory Phenomena at Higher Cognitive Levels

In many parts of this book we have argued that vision likely plays a dominant role over the other sensory modalities in driving mental imagery processes in sighted individuals. Late blind individuals relied on normal visual experience for a period of their life (usually, some years). This prior visual experience can be used by the late blind to support their haptic and auditory perception, helping them to generate a mental representation of the surrounding environment. However, late blind individuals do not receive any visual input to refresh their stored model of the visual world; hence, years of visual deprivation can affect the way in which detailed characteristics of objects, such as shapes and colors, are represented, as well as the way space is represented. In fact, there is evidence that mental imagery processes are modified during life following the dominant sensory experience, and are modulated by the inputs coming from different sensory modalities (Hollins 1985): how this happens in the late blind will be discussed below.

Visual Memories

Late blind individuals likely continue to experience visual images in their mental processes, although as the time since deficit-onset increases, haptic and auditory experiences gain in importance. For instance, in a study investigating autobiographical memories in sighted and blind individuals, late blind subjects reported predominantly visual features for childhood memories, and auditory, tactile and spatial features for more recent memories (Ogden and Barker 2001). Nonetheless, when interviewed about the dominant imagery modality they were relying on and about the mental "format" of their dreams, the majority of the late blind as well as sighted subjects nominated visual imagery (Ogden and Barker 2001).

Further support for the view that late blind subjects continue to experience visual images even after years of visual deprivation comes from data about synesthetic phenomena. Synesthesia refers to a heritable condition common to some individuals for which certain sensory stimuli elicit illusory perceptual experiences in the same or another modality (Baron-Cohen and Harrison 1996). For instance, the sight of a printed grapheme or a particular heard word may induce the perception of a particular color (e.g., Ramachandran and Hubbard 2001; Nunn, Gregory et al. 2002). At the cortical level, colored synesthetic sensations appear mediated by the activation of portion of the visual cortex (e.g., Paulesu, Harrison et al. 1995; Nunn, Gregory et al. 2002). Interestingly, synesthetic phenomena have been often reported in blind individuals (see Steven and Blakemore 2004). Already John Locke, in his *Essay Concerning Human Understanding* at the end of the seventeenth century, reported the case of a blind man who, when asked to define the type of "scarlet," replied that it was "like the sound of a trumpet" (see Baron-Cohen and Harrison 1996). Later on, other "colored" hearing experiences—such as colored pitch, colored vowel sounds, colored words and music—were reported in late blind individuals (Galton 1883; Starr 1893; Cutsforth and Wheeler 1966). More recently, Steven and Blakemore (2004) have analyzed the case of six late blind individuals who experienced synesthesia before their sight loss (note that the majority of them lost their sight quite early in life). For all these subjects the synesthetic experience took the form of colored blobs floating in space or patterns of colored dots corresponding to Braille characters. Interestingly, several of these subjects reported strong synesthesia for Braille characters but not for non-Braille tactile stimuli, suggesting that experience—and not only genetic predisposition—may play a role in the synesthetic experience of the late blind. It may be possible that some forms of synesthesia are induced by sight loss per se, as it seems to be the case of the blind man studied by Armel and Ramachandran (1999). After losing his sight, this individual started to experience synesthetic phenomena—i.e., tactile stimuli on his hand induced a sensation of "movement, expansion or jumping." These findings have been interpreted as resulting from somatosensory activity spreading in the visual cortex. Nonetheless, although occipital recruitment by non-visual sensory modalities has been consistently reported in the late blindness (Burton, Snyder et al. 2002a,b; Burton 2003; Burton, Diamond, and McDermott 2003; Burton, Sinclair, and McLaren 2004), synesthetic phenomena are experienced by only a minority of adventitiously blind individuals.

Haptic Picture Recognition

Recognizing pictures in the haptic modality implies a capacity to "visualize" how a 3D object would appear in a 2D plane. We broadly discussed how the blind perform in picture-recognition tasks in chapter 4. Here, we focus on the performance of late blind individuals. A series of experiments carried out by Heller suggest that the late blind perform better than both sighted subjects and congenitally blind individuals in tasks involving picture-perception (and associated rules such as perspective-taking and so forth), thanks to the combined advantage of increased haptic skill and the impact of prior experience with pictures. For instance, late blind participants outperformed both congenitally blind and blindfolded sighted controls in a tactile picture-identification task (Heller 1989b) and in a figure-embedded task (Heller, Wilson et al. 2003). Similarly, late blind subjects performed similar to sighted subjects in a picture perspective-taking task, whereas the early blind—although able to perform the task—were significantly slower (Heller and Kennedy 1990). Finally, late blind participants were found to perform overall better than both early blind and blindfolded sighted subjects when required to understand tangible perspective pictures of complex solid objects (Heller, Riddle et al. 2009).

Imagery and Working Memory

Even after many years of visual deprivation, imagery processes likely remain "visually" shaped. An example of this can be found in a study by Vanlierde and Wanet-Defalque (2005), in which late blind, early blind and sighted individuals were required to mentally move toward an object they had to imagine and to stop when the image was "overflowing" their reference frame. Late blind individuals successfully performed the task, which proved impossible for the early blind to complete. Moreover, late blind as well as sighted subjects were found to decrease the angular size of an imaged object with increasing distance, as in typical visual perception (while this was not the case for the early blind). These results suggest that the late blind use visual imagery processes that are similar to those of sighted subjects. Still, some differences can be observed. For instance, the late blind tended to imagine objects at a shorter distance compared to sighted subjects, possibly reflecting an interference by their extensive haptic experience of objects, that they need to integrate with their past visual experience: in fact, haptic experience is limited to peripersonal space, possibly inducing the late blind to image the objects from a closer point of view (Vanlierde and Wanet-Defalque 2005).

Visual imagery seems to be predominant in the late blind also in more active working memory tasks. For instance, when required to memorize a series of cells on a grid on the basis of verbal instructions, the late blind reported having generated a visual mental image of the grid (as did sighted controls), whereas early blind participants relied on a verbal abstract strategy (Vanlierde and Wanet-Defalque 2004).

Accordingly, in a typical mental-rotation task, late blind individuals performed similarly to sighted subjects, whereas the congenitally blind were significantly slower and less accurate, suggesting that the late blind were more efficient in generating visual analogical representations (Marmor and Zaback 1976). Using a mental scanning task (see also chapter 4), Afonso and colleagues (Afonso, Blum et al. 2010) found that late blind individuals were able to construct mental representations that preserved the metric properties of verbally described or manually handled spatial configurations, whereas this task was particularly difficult for the congenitally blind participants. Moreover, metric information was accurately represented in late blind individuals' images when learning relied on locomotor experience (a condition that resulted to be difficult for the sighted participants but in which the congenitally blind performed particularly well), although the late blind took longer to review a representation based on locomotor experience than one based on verbal inputs.

Spatial Reference Frames

Early blind individuals tend to rely on a body-centered reference frame in representing the external environment (see chapter 5). Is this the case of late blind individuals as well? Available evidence suggests that the late blind rely on an allocentric external reference frame in encoding the position of objects and in navigation, although the egocentric component likely plays a larger role in their spatial representations compared to the sighted. For instance, late blind and sighted subjects, but not congenitally blind subjects, were impaired in a tactile-discrimination task requiring subjects to judge the temporal order of two tactile stimuli, one presented at each hand, when their hands were crossed over the midline, as compared to an uncrossed condition, suggesting that in sighted and late blind individuals tactile stimuli are remapped into externally defined spatial coordinates (Röder, Rösler, and Spence 2004). When this external reference frame does not match with body-centered codes—relying primarily on somatosensory and proprioceptive inputs (as in the case of uncrossed hands)—performance is affected. Since the congenitally blind lack of any prior visual experience, this conflict seems to be inexistent for them. Notably, findings in late blind individuals suggest that a shift from an egocentric to an allocentric reference frame occurs before the age of 12 years (Röder, Rösler, and Spence 2004; Röder, Krämer, and Lange 2007).

In pointing and parallel-setting tasks, introducing a delay between the stimulus presentation and test usually induces a shift from an egocentric to an allocentric representation in sighted subjects, but not in the early blind (see chapter 5; Gaunet and Rossetti 2006; see also, Rossetti, Gaunet, and Thinus-Blanc 1996; Postma, Zuidhoek et al. 2008). Interestingly, late blind individuals' responses appear to be halfway between those of the blindfolded controls and those of the early blind. For instance, in a parallel-setting task requiring subjects to rotate a test bar in order to put it parallel to a previously touched reference-bar orientation, the late blind and blindfolded sighted became more accurate in a delayed condition, but such improvement was higher for the blindfolded sighted than for the late blind, indicating that the ability to generate allocentric representations benefits from being *continuously* exposed to normal visual stimulation (Postma, Zuidhoek et al. 2008). Accordingly, in a task requiring subjects to lateralize auditory, tactile or bimodal audiotactile stimuli, late blind participants showed an intermediate pattern of performance between the scores obtained by early blind and those obtained by sighted participants (Collignon, Charbonneau et al. 2009). In particular, whereas the early blind were overall faster than the sighted controls, no statistical difference was reported between early blind and late blind participants or between late blind and sighted controls. The results by Collignon et al. (Collignon, Charbonneau et al. 2009) suggest that vision may not only be necessary for the generation but also for the maintenance of an automatic remapping of spatial representations based upon touch/proprioception in external spatial coordinates (for a discussion on the effect of blindness on the use of a common spatial reference frame for multisensory interaction, see chapter 2).

Finally, in tasks measuring the capacity to mentally rotate spatial configurations of objects, late blind perform better than congenitally blind participants (Pasqualotto and Newell 2007), and demonstrate an ability—as well as sighted subjects—to compensate for the viewpoint-change due to the observer's active locomotion.

Navigation

It has been hypothesized that an early coordination between visual inputs and kinesthetic, vestibular and auditory concurrent information allows a more precise navigation even in darkness (Rieser, Hill et al. 1992). Early blind individuals tend to rely on route-like representations in navigation, although they are able to generate survey-like spatial representations if needed (see chapter 5; Noordzij, Zuidhoek, and Postma 2006; Tinti, Adenzato et al. 2006). In survey-like representations distant places are combined together into an integrated global overview of the entire environment (cf. Chown, Kaplan, and Kortenkamp 1995; Golledge 1999; Kitchin and Freundschuh 2000), whereas route-like maps represent object locations in a viewer-centered, egocentric frame of reference. How do the late blind behave in these situations? Some studies have reported that late blind individuals behave similarly to the early blind in navigation, by representing space in a route-like fashion (Noordzij, Zuidhoek, and Postma 2006). As noted by Noordzij et al. (Noordzij, Zuidhoek, and Postma 2006), this behavior likely depends on the orientation and mobility training that both early blind and late blind receive: in fact, blind individuals are usually trained on navigational skills by receiving information about intermittent landmarks in relation to their own body position, and not about external absolute spatial relations that they cannot directly experience. However, other studies reported different results. For instance, Rieser and colleagues (Rieser, Guth, and Hill 1986) found that both late blind subjects and blindfolded sighted subjects performed better than early blind subjects in a task requiring participants to generate a survey-like representation of a series of objects and point to the other objects while standing or imagining themselves to be standing at one specific location. Moreover, the late blind were as efficient as the sighted subjects in mentally updating the target-locations during locomotion, whereas the congenitally blind were not. Accordingly, congenitally blind subjects showed a poorer knowledge of the location of a series of landmarks within their communities than the late blind and sighted controls (Rieser, Hill et al. 1992), and were less accurate than both late blind and sighted subjects in estimating Euclidean distances between locations within a familiar building (Rieser, Lockman, and Pick 1980) or in creating tactual maps of their school campus (Casey 1978). Conversely, Loomis et al. (Loomis, Klatzky et al. 1993) failed to find significant differences among early blind, late blind and blindfolded sighted subjects in a series of spatial tasks of different complexity, requiring them either to reproduce and estimate a walked distance or a turn (simple conditions), or to retrace a multi-segment route in reverse (returning directly to an origin after being led over linear segments) or to point to targets after locomotion (complex conditions, similar to the task used in Rieser, Guth, and Hill 1986). Surprisingly, Passini, Proulx, and Rainville (1990) even found an advantage of the early blind compared to the late blind and the sighted controls in a series of way-finding tasks in a labyrinthine layout. But why do some studies report differences between early and late blind and sighted subjects and others do not? As suggested by Loomis et al. (Loomis, Klatzky et al. 1993), individual variables likely play a major role: in particular, the mobility skills of the late and early blind subjects, depending on the type of training they have received, are likely to significantly affect the way blind individuals represent space (see chapter 5 of this volume).

Verbal Memory

As it has been proposed for tactile abilities (see Thinus-Blanc and Gaunet 1997; Heller, Wilson et al. 2003), one may expect that the prior visual experience combined with the acquired higher reliance on auditory information determines a double advantage for the late blind adults in cognitive tasks based on verbal information. In this regard, in a task involving auditory and semantic processes, Röder and Rösler (2003) found that the late blind performed as well as congenitally blind subjects matched for age, and better than sighted subjects when required to memorize a series of environmental sounds that had to be encoded either physically or semantically. Interestingly, further analyses showed that duration of blindness and age at blindness-onset in the late blind group were not a significant factor in determining memory performance in the late blind, whereas the absolute age at test was (see also Bull, Rathborn, and Clifford 1983, for similar results). Although at first these data seem to suggest that prior visual experience did not benefit the late blind compared to the early blind, a different interpretation is possible, which is that auditory compensation in the late blind is only partial and it is their early visual experience that allows them to perform similarly to congenitally blind (Röder and Rösler 2003).

7.4 Cortical Plasticity and Blindness Onset

In chapter 8 we will extensively deal with cortical plasticity phenomena associated to blindness, specifically distinguishing between intramodal cortical plasticity (i.e., changes in cortical networks subtending auditory and somatosensory information processing due to extensive reliance on touch and hearing in the blind) and crossmodal cortical plasticity (i.e., the recruitment of visual cortex to process tactile and auditory information in the blind). Here we anticipate part of that discussion by considering studies that have specifically investigated whether cortical reorganization is also induced by a late-acquired visual deficit.

Converging evidence based on neuroimaging (PET, fMRI) and transcranial magnetic stimulation (TMS) techniques, indicates that the brain's susceptibility to crossmodal plasticity drastically reduces after puberty. In particular, Cohen et al. (Cohen, Weeks et al. 1999) showed that repetitive TMS over primary visual cortex (V1) interfered with Braille reading in early but not in late blind subjects, suggesting that the window of opportunity for crossmodal plasticity in blind humans is limited to childhood before age 14. Using neuroimaging, Sadato et al. (Sadato, Okada et al. 2002) identified a similar cut-off, reporting that tactile discrimination activated the visual association cortex of individuals blinded before age 16 and those blinded after age 16, whereas V1 was activated only in the former group. Hence, age 14–16 seems to be a likely time-limit for the occurrence of relevant crossmodal reorganization phenomena in the brain.

Nonetheless, the fact that crossmodal plasticity may occur in sighted adults even after a short-term visual deprivation (e.g., Pascual-Leone and Hamilton 2001; Weisser, Stilla et al. 2005; Merabet, Hamilton et al. 2008)—also leading to enhanced tactile acuity (Kauffman, Théoret, and Pascual-Leone 2002; Facchini and Aglioti 2003)—suggests that crossmodal plastic changes likely occur also in case of late blindness, although they are less robust than those observed in the early blind. For instance, in a study by Burton et al. (Burton, Snyder et al. 2002a), Braille reading induced bilateral responses in visual cortex of many early blind subjects, whereas most late blind subjects showed responses only ipsilateral to the reading hand and mostly in the inferior occipital cortex. In another study, Burton et al. (Burton, Sinclair, and McLaren 2004) reported activation of striate and extrastriate parts of the visual cortex in both early and late blind participants during vibrotactile stimulation, although the involvement of visual cortex was greater in the early blind than in the late blind group. According to Burton et al. (Burton, Snyder et al. 2002a,b; Burton 2003; Burton, Diamond, and McDermott 2003; Burton, McLaren, and Sinclair 2006), response magnitudes in V1 associated to phonological and semantic processing remained approximately constant irrespective of age at blindness-onset, whereas response magnitudes in higher visual cortices declined with age at blindness-onset (Burton, Diamond, and McDermott 2003).

In fact, the visual cortex of the late blind likely maintains—at least to a certain extent—its original functionality, as demonstrated by the fact that TMS over occipital cortex can still induce visual phosphenes in the late blind (Cowey and Walsh 2000; Kupers, Fumal et al. 2006). Accordingly, Rao et al. (Rao, Nobre et al. 2007) reported the case of a sighted individual blinded late in life who started perceiving visual phosphenes in response to auditory stimuli (see also Kupers, Fumal et al. 2006).

Notably, cortical-reorganization phenomena in the late blind may occur without necessarily being reflected at the behavioral level. For instance, in a PET study investigating free-field auditory localization accuracy, Voss et al. (Voss, Gougoux et al. 2006) found enhanced occipital activation in the late blind subjects compared to sighted controls, although no behavioral advantage was associated with such activation. In a following PET study, Voss et al. (Voss, Gougoux et al. 2008) investigated the effect of early and late blindness in a sound-discrimination task, presented under both a monaural and a binaural condition. Again, no behavioral differences were reported between late blind and sighted subjects; although the late blind were shown to recruit ventral visual areas of the occipito-temporal cortices during the monaural task, whereas the sighted did not show any activation in visual areas and the early blind presented a widespread activation in striate and extrastriate cortices of the left hemisphere.

Intramodal plasticity phenomena are also likely to be weaker in late compared to early blind. In this regard, Gougoux et al. (Gougoux, Belin et al. 2009) found that vocal auditory stimuli induced a similar pattern of activation in the occipital cortex of both late and early blind subjects (i.e., crossmodal plasticity), but a stronger activation in the left superior temporal sulcus was observed in the congenitally blind group compared to the sighted and the late blind group. Accordingly, Stevens and Weaver (2009) did not find statistical differences of volume and intensity of BOLD activity in the temporal cortex between late blind and sighted subjects in a passive listening task, whereas the early blind reported reduced hemodynamic responses to auditory stimulation, likely depending on increased efficiency within the temporal cortex during listening.

A possible confusion in examining the pattern of cortical activation during tactile and auditory tasks in the late blind involves the role of visual imagery processes. In fact, while occipital activation in the early blind seems to reflect "pure" crossmodal plasticity, striate and extrastriate activation in late blind individuals might also result from visual imagery mediation (rather than from crossmodal reorganization). For instance, Buchel et al. (Buchel, Price et al. 1998) reported V1 activation in late but not congenitally blind subjects during Braille reading: when interviewed after the experiment, the late blind reported having tried to convert the Braille-dot pattern into a visual image (see Buchel, Price et al. 1998). In an fMRI study carried out by Goyal et al. (Goyal, Hansen, and Blakemore 2006) on congenitally blind, late blind and sighted subjects, a condition requiring them to tactilely perceive motion stimuli and faces was contrasted to a condition requiring that they imagine the same stimuli. Critically, subjects were specifically instructed *not* to visually imagine the objects in the "perceptual" condition. Interestingly, both the perceptual and imagery conditions induced stimulus-specific activation in the visual cortex of late blind participants, that is, hMT/V5 for motion perception and motion imagery, and FFA for face perception and face imagery. No similar localized activation foci were reported in either the early blind or the sighted participants in the perceptual condition. Critically, late blind participants reported not having tried to visualize the objects in the perceptual condition, according to the instructions received. According to Goyal et al. (Goyal, Hansen, and Blakemore 2006), when blindness occurs after a period of normal vision, extrastriate areas remain capable of processing specific visual features via imagery, but the same neural populations also become engaged during similar forms of tactile stimulation. Hence, occipital activation in the late blind might not only be induced by (either voluntary or automatic) visual imagery processes, but could also result from an enhanced direct connectivity between areas originally involved in visual and tactile processing.

8 Cortical Plasticity and Blindness

Without blindness, would he have been able to understand that invisible essence, and thus that transcendence, of the face, and hence its alterity? It's this direction he ought to pursue: appearances that are not visible . . . an elliptical light without radiance . . . the essence of a face is not a shape but the words it speaks . . . it's a thousand times less important to see a face than to listen to it.

—Bernard Henry Lévy, *Sartre: The Philosopher of the Twentieth Century*

8.1 Cortical Reorganization Phenomena

In previous chapters we have discussed sensory compensation phenomena and differences in the cognitive processes and strategies used by blind compared to sighted individuals in domains such as memory, imagery, and spatial cognition. In many circumstances, we have mentioned that such differences are associated with cortical plasticity phenomena; this plasticity itself, however, we have not discussed in-depth since those chapters specifically focused on functional aspects of such phenomena. Here we address this issue, by considering human studies that have investigated cortical plasticity phenomena in the blind population using positron emission tomography (PET), functional magnetic resonance imaging (fMRI), evoked potentials (ERPs), and transcranial magnetic stimulation (TMS).

The human brain (as well as that of other animal species) is not a predetermined agglomeration of cells, with each pursuing a specific and unchangeable function. Rather, the brain has an extraordinary capacity to reorganize itself in response to external variables, such as the quality of available sensory experience, the extent to which a specific activity (music, sport, etc.) is practiced, traumatic phenomena or, simply, development and aging. Plasticity phenomena may occur at different organizational levels of the central nervous system, from the genetic to the molecular, neural and cortical levels (see Shaw and McEachern 2001). The studies we review here essentially concern *cortical* plasticity, and specifically, *functional intramodal* and *crossmodal* reorganization phenomena (for reviews, see Grafman 2000; Röder and Neville 2003;

Sathian and Stilla 2010). Intramodal plasticity refers to changes occurring in the same cortical regions normally devoted to processing information in a specific sensory modality: in blindness, due to the combined effects of visual deprivation and enhanced auditory/tactile practice, these areas might get reorganized. The expanded representation of the reading finger in the somatosensory cortex of blind Braille readers is an example of intramodal plasticity (e.g., Pascual-Leone and Torres 1993). Conversely, crossmodal plasticity occurs when areas usually devoted to processing visual information are recruited to process tactile or auditory inputs: the often-reported activation of the occipital cortex during Braille reading in blind individuals (e.g., Sadato, Pascual-Leone et al. 1996) is a clear example of crossmodal plasticity.

Importantly, functional plasticity may be induced both by the sensorial deprivation per se and by higher practice in the spared modalities. Separating the contribution of the two factors is far from obvious. In fact, a person blinded early (or late) in life, has to massively rely on tactile and auditory information to deal with his or her everyday activities; therefore, the effects of visual deprivation and of higher tactile/auditory practice interact since the very onset of blindness. However, as we will see in the following paragraphs, studies on sighted individuals highly trained in a specific field (e.g., professional musicians: Pantev, Oostenveld et al. 1998) have allowed us to clarify the effects that intense perceptual training per se might exert on brain plasticity.

Critically, cortical reorganization can either result from an unmasking of previously silent connections and/or from a sprouting of new neural elements from those that previously existed. Recent research investigating the pattern of *connectivity* between different brain regions is shedding light on the neural pathways that mediate the functional changes in the occipital cortex of blind individuals (see Stilla, Hanna et al. 2008; Fujii, Tanabe et al. 2009), allowing us to look at the specific contributions of both thalamo-cortical and cortico-cortical connections (cf. Bavelier and Neville 2002). As we will briefly see, these mechanisms also result in morphological alterations in blind individuals, such as changes in the volume of gray and white matter, cortical surface and cortical thickness. Finally, we will report evidence suggesting that neural networks subtending social cognition normally develop despite a congenital visual deprivation.

8.2 Intramodal Cortical Plasticity in Auditory and Somatosensory Cortices

It has been demonstrated that functional brain regions may enlarge—a phenomenon also known as "map expansion"—as a result of functional requirements (see Grafman 2000). An intramodal expansion of tonotopic representations in the auditory cortex of blind individuals has been consistently reported, and this might subserve the increased auditory capacities often associated with blindness. Blind individuals are not exposed to more auditory stimulation than sighted individuals; nevertheless, in order to effectively interact with their environment, they have to rely more heavily on auditory inputs. From this perspective, behavioral relevance works as a source of use-dependent reorganization: a larger neural network is potentially more reliable than a smaller one, allowing individuals to process temporal auditory inputs at a greater speed (see Elbert, Sterr et al. 2002). For instance, Elbert et al. (Elbert, Sterr et al. 2002), using magnetic source-localization, have demonstrated that dipoles associated with low- and high-frequency tones were separated by a greater distance in both early and late blind participants than similarly recorded dipoles in sighted subjects, indicating that the increased dependence on the auditory modality in blind individuals results in an expansion of regions in the auditory cortex. An expanded tonotopic representation in blind individuals' auditory cortex is also supported by ERPs evidence, showing differences between blind and sighted individuals in the latency and refractoriness of specific ERPs components. For instance, the behavioral result of faster response times in discriminating both auditory and somatosensory stimuli in blind participants compared to sighted controls was associated to shorter latencies and shorter refractory periods for the N1-evoked-potential component in the former (Röder, Rösler et al. 1996; Röder, Rösler, and Neville 1999; Röder, Krämer, and Lange 2007), although its topographical distribution was similar in the two groups. Faster recovery of sensory ERPs has been considered an index of higher excitability of the auditory cortex and increased auditory processing rates in the blind (Stevens and Weaver 2005), and it might indeed depend on a "hypertrophy" within auditory areas (see Röder and Rösler 2004). In a recent fMRI study, Stevens and Weaver (2009) have compared cortical activation in early blind, late blind and sighted individuals during passive listening to pure tones and frequency-modulated stimuli and demonstrated that tonotopic organization (in particular, the auditory frequency mapping) in auditory areas in the superior and middle temporal lobes is not significantly altered in blind individuals. Nonetheless, in early (but not late) blind individuals the BOLD signal was weaker than in sighted participants under low-demanding listening conditions, suggesting that the early blind were able to more efficiently process the stimuli within the first stages of auditory cortical analysis. Hence, it is likely that functional responses in auditory cortical areas are altered by early visual deprivation, an intramodal form of plasticity that might account for the superior auditory performances often reported in early blind subjects (see Collignon, Voss et al. 2009).

Somatosensory cortical plasticity refers to the capacity of the sensory and motor "homunculus" to change in response to tactile experience. For instance, the repeated use of a fingertip for Braille reading induces an enlargement in the fingertip-representation within the homunculus (e.g., Pascual-Leone and Torres 1993; Sterr, Müller et al. 1999; Burton, Sinclair, and McLaren 2004). Accordingly, a TMS experiment has shown that motor-evoked potentials in the first dorsal interosseus muscle of expert Braille readers can be induced by stimulating a larger area of the motor cortex than that of the non-reading hand of the same subjects and compared to both hands of control subjects (Pascual-Leone, Cammarota et al. 1993). In this regard, Sterr et al. (Sterr, Müller et al. 1998a) demonstrated that blind subjects who use multiple fingers in Braille reading can present a disordered cortical somatotopy which is behaviorally reflected by their inaccuracy in identifying which of their (reading) fingers has been touched during a sensory-threshold task. This because the representation of the reading fingers appears "fused" together at the cortical level due to the recurrent, simultaneous stimulation of these fingers during reading: this change in the somatotopy of reading fingers may allow Braille patterns to be processed more holistically and at a greater speed, and yet prove "maladaptive" for other tasks (Sterr, Müller et al. 1998a; Sterr, Green, and Elbert 2003).

Intramodal plasticity phenomena in blindness are likely to depend both on practices with tactile modality and on visual deprivation per se. In fact, intramodal plasticity phenomena may be induced by intense perceptual training (as in the case of professional musicians) in the absence of any sensorial deprivation, both in adult individuals and children (see Pantev, Oostenveld et al. 1998; Trainor, Shahin, and Roberts 2003; Lappe, Herholz et al. 2008; Hyde, Lerch et al. 2009). In this regard, dystonia (e.g., a movement-disorder that causes involuntary contractions of muscles, see Pujol, Roset-Llobet et al. 2000) is a clear example of maladaptive plasticity comparable to that described for blind, multi-finger Braille readers by Sterr et al. (Sterr, Müller et al. 1998a). Critically, practice-induced plasticity within sensory systems does not always co-occur with increased cortical representation, but might also be subtended by a change in the firing pattern of the involved neural populations (see Röder, Rösler, and Neville 2001).

According to some authors (see Goldreich and Kanics 2003, 2006), use-dependent intramodal cortical plasticity—although important—is an unlikely explanation for superior acuity in the spared senses which is often shown by blind individuals, as for instance demonstrated by the lack of any significant correlation between practice with Braille reading (e.g., hours of daily reading, age at learning, years since learning) and tactile acuity among blind readers (e.g., Van Boven, Hamilton et al. 2000; Goldreich and Kanics 2003, 2006; Legge, Madison et al. 2008; also see chapter 2 of this volume). Hence, it has been proposed that crossmodal plasticity phenomena play a major role in leading to superior tactile and auditory abilities in blind individuals.

8.3 Crossmodal Plasticity: Occipital Cortex Recruitment by Tactile and Auditory Processing

An extraordinary finding of the last decades has been that the same occipital areas that in sighted subjects subserve visual processing are recruited in blind individuals during tactile and auditory encoding. Pioneering research on this topic has been carried out by Wanet-Defalque and colleagues (e.g., Wanet-Defalque, Veraart et al. 1988), who measured glucose metabolism in blind individuals, finding that glucose utilization in striate and prestriate cortical regions was higher in early blind subjects compared to sighted subjects both at rest (see also Arno, De Volder et al. 2001) and during object manipulation and auditory tasks (see also Veraart, De Volder et al. 1990). Following these early observations, several studies employing different tactile and auditory discrimination tasks have consistently reported visual areas activation in blind humans. Critically, visual areas recruitment for non-visual processing in blind individuals is not just epiphenomenal: in fact, the degree of visual recruitment has often been found to correlate with behavioral performance, both for tactile and auditory tasks (see Gougoux, Zatorre et al. 2005; Stilla, Hanna et al. 2008); accordingly, TMS experiments have revealed the causal role of visual areas for tactile and auditory processing in the blind (e.g., Cohen, Celnik et al. 1997; Collignon, Lassonde et al. 2007).

Tactile Discrimination and Braille Reading

Sadato and colleagues, in a series of PET (e.g., Sadato, Pascual-Leone et al. 1996, 1998) and fMRI (e.g., Sadato and Hallett 1999; Sadato, Okada et al. 2002) studies, demonstrated that Braille reading as well as other active tactile discrimination tasks (discrimination of angle, width, and Roman embossed characters) activated the occipital, striate cortex (areas V1 and V2) in early and congenitally blind participants. Using EEG, Uhl et al. (Uhl, Franzen et al. 1991, 1993) demonstrated that tactile imagery or Braille reading in blind subjects induced task-related activation in the occipital cortex, suggesting that the somatosensory input was redirected toward occipital areas; these results were later confirmed using SPECT and regional cerebral flow measurement (Uhl, Podreka, and Deecke 1994). Burton and colleagues using fMRI demonstrated occipital activation in early and late blind subjects both during embossed uppercase-letters reading (Burton, McLaren, and Sinclair 2006) and Braille reading (Burton, Snyder et al. 2002a).

The *causal* role of visual areas activation during tactile processing in blind subjects has been demonstrated by single-case studies and TMS experiments. In particular, Hamilton et al. (Hamilton, Keenan et al. 2000) have reported that an infarction of the bilateral occipital cortex induced alexia in an early blind Braille-reader woman. This woman was congenitally blind and learned Braille when she was six years old; at the age of sixty-three, she suffered bilateral occipital ischemic strokes. Critically, after these episodes, she was still able to detect tactile stimuli without any relevant loss in her tactile sensitivity; however, she was unable to *recognize* Braille characters. This finding has been taken as evidence for the causal role of the occipital cortex in Braille reading.

Support for this view comes from studies using TMS. If PET, fMRI, and ERPs can provide detailed correlational observations, TMS allows us to investigate the need of a specific cortical region for a particular task, by inducing a sort of reversible "virtual lesion" (Walsh and Cowey 2000; see also Walsh and Pascual-Leone 2003). Although the "virtual lesion" approach is only one of the possible uses of TMS (see, for instance, TMS state-dependency paradigms: Silvanto, Muggleton, and Walsh 2008; Silvanto and Pascual-Leone 2008), it has been the most employed in studying cortical plasticity phenomena in blindness. Cohen et al. (Cohen, Celnik et al. 1997) used trains of repetitive TMS (10 Hz) to investigate the specific contribution of visual cortices in tactile discrimination tasks (e.g., Braille and embossed Roman-letters reading) in both sighted and blind subjects. When TMS was applied over occipital cortex, blind Braille readers' accuracy was significantly affected, inducing distorted somatosensory perceptions such as "missing dots," "phantom dots," and confusing sensations. Conversely, the same stimulation did not impair sighted individuals' performance when tactilely discriminating embossed Roman letters: sighted subjects' performance was instead affected when TMS was delivered over the somatosensory cortex (Cohen, Celnik et al. 1997). In a following TMS investigation, it was demonstrated that the occipital cortex is specifically involved in the "perception" of tactile stimuli (i.e., ability to recognize the tactile stimuli such as Braille dot-patterns) rather than in the "detection" of the same stimuli (i.e., simply experience a tactile sensation), and that the contribution of visual cortex to tactile processing occurs at a later stage than that of the somatosensory cortex (Hamilton and Pascual-Leone 1998; see also Théoret, Merabet, and Pascual-Leone 2004).

Occipital activation in blind subjects during Braille reading might potentially depend on both sensory and higher-order (language-related) cognitive factors (see Stilla, Hanna et al. 2008). For instance, in a PET study by Buchel et al. (Buchel, Price et al. 1998), no V1 activation was reported in the early blind when subtracting activation in an auditory-word task from that in a Braille-reading task, suggesting that early visual cortex recruitment during Braille reading might actually reflect linguistic processing (see also Röder, Stock et al. 2002; Burton, Diamond, and McDermott 2003; Amedi, Floel et al. 2004; Burton, McLaren, and Sinclair 2006). On this regard, it is worth mentioning that Gizewski et al. (Gizewski, Timmann, and Forsting 2004) reported also activation of cerebellum-specific regions in blind subjects due to the symbolic/language aspects inherent to Braille reading.

Nevertheless, primary visual cortices might also be activated by tactile-discrimination tasks without any phonological or semantic encoding (e.g., Sadato, Okada et al. 2002; Gizewski, Gasser et al. 2003). Accordingly, using fMRI, Stilla and colleagues (Stilla, Hanna et al. 2008) found that visual cortical areas (including the right lateral occipital complex, bilateral foci in the fusiform gyrus and right V3A) were activated during a (micro-)spatial tactile-discrimination task with no linguistic components compared to a temporal tactile-discrimination task in blind but not in sighted subjects (see also Stilla, Deshpande et al. 2007). Moreover, such activation was functionally relevant, since activation magnitudes in many of these foci correlated to tactile acuity. Similarly, Burton et al. (Burton, Sinclair, and McLaren 2004) reported activation of striate and extrastriate parts of visual cortex in blind participants during a passive tactile task, requiring subjects to judge whether paired vibrations (25 and 100 Hz) delivered to the right index finger differed in frequency.

TMS studies also support the involvement of occipital cortex in tactile processing per se in the blind. Ptito et al. (Ptito, Fumal et al. 2008), for example, have shown that effectors (such as the Braille-reading fingers) heavily used in tactile discrimination by blind subjects are somatotopically represented in their visual cortex: in fact, TMS applied over the occipital cortex induced tactile sensations in blind readers' fingers in the absence of any real tactile inputs. In contrast, the same stimulation only induced phosphene perception in control sighted subjects.

The results by Stilla et al. (Stilla, Hanna et al. 2008) and by Burton et al. (Burton, Sinclair, and McLaren 2004) are also critical in showing that visual cortex activation in blind individuals does not only occur during *active* tactile experience (such as in Braille reading) but also during *passive* tactile stimulation. Results have been controversial on this point: for instance, Sadato et al. (Sadato, Pascual-Leone et al. 1996) found that passive tactile stimulation did not induce activation in the primary visual cortices of blind subjects (Sadato, Pascual-Leone et al. 1996). In following studies either active touch was involved, so that the effects of hand movement and tactile stimulation were difficult to disentangle (Sadato, Okada et al. 2002; Gizewski, Gasser et al. 2003), or passive stimulation characterized by uncontrolled manual application of the stimuli was used, making it difficult to draw general conclusions (Uhl, Franzen et al. 1991, 1993). Overall, it is likely that some sort of tactile discrimination is required to induce activation in the occipital cortex of the blind: in fact, merely stimulating a cutaneous nerve electrically does not activate visual cortex in blind individuals (Gizewski, Gasser et al. 2003). Accordingly, amplitudes of ERPs recorded in the occipital pole of blind subjects are affected by the amount of manipulation required by the task (Rösler, Röder et al. 1993). As suggested by Röder and Rösler (2004), occipital activation in the blind is likely to be monotonically related to the required processing effort and always goes together with an equivalent amplitude covariation at other scalp sites (Röder, Rösler et al. 1996).

Some important findings with sighted individuals should not be ignored, as they shed light on the nature of plastic mechanisms (e.g., the extent to which they are use-dependent or induced by visual deprivation per se) occurring in the case of blindness. In particular, there is evidence that crossmodal reorganization phenomena may be induced even by a short-term reversible visual deprivation or by training per se in sighted subjects as well. Boroojerdi et al. (Boroojerdi, Bushara et al. 2000) found that visual cortex excitability increased after 60 minutes without vision, and Merabet et al. (Merabet, Hamilton et al. 2008) found that occipital cortex responded to tactile stimulation after subjects had been blindfolded for five days, a result that was accompanied by increased tactile acuity in these subjects. Interestingly, sighted people show increased tactile acuity even after 90 minutes of visual deprivation (Facchini and Aglioti 2003). There is evidence that training per se might also induce some form of crossmodal plasticity. For instance, Pantev and colleagues (Pantev, Ross et al. 2003) reported that when the lips of trumpet players were stimulated while being presented at the same time with a trumpet tone, activation in the somatosensory cortex increased more than during the sum of the separate lip and trumpet-tone stimulations, indicating that somatosensory cortices of these players had learned to respond to auditory stimuli.

Auditory Tasks

The occipital cortex in blind individuals is also robustly recruited by auditory processing, especially in situations requiring that they localize sound sources (see Collignon, Voss et al. 2009, for a review). In fact, different ERP studies have recorded changes in the topography of auditory-related potentials in blind subjects, indicating a shift toward more posterior (occipital) regions (see Kujala, Alho et al. 1992; Kujala, Alho et al. 1995; Liotti, Ryder, and Woldorff 1998; Röder, Teder-Salejarvi et al. 1999). For instance, Leclerc et al. (Leclerc, Saint-Amour et al. 2000) measured auditory ERPs during a free-field sound-localization paradigm and found that in blind subjects the N1 and P3 components not only peaked at their usual position but were also present over occipital regions, suggesting that blind subjects' occipital cortex might be involved in very early stages of auditory processing (at around 100 ms after sound presentation). In an another ERP study, Van der Lubbe, Van Mierlo, and Postma (2009) confirmed an enlarged posterior negativity for the blind compared to controls in a task requiring them to judge tactile and auditory stimuli duration. Neuroimaging techniques support these findings. In fact, using PET, Weeks and colleagues (Weeks, Horwitz et al. 2000) found that binaural auditory localization activated in blind subjects occipital-association areas (in particular, the right dorsal extrastriate cortex) originally intended for the dorsal stream visual processing. Similarly, in another PET study, Arno et al. (Arno, De Volder et al. 2001) reported activation in extrastriate visual cortices of blind participants in a pattern-recognition task in which a sensory substitution device translating visual information into sounds was used.

Visual recruitment in the blind may be particularly important for the processing of specific features of the auditory input, such as spectral cues, that are critical under monaural sound-localization conditions. Accordingly, Gougoux et al. (Gougoux, Zatorre et al. 2005) found only a small area of activation in the ventral visual area in binaural sound localization in early blind subjects, which conversely showed a robust occipital activation under monaural sound localization. Notably, though, activation in the occipital cortex during monaural stimulation was only reported in those blind subjects who also showed superior monaural sound-localization performance, suggesting that the occipital recruitment was indeed functionally relevant (Gougoux, Zatorre et al. 2005). Similar results have also been obtained by Voss et al. (Voss, Gougoux et al. 2008), who investigated the effects of early and late blindness in a sound-discrimination task, presented under both a monaural and a binaural condition. No behavioral differences were reported between groups in the binaural condition (although such condition induced activation in striate and extrastriate cortex of the early blind subjects). Conversely, in the monaural task, a subgroup of early blind subjects did show significantly enhanced accuracy: such a behavioral effect was associated with elevated activity within the (left) dorsolateral extrastriate cortex of these subjects. Accordingly, Collignon et al. (Collignon, Lassonde et al. 2007) found that repetitive TMS over (right) dorsal extrastriate areas affected auditory spatial location and the recognition of bidimensional shapes using a vision-to-audition translating device in early blind subjects (see also Merabet, Battelli et al. 2009), whereas other tasks, such as pitch and intensity judgments, were not affected. In a subsequent investigation, Collignon et al. (Collignon, Davare et al. 2009) showed that TMS over the right occipital cortex of the early blind disrupted the spatial processing of sounds in the left hemispace even when TMS was given 50 ms after the stimulus presentation, supporting the view that the occipital cortex in the blind is involved at the very first stages of auditory processing (see also Leclerc, Saint-Amour et al. 2000).

Occipital recruitment in blind subjects can also be induced by the processing of non-spatial features of the auditory input. For instance, a single-case fMRI study carried out by Hertrich et al. (Hertrich, Dietrich et al. 2009) has analyzed the enhanced speech-perception capabilities in a blind listener, finding that they were associated with the activation of the fusiform gyrus and primary visual cortex. According to Hertrich et al. (Hertrich, Dietrich et al. 2009), the left fusiform gyrus, known to be involved in phonological processing, may provide the functional link between the auditory and visual systems. Interestingly, Gaab and colleagues (Gaab, Schulze et al. 2006) have compared the neural correlates of absolute pitch perception (see chapter 2) in a group of blind and sighted musicians, reporting that the former rely on a different neural network in pitch-categorization, including visual association areas (see also Hamilton, Pascual-Leone, and Schlaug 2004), thus possibly explaining the higher incidence of *absolute pitch* in blind compared to sighted musicians (Hamilton, Pascual-Leone, and Schlaug 2004; Pring, Woolf, and Tadic 2008).

Still, intramodal plasticity (or at least plasticity in already dedicated pathways) may be more critical than crossmodal plasticity in the processing of specific auditory stimuli, such as voices (Gougoux, Belin et al. 2009). In this regard, whereas studies in sighted individuals have shown that the auditory cortex along the *anterior* superior temporal sulcus (STS) contains voice-selective regions specifically tuned to vocal sounds (Belin, Zatorre, and Ahad 2002), Gougoux et al. (Gougoux, Belin et al. 2009) have shown that when cortical activation for non-vocal stimuli was subtracted from activation for vocal stimuli (both types of auditory stimuli eliciting activation in striate and extrastriate areas), congenitally blind subjects showed activation along left posterior STS but no specific recruitment of the occipital cortex (although there was a tendency for voice to activate the fusiform cortex bilaterally). Interestingly, Gougoux et al. (Gougoux, Belin et al. 2009) also found that the activation of auditory areas during natural sounds listening was weaker in both late and early blind compared to sighted subjects. This suggests that in blind individuals the recruited visual areas might take over part of the auditory processing at the expense of normal auditory areas. In fact, similar findings have also been reported for tactile and higher-level cognitive tasks. For instance, TMS over somatosensory cortices affected accuracy in tactile-discrimination tasks in sighted but not in early blind subjects (Cohen, Celnik et al. 1997); and Amedi and colleagues (Amedi, Floel et al. 2004) found that TMS applied over inferior prefrontal cortices affected verb generation in sighted but not in early blind subjects: when TMS was delivered over the occipital cortex though, performance of the early blind was impaired both in tactile discrimination and verb generation (Cohen, Celnik et al. 1997; Amedi, Floel et al. 2004).

In line with this, it is worth mentioning that multisensory areas are also susceptible to plasticity phenomena. In the ERP studies carried out by Röder and colleagues, the authors reported differences in the scalp topography for the N2 component, which was shifted more posteriorly in blind participants compared to the sighted controls (e.g., Röder, Rösler, and Neville 1999; see also Kujala, Alho et al. 1995; Liotti, Ryder, and Woldorff 1998). Multisensory areas of the temporo-parietal junction and the parietal lobe contribute to the generation of the N2: according to Röder et al. (Röder, Rösler, and Neville 1999), these multimodal areas would be "colonized" by auditory (and somatosensory) inputs in case of blindness, explaining the difference in the scalp distribution of this component, and the enhanced performance in many auditory tasks often reported in blind subjects (see Collignon, Voss et al. 2009, for a review).

Notably, as is the case with tactile discrimination, the auditory task needs to be sufficiently demanding in order to induce significant activation in the occipital cortex of blind individuals: in fact, simply listening to a sound might not result in occipital activation in blind subjects (see Arno, De Volder et al. 2001). Accordingly, Kujala et al. (Kujala, Palva et al. 2005) found that visual areas in the blind were not activated by the mere presence of sound, but were involved in the attentive processing of changes in the auditory environment, which is important in detecting potentially dangerous or other important events in the surroundings.

Finally, it should be stressed that visual cortex crossmodal plasticity in the blind does not rely upon Braille literacy. In fact, Burton and McLaren (2006) reported occipital activation in two Braille-naïve late blind subjects during phonological and semantic tasks with auditory presentation of words; similarly, Sadato et al. (Sadato, Okada et al. 2004) reported visual cortex activation during a tactile-discrimination task in two late blind subjects who had no knowledge of Braille.

The Dorsal, Ventral, and Motion "Visual" Pathways in Blindness

The pattern of activation found in the occipital cortex of blind individuals during auditory and tactile tasks is functionally highly specific. For instance, the foci for enhanced right occipital activation in the congenitally blind reported by Weeks et al. (Weeks, Horwitz et al. 2000) in their auditory spatial-localization task were in similar locations as those reported in previous PET studies for visual-spatial (Haxby, Horwitz et al. 1994) and visual-motion processing (Watson, Myers et al. 1993) in sighted individuals (see also Arno, De Volder et al. 2001).

In particular, it is well known that in sighted subjects, visual information processing can be mediated by two distinct pathways (Ungerleider and Mishkin 1982): a dorsal pathway, which projects from early visual areas to the posterior parietal cortex, and which is involved in space perception (i.e., "where") and action control (see Goodale and Milner 1992; Milner and Goodale 1995); and a ventral pathway, which projects from early visual areas to the inferotemporal cortex, and which is involved in object-identity computation (i.e., "what"). These pathways seem to mediate similar functions in blind individuals.

Regarding the dorsal ("where"/action) stream, Fiehler et al. (Fiehler, Burke et al. 2009) using fMRI found overlapping activations in the dorsal pathway in congenitally blind subjects and sighted controls associated to kinesthetically guided hand movements and working memory maintenance of kinesthetic information. Accordingly, Garg et al. (Garg, Schwartz, and Stevens 2007) reported increased activation in the frontal eye fields (an area of the dorsal fronto-parietal pathway) both in sighted and congenitally blind subjects during a spatial-attention task. Vanlierde et al. (Vanlierde, De Volder et al. 2003) and Bonino et al. (Bonino, Ricciardi et al. 2008) also reported a similar activation in the dorsal pathway in early blind and sighted individuals while performing a spatial-imagery task on the basis of either auditory or tactile inputs, supporting the view of a supramodal organization of the dorsal stream developing even in the absence of vision (but see Burton, Sinclair, and Dixit 2010).

Similar results have been reported for the ventral ("what") pathway. Pietrini et al. (Pietrini, Furey et al. 2004) reported that tactile object-perception evoked category-related patterns of response in temporal extrastriate cortex of blind individuals similar to those shown by sighted individuals during visual and haptic exploration of the same objects, suggesting that the development of topographically organized, category-related representations in extrastriate visual cortex does not require visual experience (see figure 8.1 [plate 1]).

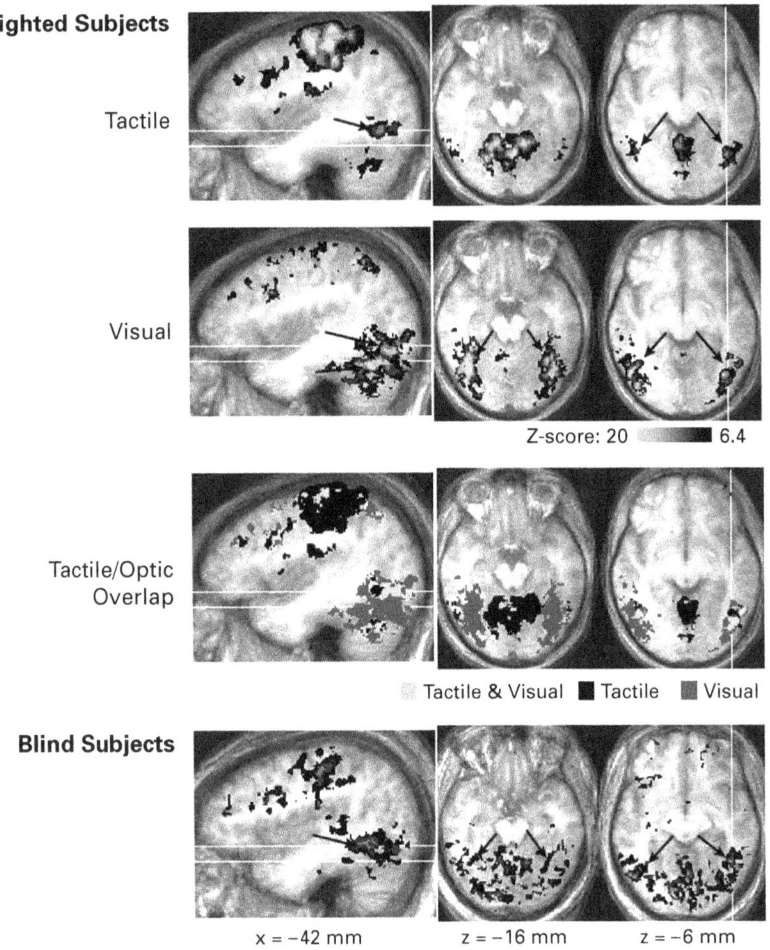

Figure 8.1
Brain areas that responded during tactile and/or visual object-perception in sighted subjects and during tactile perception in blind subjects in the study by Pietrini et al. (Pietrini, Furey et al. 2004). Sagittal and axial images from group Z-score maps of activated areas are shown for the sighted and blind subjects. The inferior temporal (IT) and ventral temporal (VT) regions activated by tactile and visual object-perception are indicated. The tactile/visual overlap map shows the areas activated by both tactile and visual perception (shown in yellow), as well as the areas activated only by tactile (red) and visual (green) perception. The white lines in the sagittal images correspond to the locations of the axial slices and, similarly, the white line in the axial slice indicates the location of the sagittal section. (See plate 1.)
Reprinted from Pietrini, Furey et al., "Beyond sensory images: Object-based representation in the human ventral pathway," *Proceedings of the National Academy of Sciences of the United States of America* 101(15) (2004): 5658–5663. (© 2004. Reprinted by permission of the National Academy of Sciences of the United States of America)

Critically, Mahon, Caramazza, and colleagues (Mahon, Anzellotti et al. 2009) demonstrated that the classical medial-to-lateral organization of the ventral stream, reflecting preferences for nonliving and living stimuli (see Martin 2007), respectively, also develops in congenitally blind individuals. Although only three blind individuals took part in this study (Mahon, Anzellotti et al. 2009), its findings are critical in suggesting that the organization of object-representations within the ventral system is not entirely shaped by visual similarities between objects (as has been suggested: Haxby, Gobbini et al. 2001) but also by dimensions of similarities that cannot be reduced to the visual experience (e.g., Caramazza and Mahon 2003; Mahon, Milleville et al. 2007). In other words, the human brain may possess an innate architecture disposed to handle information and process items from different conceptual domains independently from sensory and motor experience (Mahon, Anzellotti et al. 2009).

Moreover, areas devoted to processing visual motion information maintain their functions in case of blindness. In fact, both tactile motion and auditory motion have been found to induce in blind subjects (and sight-recovery subjects) activation of the hMT/V5 complex, a region normally involved in visual motion processing (Bedny, Konkle et al. in press; Poirier, Collignon et al. 2006; Ricciardi, Vanello et al. 2007; Ptito, Matteau et al. 2009; Matteau, Kuipers et al. 2010; Wolbers, Zahoriz, and Giudice 2010; see also Saenz, Lewis et al. 2008) (see figure 8.2 [plate 2]). Notably, the involvement of MT in processing of auditory motion critically depends on the age at blindness onset (see Bedny, Konkle et al. in press).

Nonetheless, blindness—at least to a certain extent—affects the functioning of these established networks. For instance, a TMS study by Collignon et al. (Collignon, Davare et al. 2009) has demonstrated a reorganization of the occipito-parietal stream for auditory spatial processing in early blind individuals: in particular, stimulating the right IPS (known to be critically involved in the spatial localization of sound in sighted subjects) with TMS at a specific time-window, known to interfere with sound-localization in the sighted (Collignon, Davare et al. 2008), did not significantly affect performances of the early blind subjects.

Occipital Recruitment in Blind Individuals: Task-dependent and Modality-specific Effects

An important aspect to be clarified when considering the recruitment of the occipital cortex by auditory and tactile processing is whether such recruitment is modality-specific. In fact, this may not be the case: ERP studies have reported that both auditory and tactile-evoked components showed enhanced posterior negativity in blind subjects compared to sighted controls in oddball tasks (Kujala, Alho et al. 1995; Röder, Rösler et al. 1996). Van der Lubbe et al. (Van der Lubbe, Van Mierlo, and Postma 2009) have specifically addressed this issue by measuring ERPs during an auditory or tactile duration-discrimination task in early blind and sighted subjects. Again, no support for a modality-specificity involvement of occipital cortex in the early blind group was

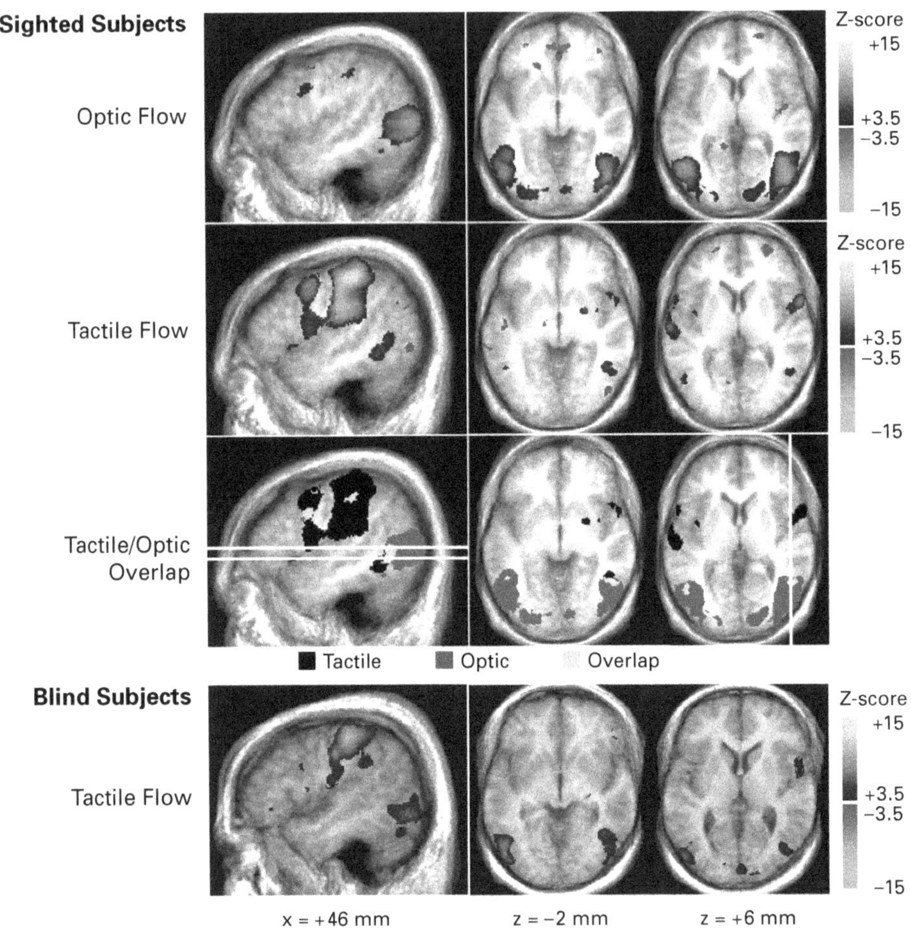

Figure 8.2

Brain areas that responded during tactile or optic flow perception in sighted subjects and during tactile flow-perception in blind subjects in the study by Ricciardi et al. (Ricciardi, Vanello et al. 2007). Sagittal and axial images from group Z-score maps of activated areas are shown for the sighted and blind subjects. The tactile/visual overlap map shows the areas activated by both tactile and optic flow perception (shown in yellow), as well as the areas activated only by tactile (red) and optic (green) perception. The white lines in the sagittal image correspond to the locations of the axial slices, and similarly, the white line in the axial slice indicates the location of the sagittal section. (See plate 2.)

Reprinted from Ricciardi, Vanello et al., "The effect of visual experience on the development of functional architecture in hMT+," *Cerebral Cortex* 17(12) (2007): 2933–2939. (Reprinted by permission of Oxford University Press) reported. Accordingly, Weaver and Stevens (2007) using fMRI identified several areas of the occipital cortex of the blind that responded similarly to auditory and tactile inputs. Overall, these findings suggest that the recruitment of the occipital cortex in the blind is "supramodal" rather than modality-specific.

Interestingly though, when some visual capacity is preserved, the visual cortex exhibits a retinotopically specific segregation of functions for vision and touch. The case of a visually impaired man tested by Cheung and colleagues (Cheung, Fang et al. 2009) is paradigmatic on this regard. The patient "S" had normal visual development until age 6, but thereafter suffered from severe visual acuity reduction due to corneal opacification, with no evidence of visual field loss. Due to these particular circumstances, S can both read print visually and Braille by touch. Cheung and colleagues (Cheung, Fang et al. 2009) have found that tactile information processing activates in S populations of neurons in the visual cortex usually subtending foveal representation in normally sighted subjects, whereas visual information activates neurons normally devoted to represent peripheral visual information. Importantly, a control experiment showed that tactile-induced activation in the occipital cortex is not due to visual imagery processes in S. Hence, S's visual cortex exhibits a retinotopically specific segregation of functions for vision and touch: only those visual neurons that are not critical for S's remaining low-resolution vision are recruited for tactile processing. S's case is of critical importance, since it shows that cortical plasticity might work at a highly specific scale and has important implications for sight-restoration procedures.

It is worth noticing that even in case of a total visual deprivation, the topography of the occipital activation may vary depending on the task used: for instance, parts of visual cortex involved in somatosensory processing differ from those engaged during semantic/language tasks (see Amedi, Raz et al. 2003). In this regard, there seems to be some evidence (although controversial) for hemispheric effects in the recruitment of the occipital cortex in blind individuals for non-visual processing. In fact, it has been proposed that the right visual cortices may be more likely involved in spatiotemporal judgments and the left visual cortices may be more likely involved in "identity" judgments (see Van der Lubbe, Van Mierlo, and Postma 2009). Unfortunately, intrinsic limits of neuroimaging techniques (i.e., spatial and temporal resolution, averaging across subjects) have not allowed so far to perfectly determine which specific regions of the visual cortex are activated during a particular task, thus also accounting for possible discrepancies across different studies. Moreover, not all early blind subjects show similar crossmodal effects: for instance, in the study by Van der Lubbe et al. (Van der Lubbe, Van Mierlo, and Postma 2009) recruitment of posterior areas was found during an auditory duration-discrimination task in some but not all early blind subjects, and such activation was related to their performance level. Similarly, Gougoux et al. (Gougoux, Zatorre et al. 2005), Voss et al. (Voss, Gougoux et al. 2008), and Amedi et al.

(Amedi, Raz et al. 2003) observed that extra recruitment of posterior areas varied in the blind group depending on the individual level of performance.

Occipital Recruitment during Non-visual Processing in Sighted Individuals

At this stage of the discussion, it is important to briefly mention that visual cortex activation has also been reported in sighted individuals during tactile and auditory tasks (see Sathian 2005 for a review). In particular, tactile-discrimination tasks, such as grating-orientation, have been found to induce occipital activation in sighted individuals (Sathian, Zangaladze et al. 1997; Zangaladze, Epstein et al. 1999; Sathian and Zangaladze 2001; but see Sadato, Okada et al. 2002; Harada, Saito et al. 2004); similarly, when sighted individuals explore objects with their hands, parts of the visual cortex, including the lingual gyrus, fusiform gyri and even the peripheral field representation in the primary visual cortex, are likely to activate (see Deibert, Kraut et al. 1999; James, Humphrey et al. 2002). Furthermore, tactile and auditory motion stimuli have been shown to affect activation of area hMT/V5 in sighted individuals (Bedny, Konkle et al. in press; Hagen, Franzén et al. 2002; Lewis, Beauchamp, and DeYoe, 2000; Ricciardi, Vanello et al. 2007). Accordingly, spatial processing of sounds have been found to involve posterior parietal and extrastriate occipital cortex in normally sighted individuals (see Lewald, Foltys, and Töpper 2002; Lewald, Meister et al. 2004; Zimmer, Lewald et al. 2004; Poirier, Collignon et al. 2005; Collignon, Davare et al. 2008).

In fact, in the case of sighted subjects, much of the visual cortex activation during auditory and tactile processing depends on visual imagery mechanisms (see Sathian 2005 for a review), which are known to activate early visual cortices in a retinotopic organized fashion (e.g., Slotnick, Thompson, and Kosslyn 2005). Since sighted participants mainly rely on vision in spatial cognition and object identification, they are likely to translate haptically perceived stimuli into a visual mental representation (e.g., Cattaneo and Vecchi 2008); such visual imagery activity would then result in early visual cortex activation. Support for this hypothesis comes from studies that have compared macrospatial tasks (i.e., requiring discrimination of relatively large-scale features such as global stimulus form and orientation) with microspatial tasks (e.g., grating groove-width discrimination and gap detection), showing that the former preferentially involve visual cortical processing and induce a greater tendency to evoke visual imagery (e.g., Sathian, Zangaladze et al. 1997; Zangaladze, Epstein et al. 1999; Sathian and Zangaladze 2001; Stoesz, Zhang et al. 2003).

Nonetheless, not all the activation in primary visual areas of sighted individuals during non-visual tasks can be attributed to visual imagery processes. For instance, using TMS, Collignon et al. (Collignon, Davare et al. 2008; Collignon, Davare et al. 2009) demonstrated that the occipital cortex is already involved in sound localization 50 ms after stimulus presentation—even earlier than the parietal cortex—both in sighted and blind participants. Such early recruitment of the visual cortex and the nature of the task used rule out a possible role of visual imagery processes in sighted participants. In fact, such early occipital activation in blind and sighted subjects is likely to have a different functional meaning: in the case of sighted individuals, visual-cortices activation may be important for the calibration of head-centered sound coordinates with respect to the position of the eyes in the orbit (see Zimmer, Lewald et al. 2004), whereas in early blind subjects (see Collignon, Davare et al. 2009) it is likely to depend on sound processing per se and hence on a true crossmodal reorganization, given that obviously the blind do not need eyes-head calibration. Accordingly, in a PET study, Gougoux et al. (Gougoux, Zatorre et al. 2005) found that the level of functional activation of occipital areas correlated with sound-localization accuracy in blind but not in sighted subjects. Similarly, others have favored the idea that occipital areas engagement during haptic shape-perception reflects a multisensory shape representation rather than the activation of a corresponding visual image (e.g., Amedi, Malach et al. 2001; Amedi, Jacobson et al. 2002; James, Humphrey et al. 2002; Pietrini, Furey et al. 2004).

Crossmodal Plasticity, Sensory Substitution, and Visual Prostheses

Crossmodal plasticity phenomena associated with blindness are extremely important for research on sensory substitution devices (SSDs) and neuroprostheses. As already reported in chapter 5, "sensory substitution" refers to the use of one sensory modality to provide information normally conveyed by another sense (see Bach-y-Rita, Collins et al. 1969; Poirier, De Volder, and Scheiber 2007, for reviews). In case of blindness, artificial devices have been developed in order to acquire visual information and translate it into a meaningful signal for the auditory and tactile systems. Indeed, converging evidence indicates that—after proper training—these devices allow blindfolded sighted and blind individuals to discriminate pattern orientations, and recognize visual patterns or graphic representations of objects (Epstein, Hughes et al. 1989; Arno, Capelle et al. 1999; Cronly-Dillon, Persaud, and Gregory 1999; Sampaio, Maris, and Bach-y-Rita 2001; Arno, Vanlierde et al. 2001; Poirier, Richard et al. 2006). Recent findings suggest that visual-to-auditory SSD may enable blind individuals to acquire the rules of visual depth and use them efficiently to interact with their environment (Renier and DeVolder 2010).

Sensory substitution devices are not invasive and do not directly stimulate visual organs; in contrast, neuroprostheses—developed in bioengineering and microtechnology research—are based upon focal electrical stimulation of intact visual structures in order to evoke the sensation of visual *qualia*, i.e., discrete points of light, also called "phosphenes" (see Merabet, Rizzo et al. 2005, for a review). Thanks to these devices, it has been hypothesized that we can induce the perception of shapes and images in

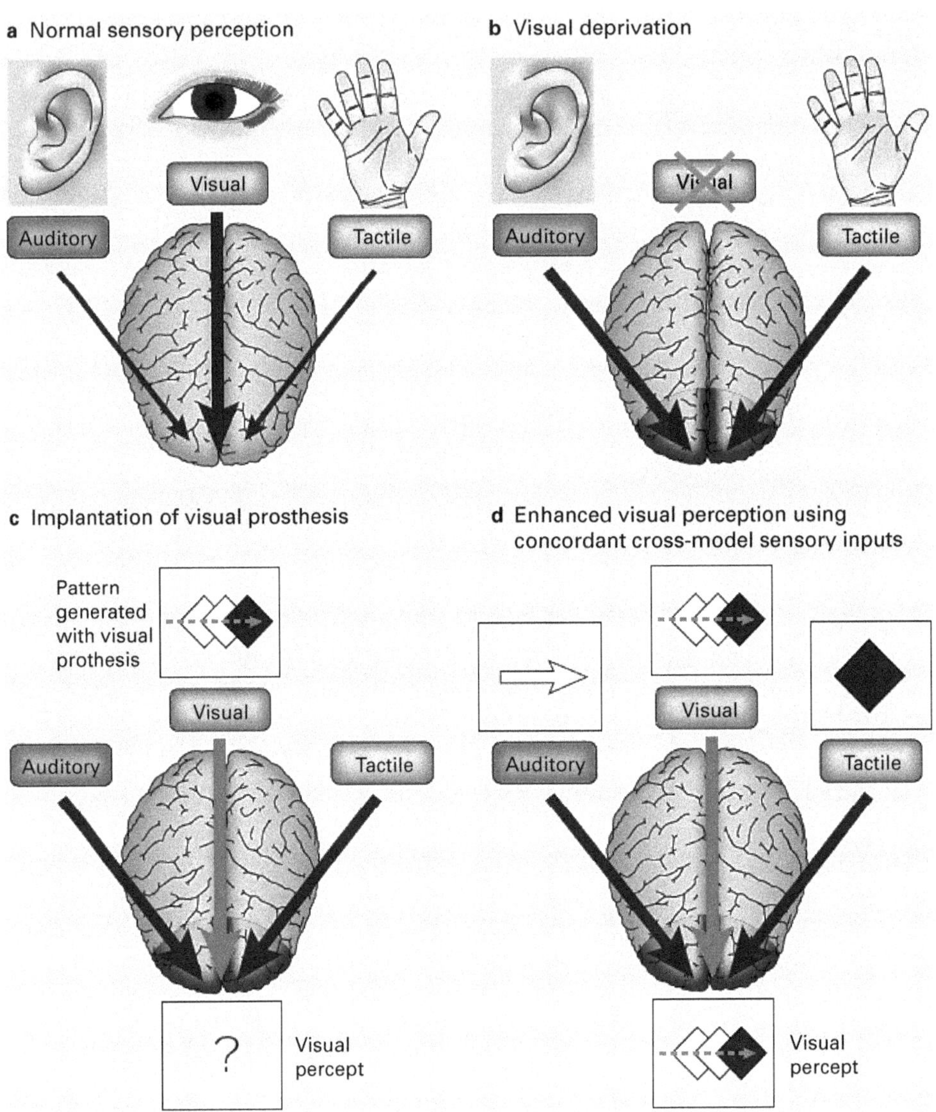

Figure 8.3

The multimodal nature of our sensory world and its implications for implementing a visual prosthesis to restore vision as discussed by Merabet et al. (Merabet, Rizzo et al. 2005). (A) Under normal conditions, the occipital cortex receives predominantly visual inputs but perception is also highly influenced by crossmodal sensory information obtained from other sources (for example, touch and hearing). (B) Following visual deprivation, neuroplastic changes occur such that the visual cortex is recruited to process sensory information from other senses (illustrated blind individuals (see figure 8.3 [plate 3]). Visual prosthetic devices may directly stimulate the visual cortex (although this technique suffers of severe limitations, such as being very invasive and likely inducing the risk of focal seizures) or the optic nerve, or can be implanted at the level of the retina (see Merabet, Rizzo et al. 2005).

It is beyond the scope of this section to provide exhaustive and technical details of current methods of restoring vision. However, the development of neuroprostheses may be very important for the investigation of crossmodality and neural plasticity. In fact, crossmodal changes occurring in the occipital cortex of the blind are functionally adaptive, but they can also represent an obstacle for the later implantation of prosthetic devices. We described above the TMS study carried out by Cohen et al. (Cohen, Celnik et al. 1997): Cohen et al. found that TMS over the occipital cortex induced erroneous and even phantom tactile sensations in the blind and did not result in any visual perception. In a similar vein, visual cortical prostheses might result in tactile (or synesthetic tactile-visual) percepts, rather than in meaningful vision. Therefore, it would be naïve to expect that the re-introduction of a sensory input by itself would be sufficient to restore a flawless sensory perception: furthermore, simple light-pattern sensations would not necessarily result in meaningful vision, as is also demonstrated by cases of patients who underwent cataract removals after years of blindness (see chapter 4). Indeed, a complete development of the visual system based upon prior visual experience is likely to be necessary for an individual to interpret signals conveyed by visual neuroprostheses in a correct and meaningful way.

Visual prosthetic devices may thus be useful for acquired blindness but not for congenital and early blindness. Moreover, rehabilitation with a visual neuroprosthesis

by larger arrows for touch and hearing). This might be through the potential "unmasking" or enhancement of connections that are already present. (C) After neuroplastic changes associated with vision loss have occurred, the visual cortex is fundamentally altered in terms of its sensory processing, so that simple reintroduction of visual input (by a visual prosthesis) is not sufficient to create meaningful vision (in this example: a pattern encoding a moving diamond figure is generated with the prosthesis). (D) To create meaningful visual percepts, a patient who has received an implanted visual prosthesis can incorporate concordant information from remaining sensory sources. In this case, the directionality of a moving visual stimulus can be presented with an appropriately timed directional auditory input and the shape of the object can be determined by simultaneous haptic exploration. In summary, modification of visual input by a visual neuroprosthesis in conjunction with appropriate auditory and tactile stimulation could potentially maximize the functional significance of restored light-perceptions and allow blind individuals to regain behaviorally relevant vision. (See plate 3.)
Reprinted from Merabet, Rizzo et al., "What blindness can tell us about seeing again: Merging neuroplasticity and neuroprostheses," *Nature Reviews. Neuroscience*, 6(1) (2005): 71–77. (© 2005. Reprinted by permission of Macmillan Publishers Ltd.)

should be supported by a continuous matching between visual sensations and tactile and auditory inputs in order to maximize the relearning process that is necessary to regain sight (Merabet, Rizzo et al. 2005).

8.4 Cortical Plasticity and Higher Cognitive Functions: Language and Memory

Several studies suggest that in the blind the deafferented visual cortex might be engaged in high-level cognitive processes, such as those mediating language comprehension and memory. For instance, using fMRI, Burton et al. (Burton, Snyder et al. 2002b) studied this possible occipital recruitment during a covert generation of verbs to heard nouns in sighted and blind individuals. The control task required passive listening to indecipherable sounds (reverse words) matched to the nouns in sound intensity, duration and spectral content. Blind and sighted subjects showed similar activation of language areas; nonetheless, blind individuals also showed a bilateral, left-dominant activation of visual cortices, mainly overlapping with that reported during Braille reading in previous studies (see Burton, Snyder et al. 2002a). In a following fMRI study, Burton, Diamond and McDermott (2003) investigated semantic-related and phonological-related cortical activation in early and late blind subjects during language processing, and found significant activations in the occipital (including V1), parietal and temporal components of the visual cortex. Such activation was greater in early than in late blind subjects and, critically, was greater for semantic than for phonological processing. Accordingly, when listening to sentences that varied for syntactic complexity and that were either semantically meaningful or meaningless, congenitally blind subjects were found to activate not only left perysilvian areas usually associated with language, but also the homologous right hemisphere structures and extrastriate and striate regions (Röder, Stock et al. 2002). Notably, the amplitude of the homodynamic response in occipital areas varied as a function of syntactic and semantic processing demands, indicating that the occipital cortex was functionally involved in language processing.

Occipital recruitment in blind individuals has also been reported in memory tasks. For instance, Amedi et al. (Amedi, Raz et al. 2003), using fMRI, found an extensive occipital activation (involving V1) in blind but not in sighted subjects, during both Braille reading, a verbal-memory task and an auditory verb-generation task. Critically, occipital activation correlated with the superior verbal memory performance in the blind group, and was topographically specific: in fact, anterior regions showed a preference for tactile Braille reading, whereas the posterior regions were more active during the verbal-memory and verb-generation tasks. In a following fMRI study, Raz et al. (Raz, Amedi, and Zohary 2005) confirmed that V1 activation in congenitally blind humans is associated with episodic retrieval. In particular, in Raz and colleagues' study, a series of words were auditorily presented to congenitally blind and sighted subjects who had to judge whether these words had already been presented in an earlier experimental session. Memory retrieval induced occipital activation in blind but not in sighted subjects, with the extent of such activation being greater during the retrieval task than during a phonological control task, and significantly correlating with episodic retrieval (Raz, Amedi, and Zohary 2005). The findings by Raz et al. (Raz, Amedi, and Zohary 2005) indicate that the occipital cortex in the blind is involved not only in semantic processing (see Amedi, Raz et al. 2003) but also in long-term memory retrieval.

TMS experiments have confirmed the causal role of visual areas for language and memory processes in blind individuals. Amedi et al. (Amedi, Floel et al. 2004) found that rTMS over the occipital pole impaired performance in a verb-generation task in blind subjects but not in sighted controls. Notably, rTMS over left occipital cortices most commonly induced semantic errors in the blind, indexing a role of the deafferented visual cortex in high-level verbal processing. Kupers et al. (Kupers, Pappens et al. 2007) reported that rTMS over occipital regions but not over S1 significantly affected blind subjects' Braille-reading accuracy and abolished an improvement in reading speed following the repetitive presentation of the same word list, suggesting a role of the visual cortex in repetition priming. Repetition priming is an implicit form of memory: therefore, the results by Kupers et al. (Kupers, Pappens et al. 2007) suggest that the occipital cortex of early blind subjects plays a role in the generation of implicit memory traces of Braille stimuli as a result of prior encounter with these words.

Lateralization of Language and Blindness

A long-debated issue concerns the possible effects that blindness has on the typical hemispheric lateralization of language functions. It has been suggested that language processes are more bilaterally organized in blind subjects than in sighted controls, and this because the lack of visual-spatial input in the blind may result in less interhemispheric competition, thus favoring a bilateral representation of language. In fact, available evidence suggests left-lateralized language functions in blind subjects, although the right hemisphere's involvement in language processes is likely greater in blind than in sighted subjects. For instance, Hugdahl et al. (Hugdahl, Ek et al. 2004) in a dichotic listening paradigm found that blind individuals, as sighted ones, performed better for stimuli presented to the right ear, but they were better than sighted subjects for left ear when allocating attention. Semenza et al. (Semenza, Zoppello et al. 1996) in a dichaptic scanning of Braille letters reported a right-hand (left-hemisphere) advantage for linguistic processing of the stimuli, suggesting left-lateralized linguistic functions in the blind. Accordingly, left-hemispheric lesions have resulted in aphasia in Braille blind readers (Signoret, van Eeckhout et al. 1987; Fisher and Larner 2008). Nonetheless, electrophysiological measures which index lexical processing provided evidence for a bilateral rather than left-lateralized cerebral organization of language in congenitally blind adults (Röder, Rösler, and Neville 2000). These findings were confirmed by a subsequent fMRI study (Röder, Stock et al. 2002) in which reading sentences of different syntactic difficulties elicited in congenitally blind not only activation in left perysilvian areas usually associated with language, but also activity in the homologous right-hemisphere structures and in extrastriate and striate regions.

In fact, it is possible that the use of Braille, similar to the use of sign language in the deaf (Neville, Bavelier et al. 1998), results in a stronger engagement of the right hemisphere for language processing, because Braille relies more upon spatial components than printed or spoken language. Accordingly, a large body of evidence indicates a right-hemispheric dominance for auditory *spatial* processing both in blind (Weeks, Horwitz et al. 2000; Voss, Lassonde et al. 2004; Gougoux, Zatorre et al. 2005) and sighted subjects (Griffiths, Rees et al. 1998; Lewald, Foltys, and Töpper 2002; Zatorre, Belin, and Penhune 2002). The role of Braille reading in reducing language lateralization is supported by the finding that the right-ear/left-hemisphere advantage decreased at the increasing of proficiency in Braille reading, while illiterate blind adults showed the normal left-right asymmetry (Karavatos, Kaprinis, and Tzavaras 1984). Hand-preference in Braille reading has also been extensively studied, possibly offering an insight into language lateralization: however, early studies have led to different results, some of them reporting superior performances for the left hand (Hermelin and O'Connor 1971; Rudel, Denckla, and Spalten 1974), some for the right hand (Fertsch 1947). Millar (1984) suggested that there is not, in absolute terms, a "preferred" hand for Braille reading (Millar 1984), but hand advantages likely depend on a combination of task demands and individuals' strategies preference.

8.5 Mechanisms Mediating Intramodal and Crossmodal Plasticity

We have already mentioned that map expansion in the somatosensory cortex (intramodal plasticity) might be induced by an intense training period in sighted individuals (see Elbert, Pantev et al. 1995). Evidence from longitudinal studies on Braille learning suggest that intramodal plastic changes may occur at two different stages: during the first six months there would be a rapid and robust enlargement of cortical representation, likely mediated by the unmasking of existing connections and changes in synaptic efficacy; further, a second more stable phase would follow in which structural changes at multiple neural levels take place (see Théoret, Merabet, and Pascual-Leone 2004).

The neural basis for crossmodal plasticity is more controversial. It has been proposed that the recruitment of visual cortices for tactile processing might occur by way of two distinct mechanisms: the formation of new thalamo-cortical pathways or the strengthening of existing cortico-cortical pathways (see Bavelier and Neville 2002; Sadato 2005; Ptito, Fumal et al. 2008, for discussions). Although the thalamus is the first level of processing where visual and tactile inputs converge, at the thalamic level the tactile and visual inputs still remain segregated. Only the contralateral side of the body is represented in the thalamus, and the lateral geniculate nucleus relays inputs only to the cortex of the same hemisphere: therefore, the finding that tactile stimulation of the right hand of blind subjects induced a bilateral activation in V1 (Pons 1996; Sadato, Pascual-Leone et al. 1996, 1998; Sadato, Okada et al. 2002) speaks against a crossmodal reorganization at the thalamic level (see Sadato 2005 for a discussion). And further, more recent studies using diffusion-tensor imaging (Shimony, Burton et al. 2006) or voxel-based morphometry (Schneider, Kupers, and Ptito 2006) showed atrophy of the geniculo-cortical tract in early blind subjects (but preservation of connections between the visual cortex and prefrontal and temporal cortices). Still, the possible role played by the generation of new thalamo-cortical pathways cannot be completely excluded, finding support in animal studies (Sur, Garraghty, and Roe 1988; Ptito, Giguère et al 2001) and in other recent connectivity studies (see Liu, Yu et al. 2007).

In general, the cortico-cortical hypothesis has received stronger support. Tactile information reaches the occipital cortex via existing cortico-cortical pathways likely involving multisensory regions in the parietal lobe (Sadato, Pascual-Leone et al. 1996; Bavelier and Neville 2002; Ptito and Kupers 2005). Accordingly, in a TMS-PET combined study, Wittenberg et al. (Wittenberg, Werhahn et al. 2004) reported that TMS over the primary somatosensory cortex induced a significant rCBF increase in the occipital cortex in early blind but not in blindfolded sighted controls. In particular, cortico-cortical connections relevant for visual cortex recruitment in tactile tasks likely involve a pathway that goes from the somatosensory cortex to parietal areas (such as VIP or area 7 or both), to areas MT and V3, and finally reaches the visual cortex (Ptito, Fumal et al. 2008). The pattern is similar for occipital recruitment by auditory processing. In this regard, Weeks et al. (Weeks, Horwitz et al. 2000) showed that activity in the right occipital cortex during auditory localization was highly correlated with activity in the right posterior parietal region in blind but not in sighted participants (where a negative correlation was reported). Accordingly, in an EEG study, Leclerc et al. (Leclerc, Segalowitz et al. 2005) found that oscillations in the theta, alpha and beta frequency bands in fronto-central and occipital electrodes were linked during the task to a larger extent in early blind subjects than in sighted controls, suggesting enhanced connectivity between auditory and visual brain regions in the early blind (Leclerc, Segalowitz et al. 2005). Noppeney et al. (Noppeney, Friston, and Price 2003) have shown increased effective connectivity between occipital regions and the prefrontal and temporal regions involved in semantic processes, shedding light on the mechanisms which mediate the occipital recruitment for high-level cognitive processes. Accordingly, a recent fMRI study investigating cortical activation associated with the tactile reading of words in Braille, print on palm, and a haptic form of American Sign Language revealed enhanced occipito-temporal cortical connections within the left hemisphere in an early blind and congenitally deaf individual that was not observed in the control subject (Obretenova, Halko, et al. 2010).

Hence, when bottom-up processing is interrupted as in blindness, tactile and auditory processes but also higher-level cognitive functions, might expand into visual cortices mainly through polysensory areas (see Sadato 2005), but also by means of direct feedforward afferences arising from auditory and somatosensory cortices. In fact, studies on normally sighted subjects have suggested that direct pathways between "low-level" sensory-specific cortices may exist and play a role in crossmodal interactions (e.g., Martuzzi, Murray et al. 2007; for review, see Driver and Noesselt 2008). Accordingly, TMS delivered over the occipital cortex at a delay of 60 ms after stimulus-onset impaired the discrimination of tactile stimuli in early blind subjects (Pascual-Leone, Amedi et al. 2005), and delivering TMS over the occipital cortex 50 ms after an auditory stimulus disrupted blind individuals' performance in sound-localization (Collignon, Lassonde et al. 2007; Collignon, Davare et al. 2009). The early occurrence of such effects demonstrates that some direct connections between putative "unimodal" areas are likely to play a role in the crossmodal recruitment of the visual cortex in blindness.

It is worth mentioning that the "positive" occipital activation in blind subjects reported by several studies comparing cortical activation patterns in the sighted and the blind might indeed reflect a reduced inhibition or deactivation in visual regions that has, in turn, been observed in sighted subjects during non-visual tasks (Röder and Rösler 2004). In fact, deactivation in other sensory cortices that are irrelevant to the task at hand has been consistently reported in sighted individuals (Laurienti, Burdette et al. 2002; Azulay, Striem, and Amedi 2009). Studies in functional connectivity between sensory cortices have confirmed that visual deprivation modifies the inter-regional "negative" connectivity and hence the "boundary" between regions processing one kind of sensory input and another (Fujii, Tanabe et al. 2009). Hence, the mechanisms "suppressing" the visual cortex might not properly develop in case of blindness, due to the competitive imbalance caused by the loss of visual input.

8.6 Structural Changes Induced by Blindness

Together with the functional changes we have described above, blindness also induces structural changes in cortical and subcortical regions. In a voxel-based morphometry study, Noppeney et al. (Noppeney, Friston et al. 2005) showed that early blind individuals presented a reduced gray-matter volume in visual areas (atrophy of the optic chiasm and optic radiation was also observed), likely reflecting changes in synaptic density, dendritic spine numbers, and axonal arborizations. Gray-matter volume was particularly reduced in *early* visual areas, suggesting that the early visual cortex may only benefit by limited crossmodal plasticity, hence being more susceptible to disuse-atrophy (see also Buchel, Price et al. 1998) compared to extrastriate associative cortices, which are more readily recruited by non-visual processing by means of crossmodal connections. In one of the few studies investigating blindness-induced changes in white matter, Shu et al. (Shu, Li et al. 2009) reported that significant alterations in white matter in the early blind were restricted to the geniculocalcarine tract and its adjacent regions. According to Shu et al. (Shu, Li et al. 2009) these alterations likely depended on both transneural degeneration secondary to the pathology in the retina and the optic nerve, and on immaturity of the visual system due to altered visual experience during critical periods of neurodevelopment.

Volumetric atrophy in visual areas of blind subjects may depend on both reduced cortical thickness and reduced surface area (the two likely reflecting different developmental mechanisms). Interestingly, Park et al. (Park, Lee et al. 2009) reported that volumetric atrophies in primary and associative cortices of congenitally blind subjects mainly depended on a decreased cortical surface area despite increased cortical thickness. According to Park et al. (Park, Lee et al. 2009), increased thickness at the primary visual cortex in congenitally blind individuals is due to visual loss during the developmental stage rather than to use-driven atrophy or compensatory plasticity at adult ages, since the reverse pattern—i.e., a tendency to cortical thinning—was observed in late blind subjects (see also Jiang, Zhu et al. 2009). Interestingly, a negative correlation was reported between years of Braille reading and cortical thickness in the bilateral superior temporal gyrus of congenitally blind subjects, a correlation that was higher for the left hemisphere, suggesting compensatory plasticity in linguistic processing. A reduced synaptic pruning of redundant connections is likely to be a major factor influencing cortical thickness (see also Jiang, Zhu et al. 2009), with abnormally increased cortico-cortical connections and thalamo-cortical connections also leading to increased thickness, as demonstrated by animal studies (Berman 1991; Kingsbury, Lettman, and Finlay 2002; Karlen, Kahn, and Krubitzer 2006).

Structural changes in non-visual areas have also been consistently reported in blind individuals. For instance, Park et al. (Park, Lee et al. 2009) found evidence of cortical thinning in the somatosensory cortex and in the right superior temporal lobe of blind subjects, possibly related to their increased tactile and auditory performance (see Hyde, Lerch et al. 2007). Accordingly, Noppeney et al. (Noppeney, Friston et al. 2005) reported an increase of white-matter tracts associated with primary somatosensory and motor cortices, indicating experience-dependent plasticity in these areas.

Local structural differences in the hippocampus of blind individuals relative to sighted individuals have also been reported. In particular, Leporé et al. (Leporé, Shi et al. 2009) reported significant anatomical differences but only in the right hippocampus: anterior regions (head/body) showed increased displacement in the blind with respect to the average template while more posterior ones (body/tail) showed decreased displacement compared to sighted controls, though this second effect was not as strong as the result in the anterior regions. Accordingly, Fortin et al. (Fortin, Voss et al. 2008) showed that the rostral portion (head) of the hippocampus (both left and right) was larger in blind individuals, and Chebat et al. (Chebat, Rainville et al. 2007) showed that the caudal portion (tail) of the right hippocampus was smaller in the blind.

Finally, a recent study using diffusion tensor tractography (Shu, Liu et al. 2009) revealed that, compared with the normal controls, the early blind subjects showed disrupted global anatomical connection patterns, such as lower degree of connectivity, a longer characteristic path length, and a lower global efficiency, especially in the visual cortex; nonetheless, some regions with motor or somatosensory function were found to have increased connections with other brain regions, suggesting experience-dependent compensatory plasticity in the early blind.

8.7 Social Cognition in the Blind Brain

The phrase "theory of mind" refers to the ability to attribute mental states to other individuals, and hence to understand them as intentional agents (see Leslie, Friedman, and German 2004). A critical question is whether visual deprivation influences the development of such an ability. In an fMRI study carried out to address this issue, Bedny and colleagues (Bedny, Pascual-Leone, and Saxe 2009) critically reported that early blind and sighted subjects recruited the same neural network for theory of mind processing, including right and left temporo-parietal junctions, medial prefrontal cortex, precuneus and anterior temporal sulci. Hence, thinking about other people's thoughts in both sighted and blind subjects is likely to depend on abstract/amodal and propositional representations that can be acquired without first-person experience, as demonstrated by the finding that the pattern of activation in blind subjects was comparable when the described scenes referred to either other people's visual or auditory experience.

Similar results have been obtained by Ricciardi et al. (Ricciardi, Bonino et al. 2009), who used fMRI to investigate whether the "mirror neurons" system normally develops in congenitally blind individuals (see figures 8.4 and 8.5 [plate 4]). The term "mirror" is used to designate a particular set of neurons that have been originally discovered in the monkey premotor and parietal cortex, having the peculiar property of discharg-

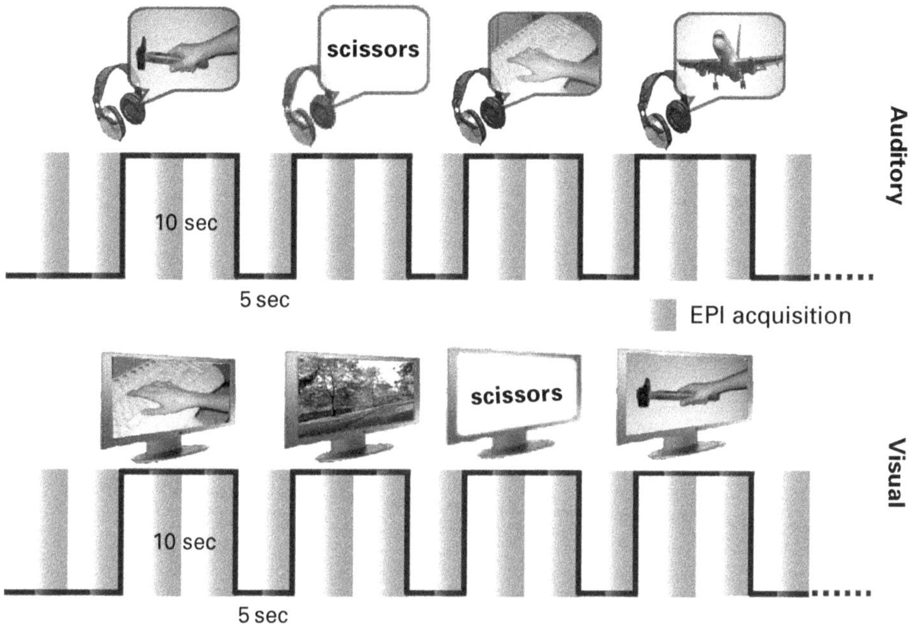

Figure 8.4
The fMRI Experimental Paradigm used by Ricciardi et al. (Ricciardi, Bonino et al. 2009). An fMRI sparse-sampling six-run block design was used to examine neural activity in congenitally blind and sighted right-handed healthy volunteers, while they alternated between the random presentation of hand-executed action or environmental sounds/movies, and the motor pantomime of a "virtual" tool or object manipulation task.
Reprinted from Ricciardi, Bonino et al., "Do we really need vision? How blind people 'see' the actions of others," *Journal of Neuroscience* 29(31) (2009): 9719–9724. (Reprinted by permission of Society for Neuroscience)

ing both when the monkey performs specific goal-directed hand or mouth actions (i.e., grasping, tearing, holding, biting, sucking) and when it observes (or listens to) another individual performing the same actions (Gallese, Fadiga et al. 1996; Rizzolatti, Fadiga et al. 1996). Critically, a similar mirror-neuron system has been discovered in humans, where it seems to be crucial in empathy and in social copnition (Rizzolatti, Fogassi, and Gallese 2001). In the study by Ricciardi et al. (Ricciardi, Bonino et al. 2009), sighted and congenitally early blind subjects had to listen to hand-executed actions or environmental sounds. In fact, a specific class of mirror neurons is known to discharge not only when the action is executed or observed, but also when its sound is heard or when the action is verbally described (Kohler, Keysers

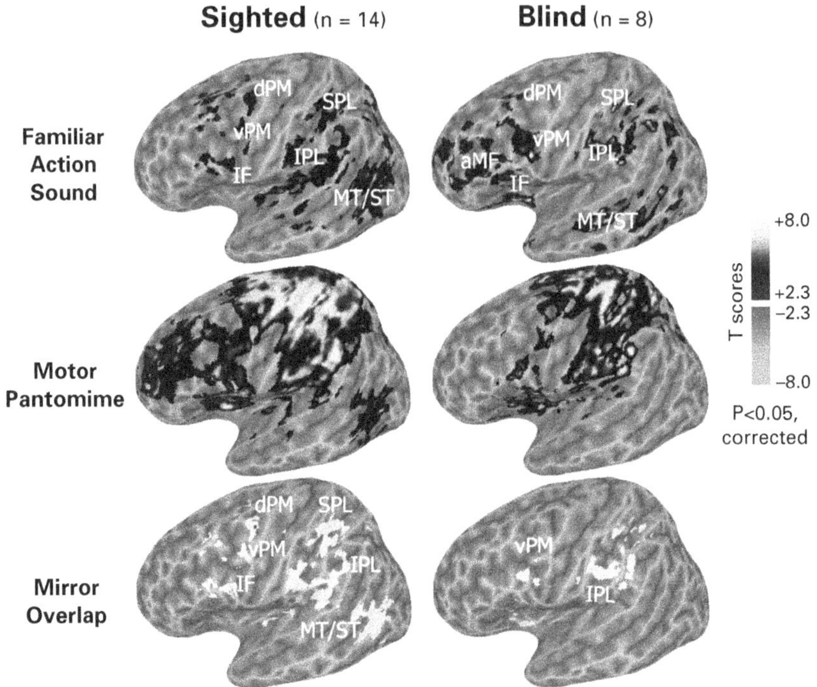

Figure 8.5

Statistical maps reported by Ricciardi et al. (Ricciardi, Bonino et al. 2009) showing activated brain regions during listening to *familiar* actions as compared to environmental sounds, and during the motor pantomime of action as compared to rest (corrected $p<0.05$). In both sighted and congenitally blind individuals, aural presentation of familiar actions as compared to the environmental sounds elicited similar patterns of activation involving a left-lateralized premotor, temporal and parietal cortical network. Hand-motor pantomimes evoked bilateral activations in premotor and sensorimotor areas. Auditory mirror voxels are shown in yellow as overlap between the two task conditions in the bottom row. Spatially normalized activations are projected onto a single-subject left-hemisphere template in Talairach space. aMF = anterior middle frontal gyrus; IF = inferior frontal gyrus; vPM = ventral premotor cortex; dPM = dorsal premotor cortex; MT/ST = middle temporal and superior temporal cortex; IPL = inferior parietal lobule; SPL = superior parietal lobule. (See plate 4.)

Reprinted from Ricciardi, Bonino et al., "Do we really need vision? How blind people 'see' the actions of others," *Journal of Neuroscience* 29(31) (2009): 9719–9724. (Reprinted by permission of Society for Neuroscience) et al. 2002). Critically, when listening to action sounds, the blind activated a left premotor-temporo-parietal network that subserved action-recognition and that substantially overlapped with the left-lateralized network elicited by auditory and visual action-related stimuli in the sighted control group. These findings by Ricciardi et al. (Ricciardi, Bonino et al. 2009) suggest that visual experience is not a prerequisite for the development of an efficient mirror-neuron system: rather, a motor representation of others' actions can be evoked through supramodal sensory mechanisms.

Conclusions

In this book we have discussed the effects that blindness and other less severe forms of visual impairment exert on perceptual and cognitive abilities. We have seen how touch and hearing capacities may gain acuity in blind individuals, reflecting real sensory improvements but also the contribution of attentional and cognitive mechanisms. We have shown how the mental world of a blind person can be as rich as that of a normally sighted person, containing vivid mental representations although these are mainly shaped by his or her dominant sensory modalities—that is, hearing and touch. Importantly, we have stressed how spatial features of objects can be efficiently extracted by touch (and hearing as well, especially for distant sources) and how mental representations of blind individuals may have an analogical spatial format. Blind individuals can produce line drawings that are easily understandable by a sighted person and are able to succeed in many imagery and working memory tasks which require that they draw spatial inferences and/or manipulate/integrate/combine different pieces of spatial information: how would this be possible if we do not assume that blind individuals experience visual-like analogical mental representations? Of course, the images generated by blind individuals mainly contain tactile and auditory details, but what should be clear after reading this book is that images in the blind do not consist of purely motor traces or auditory traces, but indeed of *analogical representations* that can be used to cope with everyday situations. The available dominant sensory experience creates differences in the spatial behavior of a blind and a sighted person: blind individuals tend to use their body as a reference frame (mainly relying on egocentric spatial representations) and to focus on near or peripersonal space—that is, on the portion of space that they can directly explore with their arm or long cane. Notably, the way spatial information is represented reflects the way it is acquired at the perceptual level, namely in a sequential fashion: for example, to go from their house to their office, blind individuals tend to generate "route-like" rather than "survey-like" types of representation, mainly relying on knowledge of landmarks. At the neurophysiological level, the gains in the auditory and tactile modalities and the differences in cognitive mechanisms often reported in blind individuals are subserved and modulated by both intramodal and crossmodal plasticity phenomena. Crossmodal plasticity affects not only sensory-specific areas, such as the visual cortex that gets recruited to process tactile or auditory information, but also supramodal areas which in sighted individuals process information regardless of its sensory format.

Throughout the book, we have tried to clarify the no less critical role of individual differences (such as locomotion abilities, Braille-reading proficiency, type of training received, nature of visual deficit, and so forth) and experimental factors (type of process involved, complexity of the tasks, and so on) in determining how well a blind (or visually impaired) person would perform in a given task. We have also stressed the critical importance of the visual deficit onset: in fact, both the age at onset of the visual deficit (i.e., congenital, a few months or years of life, or adulthood) and the duration of the visual deprivation differently affect the functional level, and modulate the robustness of compensatory phenomena at the sensory and cortical level. Finally, we have shown how visual impairment should not be considered as a unique category, since different forms of low vision are possible, mainly due to selective deficits in visual acuity or visual field, or depending upon imbalance between the two eyes, which not only result in specific perceptual limitations but also affect cognitive development.

The investigation of the psychological characteristics of blind individuals highlights that human cognitive development is not only shaped by the nature and amount of sensory experience but also presents a number of innate mechanisms and cortical networks that are able to process information in a supramodal fashion. In fact, data collected with the blind support the view that a peripheral deficit, although highly disadvantageous, does not prevent the development of high-level mechanisms such as those subserving the generation of mental representations or mediating spatial cognition, despite possible differences depending on the format of the incoming information.

Every year, we present and discuss data on blindness with students attending our psychology classes. This is a stimulating way to introduce them to theories and concepts regarding perception and to propose naïve questions (e.g., Can blind individuals imagine colors?) that may help them in understanding what memory is, how semantic representations are formed and accessed, and so on. Last year, we found out on the first day of our class that one of our students was congenitally blind. At first, we felt somehow embarrassed: how could we teach to a blind person what blindness is like? How could we talk about limits and deficits occurring in blindness in front of a blind student and her sighted mates? However, thanks to this student's contributions, that course represented one of those very fortunate and rare occasions in which teaching is supported by a first-person experience and by continuous confrontation. For instance, she spontaneously described how she usually experiences the world, noting: "I have learned to associate actions to specific sounds: for instance, I know that I shouldn't cross the street when I hear the sound of a car. Hearing helps to explore far space because by hearing it is possible to recognize sounds coming from several or many meters away, where they are coming from, and how far they are to me." Or: "Since I was a child, I have been taught how to recognize my clothes, how to read the time, and to distinguish the various coins using my hands." About colors she commented: "Colors are just verbal labels for me, but it is possible to make associations across the other senses knowing that a certain object has a specific color—for instance, since I know that the sun is yellow, I tend to associate the name 'yellow' with heat." And, about emotions: "I can recognize emotions only auditorily. I can't see tears on another person's face but I know when one is sad by listening to the particular inclinations in his or her voice." Sighted individuals are usually inclined to consider visual perception as the main—if not the unique—medium for experiencing the world. Nevertheless, throughout the book we have presented evidence that sight is not always the most accurate sensory channel; for example, attentional arousal is facilitated in the auditory modality, and texture recognition may be easier in haptic perception. The words of our blind student showed that the actual *understanding* of the physical world may not be so different in the absence of vision: spatial positions, objects' and other people's identity, emotional states—they can all be experienced through many different sensory modalities and the final outcome is identical, regardless of whether the visual channel is intact.

An outstanding example of how a "world of darkness" (in sighted people's words) may be rich and full of stimuli is represented by another congenitally blind woman. Antonella Cappabianca is a lawyer with a strong passion for horses (which she rides) and a special hobby: photography. How can a blind person enjoy taking pictures? Isn't photography quite a paradoxical hobby for a blind person? Yet her photographs have been hung in various exhibitions. In a booklet published on the occasion of one such presentation of her work, she wrote: "When I take a picture I speak the language of sighted individuals, but I reveal things about myself, because I depict only what evokes emotion in me and what I would like to tell or share with another person." Indeed, on first glance, her pictures look like the photographs that a non-professional photographer might take: a dog, a horse, a beach view. Sometimes her subjects' feet are cut from the bottom of the picture, or the "main subject" is not exactly centered. But all this would just be a superficial interpretation. Talking about a trip she took to Munich, she recalled: "When we arrived in that square, it was so beautiful that I felt I had to take a picture. . . . The sun on my face, the roaring of a fountain, happy people walking in a hurry. . . . Someone was laughing. A good smell of sweet food. But is it possible to take all this in a picture?" Perhaps it is: we see the fountain and musicians playing in the street, in her photograph, or even a watermill she "saw" in a museum. Antonella Cappabianca takes "comprehensive" pictures—she depicts odors as well as sounds, feelings, atmospheres.

Overall, the findings reported in this book suggest that the world of blind individuals is as rich as that of the sighted, or even more so: the external environment is usually shaped on sighted individuals' visual experience, yet the blind continuously translate an array of visually missing information into other sensory and cognitive codes they can interpret. Blindness is not simply "less" vision, it is an *other vision.*

References

Abel, S. M., and C. Tikuisis. 2005. Sound localization with monocular vision. *Applied Acoustics* 66 (8):932–944.

Adams, D. L., and J. C. Horton. 2002. Shadows cast by retinal blood vessels mapped in primary visual cortex. *Science* 298 (5593):572–576.

Adams, D. L., L. C. Sincich, and J. C. Horton. 2007. Complete pattern of ocular dominance columns in human primary visual cortex. *Journal of Neuroscience* 27 (39):10391–10403.

Afonso, A., A. Blum, B. F. G. Katz, P. Tarroux, G. Borst, and M. Denis. In press. Structural properties of spatial representations in blind people: Scanning images constructed from haptic exploration or from locomotion in a 3-D audio virtual environment. *Memory and Cognition.*

Ahissar, M., and S. Hochstein. 1993. Attentional control of early perceptual learning. *Proceedings of the National Academy of Sciences of the United States of America* 90 (12):5718–5722.

Alais, D., and D. Burr. 2004. The ventriloquist effect results from near-optimal bimodal integration. *Current Biology* 14 (3):257–262.

Alary, F., M. Duquette, R. Goldstein, C. E. Chapman, P. Voss, V. La Buissonnière-Ariza, and F. Lepore. 2009. Tactile acuity in the blind: A closer look reveals superiority over the sighted in some but not all cutaneous tasks. *Neuropsychologia* 47 (10):2037–2043.

Alary, F., R. Goldstein, M. Duquette, C. E. Chapman, P. Voss, and F. Lepore. 2008. Tactile acuity in the blind: A psychophysical study using a two-dimensional angle discrimination task. *Experimental Brain Research* 187 (4):587–594.

Aleman, A., L. van Lee, M. H. Mantione, I. G. Verkoijen, and E. H. de Haan. 2001. Visual imagery without visual experience: Evidence from congenitally totally blind people. *Neuroreport* 12 (11):2601–2604.

Amedi, A., A. Floel, S. Knecht, E. Zohary, and L. G. Cohen. 2004. Transcranial magnetic stimulation of the occipital pole interferes with verbal processing in blind subjects. *Nature Neuroscience* 7 (11):1266–1270.

Amedi, A., G. Jacobson, T. Hendler, R. Malach, and E. Zohary. 2002. Convergence of visual and tactile shape processing in the human lateral occipital complex. *Cerebral Cortex* 12 (11):1202–1212.

Amedi, A., R. Malach, T. Hendler, S. Peled, and E. Zohary. 2001. Visuo-haptic object-related activation in the ventral visual pathway. *Nature Neuroscience* 4 (3):324–330.

Amedi, A., R. Malach, and A. Pascual-Leone. 2005. Negative BOLD differentiates visual imagery and perception. *Neuron* 48 (5):859–872.

Amedi, A., L. B. Merabet, J. Camprodon, F. Bermpohl, S. Fox, I. Ronen, D. S. Kim, and A. Pascual-Leone. 2008. Neural and behavioral correlates of drawing in an early blind painter: A case study. *Brain Research* 1242:252–262.

Amedi, A., N. Raz, P. Pianka, R. Malach, and E. Zohary. 2003. Early "visual" cortex activation correlates with superior verbal memory performance in the blind. *Nature Neuroscience* 6 (7):758–766.

Andersen, E. S., A. Dunlea, and L. S. Kekelis. 1984. Blind children's language: Resolving some differences. *Journal of Child Language* 11:645–664.

Andersen, E. S., A. Dunlea, and L. S. Kekelis. 1993. The impact of input: Language acquisition in the visually impaired. *First Language* 13:23–49.

Anderson, R. C., E. T. Goetz, J. W. Pichert, and H. M. Halff. 1977. Two faces of the conceptual peg hypothesis. *Journal of Experimental Psychology. Human Learning and Memory* 3 (2):142–149.

Angelaki, D. E., and K. E. Cullen. 2008. Vestibular system: the many facets of a multimodal sense. *Annual Review of Neuroscience* 31:125–150.

Arditi, A., J. D. Holtzman, and S. M. Kosslyn. 1988. Mental imagery and sensory experience in congenital blindness. *Neuropsychologia* 26 (1):1–12.

Arlen, M. J. 2000. The tyranny of the visual. In *The Norton Reader: AANP*, ed. A. M. Eastman et al. New York: Norton, 1067–1074.

Armel, K. C., and V. S. Ramachandran. 1999. Acquired synesthesia in retinitis pigmentosa. *Neurocase: Case Studies in Neuropsychology, Neuropsychiatry, & Behavioural Neurology* 5 (4):293–296.

Arno, P., C. Capelle, M. C. Wanet-Defalque, M. Catalan-Ahumada, and C. Veraart. 1999. Auditory coding of visual patterns for the blind. *Perception* 28 (8):1013–1029.

Arno, P., A. G. De Volder, A. Vanlierde, M. C. Wanet-Defalque, E. Streel, A. Robert, S. Sanabria-Bohórquez, and C. Veraart. 2001. Occipital activation by pattern recognition in the early blind using auditory substitution for vision. *NeuroImage* 13 (4):632–645.

Arno, P., A. Vanlierde, E. Streel, M. C. Wanet-Defalque, S. Sanabria-Bohorquez, and C. Veraart. 2001. Auditory substitution of vision: Pattern recognition by the blind. *Applied Cognitive Psychology* 15:509–519.

Ashmead, D. H., D. L. Davis, and A. Northington. 1995. Contribution of listeners' approaching motion to auditory distance perception. *Journal of Experimental Psychology. Human Perception and Performance* 21 (2):239–256.

Ashmead, D. H., E. W. Hill, and C. R. Talor. 1989. Obstacle perception by congenitally blind children. *Perception & Psychophysics* 46 (5):425–433.

Ashmead, D. H., R. S. Wall, S. B. Eaton, K. A. Ebinger, M.-M. Snook-Hill, D. A. Guth, and X. Yang. 1998a. Echolocation reconsidered: Using spatial variations in the ambient sound field to guide locomotion. *Journal of Visual Impairment & Blindness* 92:615–632.

Ashmead, D. H., R. S. Wall, K. A. Ebinger, S. B. Eaton, M.-M. Snook-Hill, and X. Yang. 1998b. Spatial hearing in children with visual disabilities. *Perception* 27 (1):105–122.

Attneave, F., and T. E. Curlee. 1983. Locational representation in imagery: a moving spot task. *Journal of Experimental Psychology. Human Perception and Performance* 9 (1):20–30.

Auvray, M., and E. Myin. 2009. Perception with compensatory devices: From sensory substitution to sensorimotor extension. *Cognitive Science* 33 (7):1036–1058.

Axelrod, S. 1959. *Effects of Early Blindness*. New York: American Foundation for the Blind.

Azulay, H., E. Striem, and A. Amedi. 2009. Negative BOLD in sensory cortices during verbal memory: a component in generating internal representations? *Brain Topography* 21 (3–4):221–231.

Bach-y-Rita, P., C. C. Collins, F. A. Saunders, B. White, and L. Scadden. 1969. Vision substitution by tactile image projection. *Nature* 221 (5184):963–964.

Bach-y-Rita, P., and S. W. Kercel. 2003. Sensory substitution and the human-machine interface. *Trends in Cognitive Sciences* 7 (12):541–546.

Baddeley, A. D. 1986. *Working Memory*. Oxford: Oxford University Press.

Baddeley, A. 2000. The episodic buffer: A new component of working memory? *Trends in Cognitive Sciences* 4 (11):417–423.

Baddeley, A. 2003. Working memory: looking back and looking forward. *Nature Reviews. Neuroscience* 4 (10):829–839.

Baddeley, A. 2007. *Working Memory, Thought, and Action*. Oxford: Oxford University Press.

Baddeley, A. D., and J. Andrade. 2000. Working memory and the vividness of imagery. *Journal of Experimental Psychology. General* 129 (1):126–145.

Baddeley, A., and G. Hitch. 1974. Working memory. In *The Psychology of Learning and Motivation*, ed. G. Bower. New York: Academic Press, 47–89.

Baker, C. I., E. Peli, N. Knouf, and N. G. Kanwisher. 2005. Reorganization of visual processing in macular degeneration. *Journal of Neuroscience* 25 (3):614–618.

Ballesteros, S., L. Bardisa, S. Millar, and J. M. Reales. 2005. The haptic test battery: A new instrument to test tactual abilities in blind and visually impaired and sighted children. *British Journal of Visual Impairment* 23:11–24.

Ballesteros, S., and J. M. Reales. 2004. Visual and haptic discrimination of symmetry in unfamiliar displays extended in the z-axis. *Perception* 33 (3):315–327.

Barbeito, R. 1983. Sighting from the cyclopean eye: the cyclops effect in preschool children. *Perception & Psychophysics* 33 (6):561–564.

Barolo, E., R. Masini, and A. Antonietti. 1990. Mental rotation of solid objects and problem-solving in sighted and blind subjects. *Journal of Mental Imagery* 14 (3–4):65–74.

Baron-Cohen, S., and J. Harrison. 1996. *Synesthesia: Classic and Contemporary Readings*. Oxford: Blackwell.

Barrett, A. M., and S. Burkholder. 2006. Monocular patching in subjects with right-hemisphere stroke affects perceptual-attentional bias. *Journal of Rehabilitation Research and Development* 43 (3):337–346.

Barrett, B. T., A. Bradley, and P. V. McGraw. 2004. Understanding the neural basis of amblyopia. *Neuroscientist* 10 (2):106–117.

Barrouillet, P., S. Bernardin, and V. Camos. 2004. Time constraints and resource sharing in adults' working memory spans. *Journal of Experimental Psychology. General* 133 (1):83–100.

Barsalou, L. W. 1999. Perceptual symbol systems. *Behavioral and Brain Sciences* 22 (4):577–609, discussion 610–660.

Bartels, A., and S. Zeki. 2004. Functional brain mapping during free viewing of natural scenes. *Human Brain Mapping* 21:75–83.

Bartolomeo, P., and A. C. Bachoud-Lévi, J. D. Degos, and F. Boller. 1998. Disruption of residual reading capacity in a pure alexic patient after a mirror-image right-hemispheric lesion. *Neurology* 50 (1):286–288.

Bavelier, D., and H. J. Neville. 2002. Cross-modal plasticity: Where and how? *Nature Reviews. Neuroscience* 3 (6):443–452.

Bavelier, D., A. Tomann, C. Hutton, T. Mitchell, D. Corina, G. Liu, and H. Neville. 2000. Visual attention to the periphery is enhanced in congenitally deaf individuals. *Journal of Neuroscience* 20 (17):1–6.

Beaver, C. J., Q. Ji, and N. W. Daw. 2001. Layer differences in the effect of monocular vision in light- and dark-reared kittens. *Visual Neuroscience* 18 (5):811–820.

Bedny, M., A. Pascual-Leone, and R. R. Saxe. 2009. Growing up blind does not change the neural bases of Theory of Mind. *Proceedings of the National Academy of Sciences of the United States of America* 106 (27):11312–11317.

Bedny, M., T. Konkle, A. K. Pelphrey, R. Saxe, and A. Pascual-Leone. In press. Sensitive period for a vision-dominated response in human MT/MST. *Current Biology.*

Beis, J. M., J. M. Andre, A. Baumgarten, and B. Challier. 1999. Eye patching in unilateral spatial neglect: Efficacy of two methods. *Archives of Physical Medicine and Rehabilitation* 80 (1):71–76.

Belin, P., R. J. Zatorre, and P. Ahad. 2002. Human temporal-lobe response to vocal sounds. *Brain Research. Cognitive Brain Research* 13 (1):17–26.

Benedetti, L. H., and M. Loeb. 1972. A comparison of auditory monitoring performances in blind subjects with that of sighted subjects in light and dark. *Perception & Psychophysics* 11 (1): 10–16.

Berardi, N., T. Pizzorusso, and L. Maffei. 2000. Critical periods during sensory development. *Current Opinion in Neurobiology* 10 (1):138–145.

Bergen, B., and N. Chang. 2005. Embodied construction grammar in simulation-based language understanding. In *Construction Grammars: Cognitive Grounding and Theoretical Extensions*, ed. J.-O. Östman and M. Fried. Amsterdam: Benjamins, 147–190.

Berman, N. E. 1991. Alterations of visual cortical connections in cats following early removal of retinal input. *Brain Research: Developmental Brain Research* 63 (1–2):163–180.

Bertelson, P. 1999. Ventriloquism: A case of crossmodal perceptual grouping. In *Cognitive Contributions to the Perception of Spatial and Temporal Events*, ed. G. Aschersleben, T. Bachmann, and J. Müsseler. Amsterdam: Elsevier, 347–362.

Bertolo, H. 2005. Visual imagery without visual perception? *Psicológica* 26:173–188.

Bertolo, H., T. Paiva, L. Pessoa, T. Mestre, R. Marques, and R. Santos. 2003. Visual dream content, graphical representation and EEG alpha activity in congenitally blind subjects. *Brain Research: Cognitive Brain Research* 15 (3):277–284.

Bigelow, A. E. 1996. Blind and sighted children's spatial knowledge of the home environments. *International Journal of Behavioral Development* 19:797–808.

Binet, A. 1894. *Psychologie des grands calculateurset joueurs d'échecs.* Paris: Hachette.

Blanco, F., and D. Travieso. 2003. Haptic exploration and mental estimation of distances in a fictitious island: From mind's eye to mind's hand. *Journal of Visual Impairment & Blindness* 97:298–300.

Blasch, B. B., and W. R. Wiener, and R. L. Welsh, eds. 1997. *Foundations of Orientation and Mobility.* New York: American Foundation for the Blind Press.

Blauert, J. 1997. *Spatial Hearing: The Psychophysics of Human Sound Localization.* Cambridge, MA: MIT Press.

Bliss, I., and T. Kujala, and H. Hämäläinen. 2004. Comparison of blind and sighted participants' performance in a letter recognition working memory task. *Brain Research: Cognitive Brain Research* 18 (3):273–277.

Bonato, M., K. Priftis, R. Marenzi, and M. Zorzi. 2008. Modulation of hemispatial neglect by directional and numerical cues in the line bisection task. *Neuropsychologia* 46 (2):426–433.

Bonino, D., E. Ricciardi, L. Sani, C. Gentili, N. Vanello, M. Guazzelli, T. Vecchi, and P. Pietrini. 2008. Tactile spatial working memory activates the dorsal extrastriate cortical pathway in congenitally blind individuals. *Archives Italiennes de Biologie* 146 (3–4):133–146.

Booth, J. L., and R. S. Siegler. 2006. Developmental and individual differences in pure numerical estimation. *Developmental Psychology* 42 (1):189–201.

Boroditsky, L. 2000. Metaphoric structuring: Understanding time through spatial metaphors. *Cognition* 75 (1):1–28.

Boroojerdi, B., K. O. Bushara, B. Corwell, I. Immisch, F. Battaglia, W. Muellbacher, and L. G. Cohen. 2000. Enhanced excitability of the human visual cortex induced by short-term light deprivation. *Cerebral Cortex* 10 (5):529–534.

Borst, G., and S. M. Kosslyn. 2008. Visual mental imagery and visual perception: structural equivalence revealed by scanning processes. *Memory & Cognition* 36 (4):849–862.

Bower, G. H. 1972. Mental imagery and associative learning. In *Cognition in Learning and Memory*, ed. L. Gregg. London: John Wiley, 51–88.

Bowers, D., and K. M. Heilman. 1980. Pseudoneglect: effects of hemispace on a tactile line bisection task. *Neuropsychologia* 18 (4–5):491–498.

Braun, C., R. Schweizer, T. Elbert, N. Birbaumer, and E. Taub. 2000. Differential activation in somatosensory cortex for different discrimination tasks. *Journal of Neuroscience* 20 (1):446–450.

Brewer, W. F., and M. Schommer-Aikins. 2006. Scientists are not deficient in mental imagery: Galton revised. *Review of General Psychology* 10:130–146.

Brisben, A. J., S. S. Hsiao, and K. O. Johnson. 1999. Detection of vibration transmitted through an object grasped in the hand. *Journal of Neurophysiology* 81 (4):1548–1558.

Bross, M., and M. Borenstein. 1982. Temporal auditory acuity in blind and sighted subjects: A signal detection analysis. *Perceptual and Motor Skills* 55 (3):963–966.

Buchel, C., C. Price, R. S. Frackowiak, and K. Friston. 1998. Different activation patterns in the visual cortex of late and congenitally blind subjects. *Brain* 121 (3):409–419.

Bull, R., H. Rathborn, and B. R. Clifford. 1983. The voice-recognition accuracy of blind listeners. *Perception* 12 (2):223–226.

Burgess, N. 2006. Spatial memory: How egocentric and allocentric combine. *Trends in Cognitive Sciences* 10 (12):551–557.

Burgess, N. 2008. Spatial cognition and the brain. *Annals of the New York Academy of Sciences* 1124:77–97.

Burgess, N., E. A. Maguire, H. J. Spiers, and J. O'Keefe. 2001. A temporoparietal and prefrontal network for retrieving the spatial context of lifelike events. *NeuroImage* 14 (2):439–453.

Burton, H. 2003. Visual cortex activity in early and late blind people. *Journal of Neuroscience* 23 (10):4005–4011.

Burton, H., J. B. Diamond, and K. B. McDermott. 2003. Dissociating cortical regions activated by semantic and phonological tasks: An fMRI study in blind and sighted people. *Journal of Neurophysiology* 90 (3):1965–1982.

Burton, H., and D. G. McLaren. 2006. Visual cortex activation in late-onset, Braille naive blind individuals: An fMRI study during semantic and phonological tasks with heard words. *Neuroscience Letters* 392 (1–2):38–42.

Burton, H., D. G. McLaren, and R. J. Sinclair. 2006. Reading embossed capital letters: An fMRI study in blind and sighted individuals. *Human Brain Mapping* 27 (4):325–339.

Burton, H., R. J. Sinclair, and S. Dixit. 2010. Working memory for vibrotactile frequencies: Comparison of cortical activity in blind and sighted individuals. *Human Brain Mapping*.

Burton, H., R. J. Sinclair, and D. G. McLaren. 2004. Cortical activity to vibrotactile stimulation: An fMRI study in blind and sighted individuals. *Human Brain Mapping* 23 (4):210–228.

Burton, H., A. Z. Snyder, T. E. Conturo, E. Akbudak, J. M. Ollinger, and M. E. Raichle. 2002a. Adaptive changes in early and late blind: An fMRI study of Braille reading. *Journal of Neurophysiology* 87 (1):589–607.

Burton, H., A. Z. Snyder, J. B. Diamond, and M. E. Raichle. 2002b. Adaptive changes in early and late blind: An fMRI study of verb generation to heard nouns. *Journal of Neurophysiology* 88 (6):3359–3371.

Butter, C. M., and N. Kirsch. 1992. Combined and separate effects of eye patching and visual stimulation on unilateral neglect following stroke. *Archives of Physical Medicine and Rehabilitation* 73 (12):1133–1139.

Caramazza, A., and B. Z. Mahon. 2003. The organization of conceptual knowledge: The evidence from category-specific semantic deficits. *Trends in Cognitive Sciences* 7 (8):354–361.

Carlson, S., L. Hyvarinen, and A. Raninen. 1986. Persistent behavioural blindness after early visual deprivation and active visual rehabilitation: A case report. *British Journal of Ophthalmology* 70 (8):607–611.

Carpenter, P. A., and P. Eisenberg. 1978. Mental rotation and the frame of reference in blind and sighted individuals. *Perception & Psychophysics* 23 (2):117–124.

Carreiras, M. and M. Codina. 1992. Spatial cognition of the blind and sighted: Visual and amodal hypotheses. *Cahiers de Psychologie Cognitive/Current Psychology of Cognition* 12:51–78.

Carruthers, M. 1990. *The Book of Memory*. Cambridge: Cambridge University Press.

Carruthers, M. 1998. *The Craft of Thought*. Cambridge: Cambridge University Press.

Casey, S. M. 1978. Cognitive mapping by the blind. *Journal of Visual Impairment & Blindness* 72:297–301.

Castronovo, J., and X. Seron. 2007a. Numerical estimation in blind subjects: Evidence of the impact of blindness and its following experience. *Journal of Experimental Psychology: Human Perception and Performance* 33 (5):1089–1106.

Castronovo, J., and X. Seron. 2007b. Semantic numerical representation in blind subjects: The role of vision in the spatial format of the mental number line. *Quarterly Journal of Experimental Psychology* 60 (1):101–119.

Cattaneo, Z., M. Fantino, J. Silvanto, C. Tinti, A. Pascual-Leone, and T. Vecchi. 2010a. Symmetry perception in the blind. *Acta Psychologica* 134 (3):398–402.

Cattaneo, Z., M. Fantino, J. Silvanto, C. Tinti, and T. Vecchi. Under revision a. Blind individuals show pseudoneglect in bisecting numberical intervals. *Attention, Perception, and Psychophysics.*

Cattaneo, Z., M. Fantino, C. Tinti, A. Pascual-Leone, J. Silvanto and T. Vecchi. Under revision b. Spatial biases in peripersonal space in sighted and blind individuals revealed by a haptic line bisection paradigm. *Journal of Experimental Psychology: Human Perception and Performance.*

Cattaneo, Z., M. Fantino, C. Tinti, J. Silvanto, and T. Vecchi. 2010b. Crossomodal interaction between the mental number line and peripersonal haptic space representation in sighted and blind individuals. *Attention, Perception and Psychopysics* 72:885–890.

Cattaneo, Z., L. B. Merabet, E. Bhatt, and T. Vecchi. 2008. Effects of complete monocular deprivation in visuo-spatial memory. *Brain Research Bulletin* 77 (2–3):112–116.

Cattaneo, Z., J. Silvanto, A. Pascual-Leone, and L. Battelli. 2009. The role of the angular gyrus in the modulation of visuospatial attention by the mental number line. *NeuroImage* 44 (2):563–568.

Cattaneo, Z., and T. Vecchi. 2008. Supramodality effects in visual and haptic spatial processes. *Journal of Experimental Psychology. Learning, Memory, and Cognition* 34 (3):631–642.

Cattaneo, Z., T. Vecchi, C. Cornoldi, I. Mammarella, D. Bonino, E. Ricciardi, and P. Pietrini. 2008. Imagery and spatial processes in visual impairments. *Neuroscience and Biobehavioral Reviews* 32: 1346–1360.

Cattaneo, Z., T. Vecchi, M. Monegato, A. Pece, and C. Cornoldi. 2007. Effects of late visual impairment on mental representations activated by visual and tactile stimuli. *Brain Research* 1148:170–176.

Chalupa, L. M., and R. W. Williams. 1984. Organization of the cat's lateral geniculate nucleus following interruption of prenatal binocular competition. *Human Neurobiology* 3 (2):103–107.

Chao, L. L., A. Martin, and J. V. Haxby. 1999. Are face-responsive regions selective only for faces? *Neuroreport* 10 (14):2945–2950.

Chapman, C. E. 1994. Active versus passive touch: factors influencing the transmission of somatosensory signals to primary somatosensory cortex. *Canadian Journal of Physiology and Pharmacology* 72 (5):558–570.

Chatterjee, A., and M. H. Southwood. 1995. Cortical blindness and visual imagery. *Neurology* 45 (12):2189–2195.

Chebat, D. R., C. Rainville, R. Kupers, and M. Ptito. 2007. Tactile-"visual" acuity of the tongue in early blind individuals. *Neuroreport* 18 (18):1901–1904.

Chelazzi, L., E. K. Miller, J. Duncan, and R. Desimone. 2001. Responses of neurons in macaque area V4 during memory-guided visual search. *Cerebral* 11 (8):761–772.

Cheung, S. H., F. Fang, S. He, and G. E. Legge. 2009. Retinotopically specific reorganization of visual cortex for tactile pattern recognition. *Current Biology* 19 (7):596–601.

Chown, E., S. Kaplan, and D. Kortenkamp. 1995. Prototypes, Location, and Associative Networks (PLAN): Towards a unified theory of cognitive mapping. *Cognitive Science* 19:1–52.

Christou, C. G., and H. H. Bulthoff. 1999. View dependence in scene recognition after active learning. *Memory & Cognition* 27 (6):996–1007.

Ciuffreda, K. J. 1991. The Glenn A. Fry invited lecture: Accommodation to gratings and more naturalistic stimuli. *Optometry and Vision Science* 68 (4):243–260.

Clearfield, M. W., and K. S. Mix. 2001. Infants use continuous quantity—not number—to discriminate small visual sets. *Journal of Cognition and Development* 2 (3):243–260.

Clement, C. A., and R. J. Falmagne. 1986. Logical reasoning, world knowledge, and mental imagery: Interconnections in cognitive processes. *Memory & Cognition* 14 (4):299–307.

Cobb, N. J., D. M. Lawrence, and N. D. Nelson. 1979. Report on blind subjects' tactile and auditory recognition for environmental stimuli. *Perceptual and Motor Skills* 48 (2):363–366.

Cohen, L. G., P. Celnik, A. Pascual-Leone, B. Corwell, L. Falz, J. Dambrosia, M. Honda, N. Sadato, C. Gerloff, M. D. Catalá, and M. Hallett. 1997. Functional relevance of cross-modal plasticity in blind humans. *Nature* 389 (6647):180–183.

Cohen, L. G., R. A. Weeks, N. Sadato, P. Celnik, K. Ishii, and M. Hallett. 1999. Period of susceptibility for cross-modal plasticity in the blind. *Annals of Neurology* 45 (4):451–460.

Cohen, M. S., S. M. Kosslyn, H. C. Breiter, G. J. DiGirolamo, W. L. Thompson, A. K. Anderson, S. Y. Brookheimer, B. R. Rosen, and J. W. Belliveau. 1996. Changes in cortical activity during mental rotation: A mapping study using functional MRI. *Brain* 119 (1):89–100.

Colavita, F. B. 1974. Insular-temporal lesions and vibrotactile temporal pattern discrimination in cats. *Physiology & Behavior* 12 (2):215–218.

Collignon, O., G. Charbonneau, M. Lassonde, and F. Lepore. 2009c. Early visual deprivation alters multisensory processing in peripersonal space. *Neuropsychologia* 47 (14):3236–3243.

Collignon, O., M. Davare, A. G. De Volder, C. Poirier, E. Olivier, and C. Veraart. 2008. Time-course of posterior parietal and occipital cortex contribution to sound localization. *Journal of Cognitive Neuroscience* 20 (8):1454–1463.

Collignon, O., M. Davare, E. Olivier, and A. G. De Volder. 2009. Reorganisation of the right occipito-parietal stream for auditory spatial processing in early blind humans: A transcranial magnetic stimulation study. *Brain Topography* 21 (3–4):232–240.

Collignon, O., and A. G. De Volder. 2009. Further evidence that congenitally blind participants react faster to auditory and tactile spatial targets. *Canadian Journal of Experimental Psychology* 63(4): 287–293.

Collignon, O., M. Lassonde, F. Lepore, D. Bastien, and C. Veraart. 2007. Functional cerebral reorganization for auditory spatial processing and auditory substitution of vision in early blind subjects. *Cerebral Cortex* 17 (2):457–465.

Collignon, O., L. Renier, R. Bruyer, D. Tranduy, and C. Veraart. 2006. Improved selective and divided spatial attention in early blind subjects. *Brain Research* 1075 (1):175–182.

Collignon, O., P. Voss, M. Lassonde, and F. Lepore. 2009. Cross-modal plasticity for the spatial processing of sounds in visually deprived subjects. *Experimental Brain Research* 192 (3): 343–358.

Coluccia, E., I. C. Mammarella, and C. Cornoldi. 2009. Centred egocentric, decentred egocentric, and allocentric spatial representations in the peripersonal space of congenital total blindness. *Perception* 38 (5):679–693.

Connolly, A. C., L. R. Gleitman, and S. L. Thompson-Schill. 2007. Effect of congenital blindness on the semantic representation of some everyday concepts. *Proceedings of the National Academy of Sciences of the United States of America* 104 (20):8241–8246.

Connor, C. E., and K. O. Johnson. 1992. Neural coding of tactile texture: comparison of spatial and temporal mechanisms for roughness perception. *Journal of Neuroscience* 12 (9):3414–3426.

Conway, M. A., and C. W. Pleydell-Pearce. 2000. The construction of autobiographical memories in the self-memory system. *Psychological Review* 107 (2):261–288.

Cornoldi, C., B. Bertuccelli, P. Rocchi, and B. Sbrana. 1993. Processing capacity limitations in pictorial and spatial representations in the totally congenitally blind. *Cortex* 29 (4):675–689.

Cornoldi, C., D. Calore, and A. Pra-Baldi. 1979. Imagery rating and recall in congenitally blind subjects. *Perceptual and Motor Skills* 48 (2):627–639.

Cornoldi, C., A. Cortesi, and D. Preti. 1991. Individual differences in the capacity limitations of visuospatial short-term memory: Research on sighted and totally congenitally blind people. *Memory & Cognition* 19 (5):459–468.

Cornoldi, C., and R. De Beni. 1985. Effects of loci mnemonic in memorization of concrete words. *Acta Psychologica* 60:11–24.

Cornoldi, C., R. De Beni, F. Giusberti, and M. Massironi. 1998. Memory and imagery: A visual trace is not a mental image. In *Theories of Memory*, vol. 2, ed. M. Conway, S. Gathercole, and C. Cornoldi. Hove: Psychology Press, 87–110.

Cornoldi, C., R. De Beni, S. Roncari, and S. Romano. 1989. The effects of imagery instructions on totally congenitally blind recall. *European Journal of Cognitive Psychology* 1:321–331.

Cornoldi, C., C. Tinti, I. C. Mammarella, A. M. Re, and D. Varotto. 2009. Memory for an imagined pathway and strategy effects in sighted and in totally congenitally blind individuals. *Acta Psychologica* 130 (1):11–16.

Cornoldi, C., and T. Vecchi. 2000. Mental imagery in blind people: The role of passive and active visuo-spatial processes. In *Touch, Representation, and Blindness*, ed. M. E. Heller. Oxford: Oxford University Press, 143–181.

Cornoldi, C., and T. Vecchi. 2003. *Visuo-Spatial Working Memory and Individual Differences*. Hove: Psychology Press.

Correa, A., J. Lupianez, E. Madrid, and P. Tudela. 2006. Temporal attention enhances early visual processing: A review and new evidence from event-related potentials. *Brain Research* 1076 (1):116–128.

Cowan, N. 1995. *Attention and Memory: An Integrated Framework*. New York: Oxford University Press.

Cowan, N. 2005. *Working Memory Capacity*. New York: Psychology Press.

Cowey, A., and V. Walsh. 2000. Magnetically induced phosphenes in sighted, blind and blind-sighted observers. *Neuroreport* 11 (14):3269–3273.

Craig, J. C. 1999. Grating orientation as a measure of tactile spatial acuity. *Somatosensory & Motor Research* 16 (3):197–206.

Craig, J. C., and K. O. Johnson. 2000. The two-point threshold: Not a measure of tactile spatial resolution. *Current Directions in Psychological Science* 9:29–32.

Cronly-Dillon, J., K. Persaud, and R. P. Gregory. 1999. The perception of visual images encoded in musical form: A study in cross-modality information transfer. *Proceedings. Biological Sciences* 266 (1436):2427–2433.

Cuevas, I., P. Plaza, P. Rombaux, A. G. De Volder, and L. Renier. 2009. Odour discrimination and identification are improved in early blindness. *Neuropsychologia* 47 (14):3079–3083.

Cui, X., C. B. Jeter, D. Yang, P. R. Montague, and D. M. Eagleman. 2007. Vividness of mental imagery: Individual variability can be measured objectively. *Vision Research* 47 (4):474–478.

Cutsforth, T. D. and R. H. Wheeler. 1966. The synaesthesia of a blind subject with comparative data from an asynaesthetic blind subject. *American Foundation for the Blind, Research Bulletin* 12: 1–17.

D'Angiulli, A., J. M. Kennedy, and M. A. Heller. 1998. Blind children recognizing tactile pictures respond like sighted children given guidance in exploration. *Scandinavian Journal of Psychology* 39 (3):187–190.

D'Angiulli, A., and S. Maggi. 2003. Development of drawing abilities in a distinct population: Depiction of perceptual principles by three children with congenital total blindness. *International Journal of Behavioral Development* 27:193–200.

Dandona, L., and R. Dandona. 2006. What is the global burden of visual impairment? *BMC Medicine* 4:6.

Darwin, C. 1873. On the origin of certain instincts. *Nature* 7:417–418.

Davidson, P. W. 1972. Haptic judgments of curvature by blind and sighted humans. *Journal of Experimental Psychology* 93 (1):43–55.

Daw, N. W. 1995. *Visual Development*. New York: Plenum Press.

Day, S. 1995. Vision development in the monocular individual: implications for the mechanisms of normal binocular vision development and the treatment of infantile esotropia. *Transactions of the American Ophthalmological Society* 93:523–581.

De Beni, R., and C. Cornoldi. 1988. Imagery limitations in totally congenitally blind subjects. *Journal of Experimental Psychology: Learning, Memory, and Cognition* 14 (4):650–655.

de Hevia, D. M., L. Girelli, and G. Vallar. 2006. Numbers and space: a cognitive illusion? *Experimental Brain Research* 168:254–264.

De Soto, C. B., M. London, and S. Handel. 1965. Social reasoning and spatial paralogic. *Journal of Personality and Social Psychology* 2:513–521.

De Volder, A. G., H. Toyama, Y. Kimura, M. Kiyosawa, H. Nakano, A. Vanlierde, M. C. Wanet-Defalque, M. Mishina, K. Oda, K. Ishiwata, and M. Senda. 2001. Auditory triggered mental imagery of shape involves visual association areas in early blind humans. *NeuroImage* 14 (1):129–139.

Dechent, P., K. D. Merboldt, and J. Frahm. 2004. Is the human primary motor cortex involved in motor imagery? *Brain Research. Cognitive Brain Research* 19 (2):138–144.

Dehaene, S. 1992. Varieties of numerical abilities. *Cognition* 44 (1–2):1–42.

Dehaene, S. 1997. *The Number Sense*. New York: Oxford University Press.

Dehaene, S., S. Bossini, and P. Giraux. 1993. The mental representation of parity and numerical magnitude. *Journal of Experimental Psychology: General* 122:371–396.

Dehaene, S., G. Dehaene-Lambertz, and L. Cohen. 1998. Abstract representations of numbers in the animal and human brain. *Trends in Neurosciences* 21 (8):355–361.

Deibert, E., M. Kraut, S. Kremen, and J. Hart Jr. 1999. Neural pathways in tactile object recognition. *Neurology* 52 (7):1413–1417.

Dengis, C. A., T. L. Simpson, M. J. Steinbach, and H. Ono. 1998. The Cyclops effect in adults: Sighting without visual feedback. *Vision Research* 38 (2):327–331.

Dengis, C. A., M. J. Steinbach, and S. Kraft. 1992. Monocular occlusion for one month: Lack of effect on a variety of visual functions in normal adults. *Investigative Ophthalmology & Visual Science* Supplement 33:1154.

Denis, M., and S. M. Kosslyn. 1999. Scanning visual images: A window on the mind. *Cahiers de Psychologie Cognitive/Current Psychology of Cognition* 18:409–465.

Denis, S., and J. L. Boucher. 1991. Spatial representation of a two-dimensional pattern. *Canadian Journal of Psychology* 45 (3):405–414.

Desimone, R. 1996. Neural mechanisms for visual memory and their role in attention. *Proceedings of the National Academy of Sciences of the United States of America* 93 (24):13494–13499.

Déspres, O., V. Candas, and A. Dufour. 2005a. Spatial auditory compensation in early-blind humans: Involvement of eye movements and/or attention orienting? *Neuropsychologia* 43 (13):1955–1962.

Déspres, O., V. Candas, and A. Dufour. 2005b. The extent of visual deficit and auditory spatial compensation: Evidence from self-positioning from auditory cues. *Brain Research. Cognitive Brain Research* 23 (2–3):444–447.

Déspres, O., V. Candas, and A. Dufour. 2005c. Auditory compensation in myopic humans: Involvement of binaural, monaural, or echo cues? *Brain Research* 1041 (1):56–65.

Deutschlander, A., T. Stephan, K. Hüfner, J. Wagner, M. Wiesmann, M. Strupp, T. Brandt, and K. Jahn. 2009. Imagined locomotion in the blind: An fMRI study. *NeuroImage* 45 (1):122–128.

Divenyi, P. L., and I. J. Hirsh. 1974. Identification of temporal order in three-tone sequences. *Journal of the Acoustical Society of America* 56 (1):144–151.

Dodds, A. G., and D. D. Carter. 1983. Memory for movement in blind children: The role of previous visual experience. *Journal of Motor Behavior* 15 (4):343–352.

Doshi, N. R., and M. L. Rodriguez. 2007. Amblyopia. *American Family Physician* 75 (3):361–367.

Doucet, M. E., J. P. Guillemot, M. Lassonde, J. P. Gagné, C. Leclerc, and F. Lepore. 2005. Blind subjects process auditory spectral cues more efficiently than sighted individuals. *Experimental Brain Research* 160 (2):194–202.

Driver, J., and T. Noesselt. 2008. Multisensory interplay reveals crossmodal influences on "sensory-specific" brain regions, neural responses, and judgments. *Neuron* 57 (1):11–23.

Dufour, A., O. Déspres, and V. Candas. 2005. Enhanced sensitivity to echo cues in blind subjects. *Experimental Brain Research* 165 (4):515–519.

Dufour, A., and Y. Gérard. 2000. Improved auditory spatial sensitivity in near-sighted subjects. *Brain Research. Cognitive Brain Research* 10 (1–2):159–165.

Dulin, D., Y. Hatwell, Z. Pylyshyn, and S. Chokron. 2008. Effects of peripheral and central visual impairment on mental imagery capacity. *Neuroscience and Biobehavioral Reviews* 32 (8):1396–1408.

Eardley, A. F., and L. Pring. 2006. Remembering the past and imagining the future: A role for nonvisual imagery in the everyday cognition of blind and sighted people. *Memory* 14 (8):925–936.

Eardley, A. F., and L. Pring. 2007. Spatial processing, mental imagery, and creativity in individuals with and without sight. *European Journal of Cognitive Psychology* 19:37–58.

Eimer, M. 2004. Multisensory integration: How visual experience shapes spatial perception. *Current Biology* 14 (3):R115–R117.

Ek, U., S. Seregard, L. Jacobson, K. Oskar, E. Af Trampe, and E. Kock. 2002. A prospective study of children treated for retinoblastoma: Cognitive and visual outcomes in relation to treatment. *Acta Ophthalmologica Scandinavica* 80 (3):294–299.

Elbert, T., C. Pantev, C. Wienbruch, B. Rockstroh, and E. Taub. 1995. Increased cortical representation of the fingers of the left hand in string players. *Science* 270 (5234):305–307.

Elbert, T., A. Sterr, B. Rockstroh, C. Pantev, M. M. Müller, and E. Taub. 2002. Expansion of the tonotopic area in the auditory cortex of the blind. *Journal of Neuroscience* 22 (22):9941–9944.

Eldridge, R., K. O'Meara, and D. Kitchin. 1972. Superior intelligence in sighted retinoblastoma patients and their families. *Journal of Medical Genetics* 9 (3):331–335.

Epstein, W., B. Hughes, S. L. Schneider, and P. Bach-y-Rita. 1989. Perceptual learning of spatiotemporal events: Evidence from an unfamiliar modality. *Journal of Experimental Psychology. Human Perception and Performance* 15 (1):28–44.

Ernst, M. O., and H. H. Bulthoff. 2004. Merging the senses into a robust percept. *Trends in Cognitive Sciences* 8 (4):162–169.

Espinosa, M. A., S. Ungar, E. Ochaita, M. Blades, and C. Spencer. 1998. Comparing methods for introducing blind and visually impaired people to unfamiliar urban environments. *Journal of Environmental Psychology* 18:277–287.

Evans, J. S. B. T., S. E. Newstead, and R. M. J. Byrne. 1993. *Human Reasoning: The Psychology of Deduction*. Hove: Lawrence Erlbaum Associates.

Facchini, S., and S. M. Aglioti. 2003. Short term light deprivation increases tactile spatial acuity in humans. *Neurology* 60 (12):1998–1999.

Fangmeier, T., and M. Knauff. 2009. Neural correlates of acoustic reasoning. *Brain Research* 1249:181–190.

Farah, M. J., K. M. Hammond, D. N. Levine, and R. Calvanio. 1988. Visual and spatial mental imagery: Dissociable systems of representation. *Cognitive Psychology* 20 (4):439–462.

Farrell, M. J., and J. A. Thomson. 1999. On-line updating of spatial information during locomotion without vision. *Journal of Motor Behavior* 3:39–53.

Feinsod, M., P. Bach-y-Rita, and J. M. Madey. 1973. Somatosensory evoked responses: Latency differences in blind and sighted persons. *Brain Research* 60 (1):219–223.

Felleman, D. J., and D. C. Van Essen. 1991. Distributed hierarchical processing in the primate cerebral cortex. *Cerebral Cortex* 1 (1):1–47.

Fennema, E. 1979. Women and girls in mathematics—equity in mathematics education. *Educational Studies in Mathematics* 10:389–401.

Ferguson, E. S. 1977. The mind's eye: Nonverbal thought in technology. *Science* 197 (4306):827–836.

Fertsch, P. F. 1947. Hand dominance in reading Braille. *Journal of Child Psychology and Psychiatry, and Allied Disciplines* 27:367–381.

Fias, W., M. Brysbaert, F. Geypens, and G. d'Ydewalle. 1996. The importance of magnitude information in numerical processing: Evidence from the SNARC effect. *Mathematical Cognition* 2:95–110.

Fiehler, K., M. Burke, S. Bien, B. Röder, and F. Rösler. 2009. The human dorsal action control system develops in the absence of vision. *Cerebral Cortex* 19 (1):1–12.

Fiehler, K., J. Reuschel, and F. Rösler. 2009. Early non-visual experience influences proprioceptive-spatial discrimination acuity in adulthood. *Neuropsychologia* 47 (3):897–906.

Findlay, J. M., and I. D. Gilchrist. 2003. *Active Vision: The Psychology of Looking and Seeing*. Oxford: Oxford University Press.

Fine, I., A. R. Wade, A. A. Brewer, M. G. May, D. F. Goodman, G. M. Boynton, B. A. Wandell, and D. I. MacLeod. 2003. Long-term deprivation affects visual perception and cortex. *Nature Neuroscience* 6 (9):915–916.

Finke, R. A., and J. J. Freyd. 1989. Mental extrapolation and cognitive penetrability: Reply to Ranney and proposals for evaluative criteria. *Journal of Experimental Psychology. General* 118 (4):403–408.

Finke, R. A., and K. Slayton. 1988. Explorations of creative visual synthesis in mental imagery. *Memory & Cognition* 16 (3):252–257.

Fischer, M. H. 2001. Number processing induces spatial performance biases. *Neurology* 57 (5):822–826.

Fischer, M. H., A. D. Castel, M. D. Dodd, and J. Pratt. 2003. Perceiving numbers causes spatial shifts of attention. *Nature Neuroscience* 6 (6):555–556.

Fischer, M. H., N. Warlop, R. L. Hill, and W. Fias. 2004. Oculomotor bias induced by number perception. *Experimental Psychology* 51 (2):91–97.

Fisher, C. A., and A. J. Larner. 2008. Jean Langlais (1907–91): An historical case of a blind organist with stroke-induced aphasia and Braille alexia but without amusia. *Journal of Medical Biography* 16 (4):232–234.

Foree, D. D., and V. M. LoLordo. 1973. Attention in the pigeon: Differential effects of food-getting versus shock-avoidance procedures. *Journal of Comparative & Physiological Psychology* 85 (3):551–558.

Forster, B., A. F. Eardley, and M. Eimer. 2007. Altered tactile spatial attention in the early blind. *Brain Research* 1131 (1):149–154.

Fortin, M., P. Voss, C. Lord, M. Lassonde, J. Pruessner, D. Saint-Amour, C. Rainville, and F. Lepore. 2008. Wayfinding in the blind: Larger hippocampal volume and supranormal spatial navigation. *Brain* 131 (11):2995–3005.

Fournier, J. F., S. Deremaux, and M. Berniera. 2008. Content, characteristics, and function of mental images. *Psychology of Sport and Exercise* 9 (6):734–748.

Freeman, R. D., and A. Bradley. 1980. Monocularly deprived humans: Nondeprived eye has supernormal vernier acuity. *Journal of Neurophysiology* 43 (6):1645–1653.

Fujii, T., H. C. Tanabe, T. Kochiyama, and N. Sadato. 2009. An investigation of cross-modal plasticity of effective connectivity in the blind by dynamic causal modeling of functional MRI data. *Neuroscience Research* 65 (2):175–186.

Gaab, N., K. Schulze, E. Ozdemir, and G. Schlaug. 2006. Neural correlates of absolute pitch differ between blind and sighted musicians. *Neuroreport* 17 (18):1853–1857.

Gallese, V., L. Fadiga, L. Fogassi, and G. Rizzolatti. 1996. Action recognition in the premotor cortex. *Brain* 119 (2):593–609.

Gallistel, C. R., and I. I. Gelman. 2000. Non-verbal numerical cognition: From reals to integers. *Trends in Cognitive Sciences* 4 (2):59–65.

Gallistel, C. R., and R. Gelman. 1992. Preverbal and verbal counting and computation. *Cognition* 44 (1–2):43–74.

Galton, F. 1880. Statistics of mental imagery. *Mind* 5:301–318.

Galton, F. 1883. *Inquiries into Human Faculty and Its Development.* London: Macmillan.

Ganis, G., and H. E. Schendan. 2008. Visual mental imagery and perception produce opposite adaptation effects on early brain potentials. *NeuroImage* 42 (4):1714–1727.

Gardini, S., C. Cornoldi, R. De Beni, and A. Venneri. 2009. Cognitive and neuronal processes involved in sequential generation of general and specific mental images. *Psychological Research* 73 (5):633–643.

Gardini, S., R. De Beni, C. Cornoldi, A. Bromiley, and A. Venneri. 2005. Different neuronal pathways support the generation of general and specific mental images. *NeuroImage* 27 (3):544–552.

Garg, A., D. Schwartz, and A. Stevens. 2007. Orienting auditory spatial attention engages frontal eye fields and medial occipital cortex in congenitally blind humans. *Neuropsychologia* 45 (10):2307–2321.

Gaunet, F., J. L. Martinez, and C. Thinus-Blanc. 1997. Early-blind subjects' spatial representation of manipulatory space: Exploratory strategies and reaction to change. *Perception* 26 (3):345–366.

Gaunet, F., and Y. Rossetti. 2006. Effects of visual deprivation on space representation: Immediate and delayed pointing toward memorised proprioceptive targets. *Perception* 35 (1):107–124.

Gelman, R., and C. R. Gallistel. 2004. Language and the origin of numerical concepts. *Science* 306 (5695):441–443.

Gibson, G. O., and J. C. Craig. 2002. Relative roles of spatial and intensive cues in the discrimination of spatial tactile stimuli. *Perception & Psychophysics* 64 (7):1095–1107.

Gibson, J. J. 1962. Observations on active touch. *Psychological Review* 69:477–491.

Gibson, J. J. 1979. *The Ecological Approach to Visual Perception*. Boston: Houghton Mifflin.

Gilbert, C. D., and M. Sigman. 2007. Brain states: Top-down influences in sensory processing. *Neuron* 54 (5):677–696.

Gizewski, E. R., T. Gasser, A. de Greiff, A. Boehm, and M. Forsting. 2003. Cross-modal plasticity for sensory and motor activation patterns in blind subjects. *NeuroImage* 19 (3):968–975.

Gizewski, E. R., D. Timmann, and M. Forsting. 2004. Specific cerebellar activation during Braille reading in blind subjects. *Human Brain Mapping* 22 (3):229–235.

Glasauer, S., M. A. Amorim, I. Viaud-Delmon, and A. Berthoz. 2002. Differential effects of labyrinthine dysfunction on distance and direction during blindfolded walking of a triangular path. *Experimental Brain Research* 145 (4):489–497.

Goebel, R., D. Khorram-Sefat, L. Muckli, H. Hacker, and W. Singer. 1998. The constructive nature of vision: Direct evidence from functional magnetic resonance imaging studies of apparent motion and motion imagery. *European Journal of Neuroscience* 10 (5):1563–1573.

Goetz, E. T., M. Sadoski, A. G. Stricker, T. S. White, and Z. Wang. 2007. The role of imagery in the production of written definitions. *Reading Psychology* 28:241–256.

Goldenberg, G., W. Müllbacher, and A. Nowak. 1995. Imagery without perception—a case study of anosognosia for cortical blindness. *Neuropsychologia* 33 (11):1373–1382.

Goldreich, D., and I. M. Kanics. 2003. Tactile acuity is enhanced in blindness. *Journal of Neuroscience* 23 (8):3439–3445.

Goldreich, D., and I. M. Kanics. 2006. Performance of blind and sighted humans on a tactile grating detection task. *Perception & Psychophysics* 68 (8):1363–1371.

Goldreich, D., M. Wong, R. M. Peters, and I. M. Kanics. 2009. A tactile automated passive-finger stimulator (TAPS). *Journal of Visualized Experiments* 28:1374.

Golledge, R. G. 1991. Tactual strip maps as navigational aids. *Journal of Visual Impairment & Blindness* 85:296–301.

Golledge, R. G. 1999. *Wayfinding Behavior: Cognitive Mapping and Other Spatial Processes*. Baltimore: Johns Hopkins University Press.

Goltz, H. C., M. J. Steinbach, and B. L. Gallie. 1997. Head turn in 1-eyed and normally sighted individuals during monocular viewing. *Archives of Ophthalmology* 115 (6):748–750.

González, E., M. J. Steinbach, H. Ono, and N. Rush-Smith. 1992. Vernier acuity in monocular and binocular children. *Clinical Vision Sciences* 7:257–261.

González, E., M. J. Steinbach, H. Ono, and M. Wolf. 1989. Depth perception in humans enucleated at an early age. *Clinical Vision Sciences* 4:172–177.

González, E. G., J. K. Steeves, S. P. Kraft, B. L. Gallie, and M. J. Steinbach. 2002. Foveal and eccentric acuity in one-eyed observers. *Behavioural Brain Research* 128 (1):71–80.

González, E. G., J. K. E. Steeves, and M. J. Steinbach. 1998. Perceptual learning for motion-defined letters in unilaterally enucleated observers and monocularly viewing normal controls. *Investigative Ophthalmology & Visual Science* Supplement 39:S400.

González, E. G., M. Weinstock, and M. J. Steinbach. 2007. Peripheral fading with monocular and binocular viewing. *Vision Research* 47 (1):136–144.

Goodale, M. A., J. P. Meenan, H. H. Bülthoff, D. A. Nicolle, K. J. Murphy, and C. I. Racicot. 1994. Separate neural pathways for the visual analysis of object shape in perception and prehension. *Current Biology* 4 (7):604–610.

Goodale, M. A., and A. D. Milner. 1992. Separate visual pathways for perception and action. *Trends in Neurosciences* 15 (1):20–25.

Goodale, M. A., D. A. Westwood, and A. D. Milner. 2004. Two distinct modes of control for object-directed action. *Progress in Brain Research* 144:131–144.

Goodwin, G. P., and P. N. Johnson-Laird. 2005. Reasoning about relations. *Psychological Review* 112 (2):468–493.

Gothe, J., S. A. Brandt, K. Irlbacher, S. Röricht, B. A. Sabel, and B. U. Meyer. 2002. Changes in visual cortex excitability in blind subjects as demonstrated by transcranial magnetic stimulation. *Brain* 125 (3):479–490.

Gougoux, F., P. Belin, P. Voss, F. Lepore, M. Lassonde, and R. J. Zatorre. 2009. Voice perception in blind persons: A functional magnetic resonance imaging study. *Neuropsychologia* 47 (13):2967–2974.

Gougoux, F., F. Lepore, M. Lassonde, P. Voss, R. J. Zatorre, and P. Belin. 2004. Neuropsychology: Pitch discrimination in the early blind. *Nature* 430 (6997):309.

Gougoux, F., R. J. Zatorre, M. Lassonde, P. Voss, and F. Lepore. 2005. A functional neuroimaging study of sound localization: Visual cortex activity predicts performance in early-blind individuals. *PLoS Biology* 3 (2):27.

Goyal, M. S., P. J. Hansen, and C. B. Blakemore. 2006. Tactile perception recruits functionally related visual areas in the late-blind. *Neuroreport* 17 (13):1381–1384.

Grafman, J. 2000. Conceptualizing functional neuroplasticity. *Journal of Communication Disorders* 33 (4):345–355, quiz 355–356.

Grant, A. C., M. C. Thiagarajah, and K. Sathian. 2000. Tactile perception in blind Braille readers: A psychophysical study of acuity and hyperacuity using gratings and dot patterns. *Perception & Psychophysics* 62 (2):301–312.

Greenberg, D. L., and D. C. Rubin. 2003. The neuropsychology of autobiographical memory. *Cortex* 39 (4–5):687–728.

Gregory, R. 2004. The blind leading the sighted. *Nature* 430 (7002):836.

Gregory, R. L. 1980. Perceptions as hypotheses. *Philosophical Transactions of the Royal Society of London: Series B, Biological Sciences* 290 (1038):181–197.

Gregory, R. L. 1981. The 4th dimension of 3-D (2). *Perception* 10 (1):1–4.

Gregory, R. L. and J. G. Wallace. 1963. Recovery from early blindness: A case study. *Quarterly Journal of Psychology*. <http://www.richardgregory.org/papers/recovery_blind/contents.htm>.

Griffiths, T. D., G. Rees, A. Rees, G. G. R. Green, C. Witton, D. Rowe, C. Büchel, R. Turner, and R. S. J. Frackowiak. 1998. Right parietal cortex is involved in the perception of sound movement in humans. *Nature Neuroscience* 1 (1):74–79.

Grill-Spector, K., R. Henson, and A. Martin. 2006. Repetition and the brain: Neural models of stimulus-specific effects. *Trends in Cognitive Sciences* 10 (1):14–23.

Grush, R. 2000. Self, world, and space: The meaning and mechanisms of ego- and allocentric spatial representation. *Brain and Mind* 1:59–92.

Haber, R. N., L. R. Haber, C. A. Levin, and R. Hollyfield. 1993. Properties of spatial representations: Data from sighted and blind subjects. *Perception & Psychophysics* 54 (1):1–13.

Hagen, M. C., O. Franzén, F. McGlone, G. Essick, C. Dancer, and J. V. Pardo. 2002. Tactile motion activates the human middle temporal/V5 (MT/V5) complex. *European Journal of Neuroscience* 16 (5):957–964.

Hager-Ross, C., and R. S. Johansson. 1996. Nondigital afferent input in reactive control of fingertip forces during precision grip. *Experimental Brain Research* 110 (1):131–141.

Hall, C., D. Mack, A. Paivio, and H. A. Hausenblas. 1998. Imagery use by athletes: Development of the Sport Imagery Questionnaire. *International Journal of Sport Psychology* 29:73–89.

Hall, E. C., and K. J. Ciuffreda. 2002. Fixational ocular motor control is plastic despite visual deprivation. *Visual Neuroscience* 19 (4):475–481.

Hall, E. C., J. Gordon, L. Hainline, I. Abramov, and K. Engber. 2000. Childhood visual experience affects adult voluntary ocular motor control. *Optometry and Vision Science* 77 (10):511–523.

Hall, J. C. 2002. Imagery practice and the development of surgical skills. *American Journal of Surgery* 184:465–470.

Halpern, A. R., and R. J. Zatorre. 1999. When that tune runs through your head: A PET investigation of auditory imagery for familiar melodies. *Cerebral Cortex* 9 (7):697–704.

Hamilton, R., J. P. Keenan, M. Catala, and A. Pascual-Leone. 2000. Alexia for Braille following bilateral occipital stroke in an early blind woman. *Neuroreport* 11 (2):237–240.

Hamilton, R. H., and A. Pascual-Leone. 1998. Cortical plasticity associated with Braille learning. *Trends in Cognitive Sciences* 2:168–174.

Hamilton, R. H., A. Pascual-Leone, and G. Schlaug. 2004. Absolute pitch in blind musicians. *Neuroreport* 15 (5):803–806.

Harada, T., D. N. Saito, K. Kashikura, T. Sato, Y. Yonekura, M. Honda, and N. Sadato. 2004. Asymmetrical neural substrates of tactile discrimination in humans: A functional magnetic resonance imaging study. *Journal of Neuroscience* 24 (34):7524–7530.

Harris, L. R., and M. Cynader. 1981. The eye movements of the dark-reared cat. *Experimental Brain Research* 44 (1):41–56.

Harwerth, R. S., and E. L. Smith III, G. C. Duncan, M. L. Crawford, and G. K. von Noorden. 1986. Effects of enucleation of the fixating eye on strabismic amblyopia in monkeys. *Investigative Ophthalmology & Visual Science* 27 (2):246–254.

Hatwell, Y. 2003. *Psychologie cognitive de la cécité précoce*. Paris: Dunod.

Haxby, J. V., M. I. Gobbini, M. L. Furey, A. Ishai, J. L. Schouten, and P. Pietrini. 2001. Distributed and overlapping representations of faces and objects in ventral temporal cortex. *Science* 293 (5539):2425–2430.

Haxby, J. V., B. Horwitz, L. G. Ungerleider, J. M. Maisog, P. Pietrini, and C. L. Grady. 1994. The functional organization of human extrastriate cortex: A PET-rCBF study of selective attention to faces and locations. *Journal of Neuroscience* 14 (11/1):6336–6353.

Heffner, R. S., and H. E. Heffner. 1992. Hearing in large mammals: Sound-localization acuity in cattle (Bos taurus) and goats (Capra hircus). *Journal of Comparative Psychology* 106 (2):107–113.

Hegarty, M. 2004. Mechanical reasoning by mental simulation. *Trends in Cognitive Sciences* 8 (6):280–285.

Hegarty, M., M. A. Just, and I. R. Morrison. 1988. Mental models of mechanical systems: Individual differences in qualitative and quantitative reasoning. *Cognitive Psychology* 20 (2):191–236.

Hegarty, M., and M. Kozhevnikov. 1999. Types of visual-spatial representations and mathematical problem solving. *Journal of Educational Psychology* 91:684–689.

Held, R. 2009. Visual-haptic mapping and the origin of cross-modal identity. *Optometry and Vision Science* 86 (6):595–598.

Held, R., Y. Ostrovsky, B. deGelder, and P. Sinha. 2008. Revisiting the Molyneux question. *Journal of Vision* 8 (6):523, 523a.

Heller, M. A. 1986. Active and passive tactile braille recognition. *Bulletin of the Psychonomic Society* 24:201–202.

Heller, M. A. 1989a. Texture perception in sighted and blind observers. *Perception & Psychophysics* 45 (1):49–54.

Heller, M. A. 1989b. Tactile memory in sighted and blind observers: The influence of orientation and rate of presentation. *Perception* 18 (1):121–133.

Heller, M. A. 1992. "Haptic dominance" in form perception: Vision versus proprioception. *Perception* 21:655–660.

Heller, M. A. 2006. Picture perception and spatial cognition in visually impaired people. In *Touch and Blindness: Psychology and Neuroscience*, ed. S. Ballesteros and M. Heller. Mahwah, N.J.: Lawrence Erlbaum Associates.

Heller, M. A., D. D. Brackett, E. Scroggs, A. C. Allen, and S. Green. 2001. Haptic perception of the horizontal by blind and low-vision individuals. *Perception* 30 (5):601–610.

Heller, M. A., D. D. Brackett, E. Scroggs, H. Steffen, K. Heatherly, and S. Salik. 2002. Tangible pictures: Viewpoint effects and linear perspective in visually impaired people. *Perception* 31 (6):747–769.

Heller, M. A., J. Calcaterra, S. Green, and F. J. de Lima. 1999. The effect of orientation on braille recognition in persons who are sighted and blind. *Journal of Visual Impairment & Blindness* 93:416–419.

Heller, M. A., J. A. Calcaterra, L. A. Tyler, and L. L. Burson. 1996. Production and interpretation of perspective drawings by blind and sighted people. *Perception* 25 (3):321–334.

Heller, M. A., A. M. Kappers, M. McCarthy, A. Clark, T. Riddle, E. Fulkerson, L. Wemple, A. M. Walk, A. Basso, C. Wanek, and K. Russler. 2008. The effects of curvature on haptic judgments of extent in sighted and blind people. *Perception* 37 (6):816–840.

Heller, M. A., and J. M. Kennedy. 1990. Perspective taking, pictures, and the blind. *Perception & Psychophysics* 48 (5):459–466.

Heller, M. A., J. M. Kennedy, A. Clark, M. McCarthy, A. Borgert, L. Wemple, E. Fulkerson, N. Kaffel, A. Duncan, and T. Riddle. 2006. Viewpoint and orientation influence picture recognition in the blind. *Perception* 35 (10):1397–1420.

Heller, M. A., J. M. Kennedy, and T. D. Joyner. 1995. Production and interpretation of pictures of houses by blind people. *Perception* 24 (9):1049–1058.

Heller, M. A., T. Riddle, E. Fulkerson, L. Wemple, A. McClure Walk, S. Guthrie, C. Kranz, and P. Klaus. 2009. The influence of viewpoint and object detail in blind people when matching pictures to complex objects. *Perception* 38:1234–1250.

Heller, M. A., K. Wilson, H. Steffen, K. Yoneyama, and D. D. Brackett. 2003. Superior haptic perceptual selectivity in late-blind and very-low-vision subjects. *Perception* 32 (4):499–511.

Hering, E. [1879] 1942. *Spatial Sense and Movements of the Eye*. Baltimore: American Academy of Optometry.

Hermelin, B., and N. O'Connor. 1971. Right and left handed reading of Braille. *Nature* 231 (5303):470.

Hermens, F., A. M. Kappers, and S. C. Gielen. 2006. The structure of frontoparallel haptic space is task dependent. *Perception & Psychophysics* 68 (1):62–75.

Hertrich, I., S. Dietrich, A. Moos, J. Trouvain, and H. Ackermann. 2009. Enhanced speech perception capabilities in a blind listener are associated with activation of fusiform gyrus and primary visual cortex. *Neurocase* 15 (2):163–170.

Heyes, A. D. 1984. Sonic Pathfinder: A programmable guidance aid for the blind. *Electronics and Wireless World* 90:26–29.

Hirsch, M. J. 1959. The relationship between refractive state of the eye and intelligence test scores. *American Journal of Optometry and Archives of American Academy of Optometry* 36 (1):12–21.

Hirsh, I. J. 1988. Auditory perception and speech. In *Stevens' Handbook of Experimental Psychology*, 2nd ed., vol. 1, ed. R. J. Atkinson, G. Lindzey, and R. D. Luce. New York: John Wiley, 377–408.

Hitch, G. J., M. A. Brandimonte, and P. Walker. 1995. Two types of representation in visual memory: Evidence from the effects of stimulus contrast on image combination. *Memory & Cognition* 23 (2):147–154.

Hofman, P. M., J. G. Van Riswick, and A. J. Van Opstal. 1998. Relearning sound localization with new ears. *Nature Neuroscience* 1 (5):417–421.

Hollins, M. 1985. Styles of mental imagery in blind adults. *Neuropsychologia* 23 (4):561–566.

Hollins, M. 1986. Haptic mental rotation: More consistent in blind subjects? *Journal of Visual Impairment & Blindness* 80:950–952.

Hollins, M. 1989. *Understanding Blindness: An Integrative Approach*. Hillsdale, NJ: Lawrence Erlbaum Associates.

Hollins, M., and E. K. Kelley. 1988. Spatial updating in blind and sighted people. *Perception & Psychophysics* 43 (4):380–388.

Hollins, M., and S. R. Risner. 2000. Evidence for the duplex theory of tactile texture perception. *Perception & Psychophysics* 62 (4):695–705.

Holzinger, B. 2000. The dreams of the blind: In consideration of the congenital and adventitously blindness. *Journal of Sleep Research* 9 (Supplement 1):83.

Horton, J. C., and D. R. Hocking. 1998. Effect of early monocular enucleation upon ocular dominance columns and cytochrome oxidase activity in monkey and human visual cortex. *Visual Neuroscience* 15 (2):289–303.

Hötting, K., and B. Röder. 2004. Hearing cheats touch, but less in congenitally blind than in sighted individuals. *Psychological Science* 15 (1):60–64.

Hötting, K., and B. Röder. 2009. Auditory and auditory-tactile processing in congenitally blind humans. *Hearing Research* 258 (1–2):165–174.

Hötting, K., F. Rösler, and B. Röder. 2004. Altered auditory-tactile interactions in congenitally blind humans: An event-related potential study. *Experimental Brain Research* 159 (3):370–381.

Howard, I. P., and W. B. Templeton. 1966. *Human Spatial Orientation.* New York: John Wiley.

Hubel, D. H., and T. N. Wiesel. 1965. Binocular interaction in striate cortex of kittens reared with artificial squint. *Journal of Neurophysiology* 28 (6):1041–1059.

Hubel, D. H., and T. N. Wiesel. 1977. Ferrier lecture: Functional architecture of macaque monkey visual cortex. *Proceedings of the Royal Society of London, Series B: Biological Sciences* 198 (1130):1–59.

Hugdahl, K., M. Ek, F. Takio, T. Rintee, J. Tuomainen, C. Haarala, and H. Hämäläinen. 2004. Blind individuals show enhanced perceptual and attentional sensitivity for identification of speech sounds. *Brain Research. Cognitive Brain Research* 19 (1):28–32.

Hughes, B. 2001. Active artificial echolocation and the nonvisual perception of aperture passability. *Human Movement Science* 20 (4–5):371–400.

Hull, T., and H. Mason. 1995. Performance of blind children on digit span tests. *Journal of Visual Impairment & Blindness* 89 (2):166–169.

Hunter, I. M. L. 1954. Tactile-kinesthetic perception of straightness in blind and sighted humans. *Quarterly Journal of Experimental Psychology* 6:149–154.

Hurovitz, C., S. Dunn, G. W. Domhoff, and H. Fiss. 1999. The dreams of blind men and women: A replication and extension of previous findings. *Dreaming* 9 (2–3):183–193.

Hyde, K. L., J. Lerch, A. Norton, M. Forgeard, E. Winner, A. C. Evans, and G. Schlaug. 2009. Musical training shapes structural brain development. *Journal of Neuroscience* 29 (10):3019–3025.

Hyde, K. L., J. P. Lerch, R. J. Zatorre, T. D. Griffiths, A. C. Evans, and I. Peretz. 2007. Cortical thickness in congenital amusia: When less is better than more. *Journal of Neuroscience* 27 (47):13028–13032.

Intons-Peterson, M. J. 1996. Linguistic effects in a visual manipulation task. *Psychologische Beiträge* 38 (3–4):251–278.

Ishai, A., J. V. Haxby, and L. G. Ungerleider. 2002. Visual imagery of famous faces: effects of memory and attention revealed by fMRI. *NeuroImage* 17 (4):1729–1741.

Ishai, A., and D. Sagi. 1995. Common mechanisms of visual imagery and perception. *Science* 268 (5218):1772–1774.

Ishai, A., L. G. Ungerleider, and J. V. Haxby. 2000. Distributed neural systems for the generation of visual images. *Neuron* 28 (3):979–990.

Ishai, A., L. G. Ungerleider, A. Martin, J. L. Schouten, and J. V. Haxby. 1999. Distributed representation of objects in the human ventral visual pathway. *Proceedings of the National Academy of Sciences of the United States of America* 96 (16):9379–9384.

Ito, A., H. Kawabata, N. Fujimoto, and E. Adachi-Usami. 2001. Effect of myopia on frequency-doubling perimetry. *Investigative Ophthalmology & Visual Science* 42 (5):1107–1110.

Ittyerah, M., F. Gaunet, and Y. Rossetti. 2007. Pointing with the left and right hands in congenitally blind children. *Brain and Cognition* 64 (2):170–183.

Jacomuzzi, A., P. Kobau, and N. Bruno. 2003. Molyneux's question redux. *Phenomenology and the Cognitive Sciences* 2:255–280.

James, T. W., G. K. Humphrey, J. S. Gati, P. Servos, R. S. Menon, and M. A. Goodale. 2002. Haptic study of three-dimensional objects activates extrastriate visual areas. *Neuropsychologia* 40 (10):1706–1714.

James, W. [1890] 1950. *The Principles of Psychology*. New York: Dover.

Janson, U. 1993. Normal and deviant behavior in blind children with ROP. *Acta Ophthalmologica* Supplement 210:20–26.

Janzen, G. 2006. Memory for object location and route direction in virtual large-scale space. *Quarterly Journal of Experimental Psychology* 59 (3):493–508.

Jastrow, J. 1900. *Fact and Fable in Psychology*. New York: Houghton Mifflin.

Jeannerod, M., M. A. Arbib, G. Rizzolatti, and H. Sakata. 1995. Grasping objects: The cortical mechanisms of visuomotor transformation. *Trends in Neurosciences* 18 (7):314–320.

Jeannerod, M., J. Decety, and F. Michel. 1994. Impairment of grasping movements following a bilateral posterior parietal lesion. *Neuropsychologia* 32 (4):369–380.

Jewell, G., and M. E. McCourt. 2000. Pseudoneglect: A review and meta-analysis of performance factors in line bisection tasks. *Neuropsychologia* 38 (1):93–110.

Jiang, J., W. Zhu, F. Shi, Y. Liu, J. Li, W. Qin, K. Li, C. Yu, and T. Jiang. 2009. Thick visual cortex in the early blind. *Journal of Neuroscience* 29 (7):2205–2211.

Johansson, R. S., and J. R. Flanagan. 2009. Coding and use of tactile signals from the fingertips in object manipulation tasks. *Nature Reviews. Neuroscience* 10 (5):345–359.

Johnson-Laird, P. N. 1983. *Mental Models: Towards a Cognitive Science of Language, Inference, and Consciousness*. Cambridge: Cambridge University Press.

Johnson-Laird, P. N. 1994. Mental models and probabilistic thinking. *Cognition* 50 (1–3):189–209.

Johnson-Laird, P. N. 1998. Imagery, visualization, and thinking. In *Perception and Cognition at Century's End*, ed. J. Hochberg. San Diego: Academic Press, 441–467.

Johnson-Laird, P. N., R. M. J. Byrne, and P. Tabossi. 1989. Reasoning by model: The case of multiple quantifiers. *Psychological Review* 96:658–673.

Johnson, K. O. 2001. The roles and functions of cutaneous mechanoreceptors. *Current Opinion in Neurobiology* 11 (4):455–461.

Johnson, K. O., and J. R. Phillips. 1981. Tactile spatial resolution. I. Two-point discrimination, gap detection, grating resolution, and letter recognition. *Journal of Neurophysiology* 46 (6):1177–1192.

Jones, B. 1975. Spatial perception in the blind. *British Journal of Psychology* 66 (4):461–472.

Jones, B., and B. Kabanoff. 1975. Eye movements in auditory space perception. *Perception & Psychophysics* 17 (3):241–245.

Kainthola, S. D., and T. B. Singh. 1992. A test of tactile concentration and short-term memory. *Journal of Visual Impairment & Blindness* 86:219–221.

Kallman, H. J., and D. W. Massaro. 1979. Similarity effects in backward recognition masking. *Journal of Experimental Psychology. Human Perception and Performance* 5 (1):110–128.

Kappers, A. M. 1999. Large systematic deviations in the haptic perception of parallelity. *Perception* 28 (8):1001–1012.

Kappers, A. M. 2002. Haptic perception of parallelity in the midsagittal plane. *Acta Psychologica* 109 (1):25–40.

Kappers, A. M. 2003. Large systematic deviations in a bimanual parallelity task: Further analysis of contributing factors. *Acta Psychologica* 114 (2):131–145.

Kappers, A. M. 2004. The contributions of egocentric and allocentric reference frames in haptic spatial tasks. *Acta Psychologica* 117 (3):333–340.

Kappers, A. M. 2007. Haptic space processing—allocentric and egocentric reference frames. *Canadian Journal of Experimental Psychology* 61 (3):208–218.

Kappers, A. M., and J. J. Koenderink. 1999. Haptic perception of spatial relations. *Perception* 28 (6):781–795.

Kappers, A. M., and R. F. Viergever. 2006. Hand orientation is insufficiently compensated for in haptic spatial perception. *Experimental Brain Research* 173 (3):407–414.

Karavatos, A., G. Kaprinis, and A. Tzavaras. 1984. Hemispheric specialization for language in the congenitally blind: The influence of the Braille system. *Neuropsychologia* 22 (4):521–525.

Karlen, S. J., D. M. Kahn, and L. Krubitzer. 2006. Early blindness results in abnormal corticocortical and thalamocortical connections. *Neuroscience* 142 (3):843–858.

Kaski, D. 2002. Revision: Is visual perception a requisite for visual imagery? *Perception* 31 (6):717–731.

Kauffman, T., H. Théoret, and A. Pascual-Leone. 2002. Braille character discrimination in blindfolded human subjects. *Neuroreport* 13 (5):571–574.

Kay, L. 1985. Sensory aids to spatial perception for blind persons: Their design and evaluation. In *Electronic Spatial Sensing for the Blind*, ed. E. S. D. Warren. Dordrecht: Martinus Nijhoff, 125–139.

Kellogg, W. N. 1962. Sonar system of the blind. *Science* 137:399–404.

Kennedy, H., and A. Burkhalter. 2004. Ontogenesis of cortical connectivity. In *The Visual Neurosciences*, ed. L. M. Chalupa and J. S. Werner. Cambridge, MA: MIT Press, 146–158.

Kennedy, J. M. 1993. *Drawing and the Blind: Pictures to Touch*. New Haven: Yale University Press.

Kennedy, J. M., and I. Jurevic. 2006. Form, projection, and pictures for the blind. In *Touch and Blindness: Psychology and Neurosciences*, ed. M. Heller and S. Ballesteros. Mahwah, NJ: Lawrence Erlbaum, 73–93.

Kennett, S., M. Eimer, C. Spence, and J. Driver. 2001. Tactile-visual links in exogenous spatial attention under different postures: Convergent evidence from psychophysics and ERPs. *Journal of Cognitive Neuroscience* 13 (4):462–478.

Kerr, N. H. 1983. The role of vision in "visual imagery" experiments: evidence from the congenitally blind. *Journal of Experimental Psychology. General* 112 (2):265–277.

Kerr, N. H. 1987. Locational representation in imagery: The third dimension. *Memory & Cognition* 15 (6):521–530.

Kerr, N. H. 2000. Dreaming, imagery, and perception. In *Principles and Practice of Sleep Medicine*, 3rd. ed., vol. 6, ed. M. H. Kryger, T. Roth, and W. C. Dement. Philadelphia: W. B. Saunders, 482–490.

Kerr, N. H., D. Foulkes, and M. Schmidt. 1982. The structure of laboratory dream reports in blind and sighted subjects. *Journal of Nervous and Mental Disease* 170 (5):286–294.

Kimura, D. 1967. Functional asymmetry of the brain in dichotic listening. *Cortex* 3:163.

King, A. J., and S. Carlile. 1993. Changes induced in the representation of auditory space in the superior colliculus by rearing ferrets with binocular eyelid suture. *Experimental Brain Research* 94 (3):444–455.

King, A. J., M. E. Hutchings, D. R. Moore, and C. Blakemore. 1988. Developmental plasticity in the visual and auditory representations in the mammalian superior colliculus. *Nature* 332 (6159):73–76.

King, A. J., and C. H. Parsons. 1999. Improved auditory spatial acuity in visually deprived ferrets. *European Journal of Neuroscience* 11 (11):3945–3956.

Kingsbury, M. A., N. A. Lettman, and B. L. Finlay. 2002. Reduction of early thalamic input alters adult corticocortical connectivity. *Brain Research. Developmental Brain Research* 138 (1):35–43.

Kitchin, R., and S. Freundschuh. 2000. *Cognitive Mapping: Past, Present, and Future.* London: Routledge.

Klatzky, R. L., Y. Lippa, J. M. Loomis, and R. G. Golledge. 2002. Learning directions of objects specified by vision, spatial audition, or auditory spatial language. *Learning & Memory* 9 (6):364–367.

Klatzky, R. L., Y. Lippa, J. M. Loomis, and R. G. Golledge. 2003. Encoding, learning, and spatial updating of multiple object locations specified by 3-D sound, spatial language, and vision. *Experimental Brain Research* 149 (1):48–61.

Klatzky, R. L., J. M. Loomis, R. G. Golledge, J. G. Cicinelli, S. Doherty, and J. W. Pellegrino. 1990. Acquisition of route and survey knowledge in the absence of vision. *Journal of Motor Behavior* 22 (1):19–43.

Klatzky, R. L., J. M. Loomis, S. J. Lederman, H. Wake, and N. Fujita. 1993. Haptic identification of objects and their depictions. *Perception & Psychophysics* 54 (2):170–178.

Knauff, M., T. Fangmeier, C. C. Ruff, and P. N. Johnson-Laird. 2003. Reasoning, models, and images: Behavioral measures and cortical activity. *Journal of Cognitive Neuroscience* 15 (4):559–573.

Knauff, M., and P. N. Johnson-Laird. 2002. Visual imagery can impede reasoning. *Memory & Cognition* 30 (3):363–371.

Knauff, M., and E. May. 2006. Mental imagery, reasoning, and blindness. *Quarterly Journal of Experimental Psychology* 59 (1):161–177.

Knauff, M., and M. May. 2004. Visual imagery in deductive reasoning: Results from experiments with sighted, blindfolded, and congenitally totally blind persons. In *Proceedings of the Twenty-Sixth Annual Conference of the Cognitive Science Society*. Mahwah, N.J.: Lawrence Erlbaum.

Knudsen, E. I., and M. S. Brainard. 1995. Creating a unified representation of visual and auditory space in the brain. *Annual Review of Neuroscience* 18:19–43.

Knudsen, E. I., and P. F. Knudsen. 1985. Vision guides the adjustment of auditory localization in young barn owls. *Science* 230 (4725):545–548.

Kobayashi, M., M. Takeda, N. Hattori, M. Fukunaga, T. Sasabe, N. Inoue, Y. Nagai, T. Sawada, N. Sadato, and Y. Watanabe. 2004. Functional imaging of gustatory perception and imagery: "Top-down" processing of gustatory signals. *NeuroImage* 23:1271–1282.

Kohler, E., C. Keysers, M. A. Umiltà, L. Fogassi, V. Gallese, and G. Rizzolatti. 2002. Hearing sounds, understanding actions: Action representation in mirror neurons. *Science* 297 (5582):846–848.

Koller, G., A. Haas, M. Zulauf, F. Koerner, and D. Mojon. 2001. Influence of refractive correction on peripheral visual field in static perimetry. *Graefes Archive for Clinical and Experimental Ophthalmology* 239 (10):759–762.

Kosslyn, S. M. 1973. Scanning visual images: Some structural implications. *Perception & Psychophysics* 14 (1):90–94.

Kosslyn, S. M. 1980. *Image and Mind.* Cambridge, MA: Harvard University Press.

Kosslyn, S. M. 1994. *Image and Brain: The Resolution of the Imagery Debate.* Cambridge, MA: MIT Press.

Kosslyn, S. M. 2006. You can play 20 questions with nature and win: Categorical versus coordinate spatial relations as a case study. *Neuropsychologia* 44 (9):1519–1523.

Kosslyn, S. M., T. M. Ball, and B. J. Reiser. 1978. Visual images preserve metric spatial information: Evidence from studies of image scanning. *Journal of Experimental Psychology. Human Perception and Performance* 4 (1):47–60.

Kosslyn, S. M., G. J. DiGirolamo, W. L. Thompson, and N. M. Alpert. 1998. Mental rotation of objects versus hands: Neural mechanisms revealed by positron emission tomography. *Psychophysiology* 35 (2):151–161.

Kosslyn, S. M., G. Ganis, and W. L. Thompson. 2001. Neural foundations of imagery. *Nature Reviews. Neuroscience* 2 (9):635–642.

Kosslyn, S. M., L. L. LeSueur, I. E. Dror, and M. S. Gazzaniga. 1993. The role of the corpus callosum in the representation of lateral orientation. *Neuropsychologia* 31 (7):675–686.

Kosslyn, S. M., and K. N. Ochsner. 1994. In search of occipital activation during visual mental imagery. *Trends in Neurosciences* 17 (7):290–292.

Kosslyn, S. M., A. Pascual-Leone, O. Felician, S. Camposano, J. P. Keenan, W. L. Thompson, G. Ganis, K. E. Sukel, and N. M. Alpert. 1999. The role of area 17 in visual imagery: Convergent evidence from PET and rTMS. *Science* 284 (5411):167–170.

Kosslyn, S. M., J. M. Shephard, and W. L. Thompson. 2007. Spatial processing during mental imagery: A neurofunctional theory. In *Spatial Processing in Navigation, Imagery and Perception,* ed. F. Mast and L. Jäncke. New York: Springer, 1–16.

Kosslyn, S. M., and W. L. Thompson. 2003. When is early visual cortex activated during visual mental imagery? *Psychological Bulletin* 129 (5):723–746.

Kosslyn, S. M., W. L. Thompson, and N. M. Alpert. 1997. Neural systems shared by visual imagery and visual perception: A positron emission tomography study. *NeuroImage* 6 (4):320–334.

Kosslyn, S. M., W. L. Thompson, I. J. Kim, and N. M. Alpert. 1995. Topographical representations of mental images in primary visual cortex. *Nature* 378 (6556):496–498.

Kourtzi, Z., and K. Grill-Spector. 2005. fMRI adaptation: A tool for studying visual representations in the primate brain. In *Fitting the Mind to the World: Adaptation and Aftereffects in High-Level Vision,* ed. G. Rhodes and C. W. G. Clifford. Oxford: Oxford University Press.

Kozhevnikov, M., M. Hegarty, and R. E. Mayer. 2002. Spatial abilities in kinematics problem solving. In *Diagrammatic Representation and Reasoning*, ed. M. Anderson, B. Meyer, and P. Olivier. Berlin: Springer-Verlag, 155–171.

Kraemer, P. J., and W. A. Roberts. 1985. Short-term memory for simultaneously presented visual and auditory signals in the pigeon. *Journal of Experimental Psychology: Animal Behavior Processes* 11 (2):137–151.

Kujala, T., K. Alho, J. Kekoni, H. Hämäläinen, K. Reinikainen, O. Salonen, C. G. Standertskjöld-Nordenstam, and R. Näätänen. 1995. Auditory and somatosensory event-related brain potentials in early blind humans. *Experimental Brain Research* 104 (3):519–526.

Kujala, T., K. Alho, P. Paavilainen, H. Summala, and R. Näätänen. 1992. Neural plasticity in processing of sound location by the early blind: An event-related potential study. *Electroencephalography and Clinical Neurophysiology* 84 (5):469–472.

Kujala, T., A. Lehtokoski, K. Alhoa, J. Kekonib, and R. Näätänena. 1997. Faster reaction times in the blind than sighted during bimodal divided attention. *Acta Psychologica* 96:75–82.

Kujala, T., M. J. Palva, O. Salonene, P. Alkuf, M. Huotilainena, A. Järvinenf, and R. Näätänenb. 2005. The role of blind humans' visual cortex in auditory change detection. *Neuroscience Letters* 379 (2):127–131.

Kupers, R., A. Fumal, A. Maertens de Noordhout, A. Gjedde, J. Schoenen, and M. Ptito. 2006. Transcranial magnetic stimulation of the visual cortex induces somatotopically organized qualia in blind subjects. *Proceedings of the National Academy of Sciences of the United States of America* 103 (35):13256–13260.

Kupers, R., M. Pappens, A. Maertens de Noordhout, J. Schoenen, M. Ptito, and A. Fumal. 2007. rTMS of the occipital cortex abolishes Braille reading and repetition priming in blind subjects. *Neurology* 68 (9):691–693.

LaBerge, D. 2000. Networks of attention. In *The New Cognitive Neurosciences*, 2nd edition, ed. M. S. Gazzaniga. Cambridge, MA: MIT Press, 711–724.

Lamm, C., C. Windischberger, U. Leodolter, E. Moser, and H. Bauer. 2001. Evidence for premotor cortex activity during dynamic visuospatial imagery from single-trial functional magnetic resonance imaging and event-related slow cortical potentials. *NeuroImage* 14 (2):268–283.

Lamme, V. A., and P. R. Roelfsema. 2000. The distinct modes of vision offered by feedforward and recurrent processing. *Trends in Neurosciences* 23 (11):571–579.

Landis, B. N., C. G. Konnerth, and T. Hummel. 2004. A study on the frequency of olfactory dysfunction. *Laryngoscope* 114 (10):1764–1769.

Lange, K., and B. Röder. 2006. Orienting attention to points in time improves stimulus processing both within and across modalities. *Journal of Cognitive Neuroscience* 18 (5):715–729.

Lappe, C., S. C. Herholz, L. J. Trainor, and C. Pantev. 2008. Cortical plasticity induced by short-term unimodal and multimodal musical training. *Journal of Neuroscience* 28 (39):9632–9639.

Latini Corazzini, L., C. Tinti, S. Schmidt, C. Mirandola, and C. Cornoldi. 2010. Developing spatial knoweldge in the absence of vision: Allocentric and egocentric representations generated by blind people when supported by auditory cues. *Psychologica Belgica.*

Laurienti, P. J., J. H. Burdette, M. T. Wallace, Y. F. Yen, A. S. Field, and B. E. Stein. 2002. Deactivation of sensory-specific cortex by cross-modal stimuli. *Journal of Cognitive Neuroscience* 14 (3):420–429.

Lavie, P. 1996. *The Enchanted World of Sleep*. New Haven: Yale University Press.

LeBoutillier, N., and D. F. Marks. 2003. Mental imagery and creativity: A meta-analytic review study. *British Journal of Psychology* 94 (1):29–44.

Leclerc, C., D. Saint-Amour, M. E. Lavoie, M. Lassonde, and F. Lepore. 2000. Brain functional reorganization in early blind humans revealed by auditory event-related potentials. *Neuroreport* 11 (3):545–550.

Leclerc, C., S. J. Segalowitz, J. Desjardins, M. Lassonde, and F. Lepore. 2005. EEG coherence in early-blind humans during sound localization. *Neuroscience Letters* 376 (3):154–159.

Le Conte, J. 1881. *Sight: An Exposition of the Principles of Monocular and Binocular Vision*. London: Kegan Paul.

Le Grand, R., C. J. Mondloch, D. Maurer, and H. P. Brent. 2001. Neuroperception: Early visual experience and face processing. *Nature* 410 (6831):890.

Lederman, S. J., and R. L. Klatzky. 1987. Hand movements: A window into haptic object recognition. *Cognitive Psychology* 19 (3):342–368.

Lederman, S. J., and R. L. Klatzky. 2009. Haptic perception: A tutorial. *Attention, Perception & Psychophysics* 71 (7):1439–1459.

Lederman, S. J., R. L. Klatzky, C. Chataway, and C. D. Summers. 1990. Visual mediation and the haptic recognition of two-dimensional pictures of common objects. *Perception & Psychophysics* 47 (1):54–64.

Legge, G. E., C. Madison, B. N. Vaughn, A. M. Cheong, and J. C. Miller. 2008. Retention of high tactile acuity throughout the life span in blindness. *Perception & Psychophysics* 70 (8):1471–1488.

Leopold, D. A., M. Wilke, A. Maier, and N. K. Logothetis. 2002. Stable perception of visually ambiguous patterns. *Nature Neuroscience* 5 (6):605–609.

Leporé, N., Y. Shi, F. Lepore, M. Fortin, P. Voss, Y. Y. Chou, C. Lord, M. Lassonde, I. D. Dinov, A. W. Toga, P. M. Thompson. 2009. Pattern of hippocampal shape and volume differences in blind subjects. *NeuroImage* 46 (4):949–957.

Leslie, A. M., O. Friedman, and T. P. German. 2004. Core mechanisms in "theory of mind." *Trends in Cognitive Sciences* 8 (12):528–533.

Lessard, N., M. Paré, F. Lepore, and M. Lassonde. 1998. Early-blind human subjects localize sound sources better than sighted subjects. *Nature* 395 (6699):278–280.

LeVay, S., T. N. Wiesel, and D. H. Hubel. 1980. The development of ocular dominance columns in normal and visually deprived monkeys. *Journal of Comparative Neurology* 191 (1):1–51.

Levin, N., S. O. Dumoulin, J. Winawer, R. F. Dougherty, and B. A. Wandell. 2010. Cortical maps and white matter tracts following long period of visual deprivation and retinal image restoration. *Neuron* 65 (1):21–31.

Levy, L. M., R. I. Henkin, C. S. Lin, A. Hutter, and D. Schellinger. 1999. Odor memory induces brain activation as measured by functional MRI. *Journal of Computer Assisted Tomography* 23 (4):487–498.

Lewald, J. 2002a. Opposing effects of head position on sound localization in blind and sighted human subjects. *European Journal of Neuroscience* 15 (7):1219–1224.

Lewald, J. 2002b. Vertical sound localization in blind humans. *Neuropsychologia* 40 (12):1868–1872.

Lewald, J., G. J. Dörrscheidt, and W. H. Ehrenstein. 2000. Sound localization with eccentric head position. *Behavioural Brain Research* 108 (2):105–125.

Lewald, J., H. Foltys, and R. Töpper. 2002. Role of the posterior parietal cortex in spatial hearing. *Journal of Neuroscience* 22 (3):RC207.

Lewald, J., I. G. Meister, J. Weidemann, and R. Töpper. 2004. Involvement of the superior temporal cortex and the occipital cortex in spatial hearing: Evidence from repetitive transcranial magnetic stimulation. *Journal of Cognitive Neuroscience* 16 (5):828–838.

Lewis, J. W., M. S. Beauchamp, and E. A. DeYoe. 2000. A comparison of visual and auditory motion processing in human cerebral cortex. *Cerebral Cortex* 10:873–888.

Li, R. W., S. A. Klein, and D. M. Levi. 2008. Prolonged perceptual learning of positional acuity in adult amblyopia: Perceptual template retuning dynamics. *Journal of Neuroscience* 28 (52):14223–14229.

Liotti, M., K. Ryder, and M. G. Woldorff. 1998. Auditory attention in the congenitally blind: Where, when and what gets reorganized? *Neuroreport* 9 (6):1007–1012.

Liu, Y., C. Yu, M. Liang, J. Li, L. Tian, Y. Zhou, W. Qin, K. Li, and T. Jiang. 2007. Whole brain functional connectivity in the early blind. *Brain* 130 (8):2085–2096.

Livingstone, M., and D. Hubel. 1988. Segregation of form, color, movement, and depth: Anatomy, physiology, and perception. *Science* 240 (4853):740–749.

Locke, J. [1690] 1959. *An Essay Concerning Human Understanding*. New York: Dover.

Logie, R. H. 1995. *Visuo-Spatial Working Memory*. Hove: Lawrence Erlbaum.

Loomis, J. M. 1985. Tactile recognition of raised characters: A parametric study. *Bulletin of the Psychonomic Society* 23:18–20.

Loomis, J. M., R. L. Klatzky, and R. G. Golledge. 2001. Navigating without vision: basic and applied research. *Optometry and Vision Science* 78 (5):282–289.

Loomis, J. M., R. L. Klatzky, R. G. Golledge, J. G. Cicinelli, J. W. Pellegrino, and P. A. Fry. 1993. Nonvisual navigation by blind and sighted: Assessment of path integration ability. *Journal of Experimental Psychology. General* 122 (1):73–91.

Loomis, J. M., and S. J. Lederman. 1986. Tactual perception. In *Handbook of Perception and Human Performance,* vol. 2, ed. K. Boff, L. Kaufman, and J. Thomas. New York: Wiley.

Loomis, J. M., Y. Lippa, R. G. Golledge, and R. L. Klatzky. 2002. Spatial updating of locations specified by 3-D sound and spatial language. *Journal of Experimental Psychology: Learning, Memory, and Cognition* 28 (2):335–345.

Lopes da Silva, F. H. 2003. Visual dreams in the congenitally blind? *Trends in Cognitive Sciences* 7:328–330.

Luzzatti, C., T. Vecchi, D. Agazzi, M. Cesa-Bianchi, and C. Vergani. 1998. A neurological dissociation between preserved visual and impaired spatial processing in mental imagery. *Cortex* 34 (3):461–469.

Machilsen, B., M. Pauwels, and J. Wagemans. 2009. The role of vertical mirror symmetry in visual shape detection. *Journal of Vision* 9 (12):1–11.

Maguire, E. A., and L. Cipolotti. 1998. Selective sparing of topographical memory. *Journal of Neurology, Neurosurgery, and Psychiatry* 65 (6):903–909.

Mahon, B. Z., S. Anzellotti, J. Schwarzbach, M. Zampini, and A. Caramazza. 2009. Category-specific organization in the human brain does not require visual experience. *Neuron* 63 (3):397–405.

Mahon, B. Z., S. C. Milleville, G. A. Negri, R. I. Rumiati, A. Caramazza, and A. Martin. 2007. Action-related properties shape object representations in the ventral stream. *Neuron* 55 (3):507–520.

Majewska, A. K., and M. Sur. 2006. Plasticity and specificity of cortical processing networks. *Trends in Neurosciences* 29 (6):323–329.

Mammarella, I. C., C. Cornoldi, F. Pazzaglia, C. Toso, M. Grimoldi, and C. Vio. 2006. Evidence for a double dissociation between spatial-simultaneous and spatial-sequential working memory in visuospatial (nonverbal) learning disabled children. *Brain and Cognition* 62 (1):58–67.

Mammarella, I. C., F. Pazzaglia, and C. Cornoldi. 2008. Evidence for different components in children's visuospatial working memory. *British Journal of Developmental Psychology* 26:337–355.

Mandavilli, A. 2006. Visual neuroscience: Look and learn. *Nature* 441 (7091):271–272.

Mansouri, B., and R. F. Hess. 2006. The global processing deficit in amblyopia involves noise segregation. *Vision Research* 46 (24):4104–4117.

Marmor, G. S. 1978. Age at onset of blindness and the development of the semantics of color names. *Journal of Experimental Child Psychology* 25 (2):267–278.

Marmor, G. S., and L. A. Zaback. 1976. Mental rotation by the blind: Does mental rotation depend on visual imagery? *Journal of Experimental Psychology. Human Perception and Performance* 2 (4):515–521.

Marotta, J. J., T. S. Perrot, D. Nicolle, P. Servos, and M. A. Goodale. 1995. Adapting to monocular vision: Grasping with one eye. *Experimental Brain Research* 104 (1):107–114.

Martin, A. 2007. The representation of object concepts in the brain. *Annual Review of Psychology* 58:25–45.

Martuzzi, R., M. M. Murray, C. M. Michel, J.-P. Thiran, P. P. Maeder, S. Clarke, and R. A. Meuli. 2007. Multisensory interactions within human primary cortices revealed by BOLD dynamics. *Cerebral Cortex* 17 (7):1672–1679.

Matteau, I., R. Kupers, E. Ricciardi, P. Pietrini, and M. Ptito. 2010. Beyond visual, aural, and haptic movement perception: hMT+ is activated by electrotactile motion stimulation of the tongue in sighted and in congenitally blind individuals. *Brain Research Bulletin* 82 (5–6):264–270.

McAdams, C. J., and J. H. Maunsell. 2000. Attention to both space and feature modulates neuronal responses in macaque area V4. *Journal of Neurophysiology* 83 (3):1751–1755.

McCourt, M. E., and G. Jewell. 1999. Visuospatial attention in line bisection: Stimulus modulation of pseudoneglect. *Neuropsychologia* 37 (7):843–855.

McKee, S. P., D. M. Levi, and J. A. Movshon. 2003. The pattern of visual deficits in amblyopia. *Journal of Vision* 3 (5):380–405.

McLuhan, M. 1962. *Gutenberg Galaxy: The Making of Typographic Man.* Toronto: University of Toronto Press.

Mechelli, A., C. J. Price, K. J. Friston, and A. Ishai. 2004. Where bottom-up meets top-down: Neuronal interactions during perception and imagery. *Cerebral Cortex* 14 (11):1256–1265.

Mellet, E., N. Tzourio, F. Crivello, M. Joliot, M. Denis, and B. Mazoyer. 1996. Functional anatomy of spatial mental imagery generated from verbal instructions. *Journal of Neuroscience* 16 (20):6504–6512.

Merabet, L. B., L. Battelli, S. Obretenova, S. Maguire, P. Meijer, and A. Pascual-Leone. 2009. Functional recruitment of visual cortex for sound encoded object indentification in the blind. *Neuroreport* 20 (2):132–138.

Merabet, L. B., R. Hamilton, G. Schlaug, J. D. Swisher, E. T. Kiriakopoulos, N. B. Pitskel, T. Kauffman, and A. Pascual-Leone. 2008. Rapid and reversible recruitment of early visual cortex for touch. *PLoS ONE* 3 (8):e3046.

Merabet, L. B., J. F. Rizzo, A. Amedi, D. C. Somers, and A. Pascual-Leone. 2005. What blindness can tell us about seeing again: Merging neuroplasticity and neuroprostheses. *Nature Reviews. Neuroscience* 6 (1):71–77.

Millar, S. 1975. Visual experience or translation rules? Drawing the human figure by blind and sighted children. *Perception* 4:363–371.

Millar, S. 1976. Spatial representation by blind and sighted children. *Journal of Experimental Child Psychology* 21 (3):460–479.

Millar, S. 1984. Is there a "best hand" for Braille? *Cortex* 20 (1):75–87.

Millar, S. 1991. A reverse lag in the recognition and production of tactual drawings: Theoretical implications for haptic coding. In *The Psychology of Touch*, ed. M. A. Heller and W. Schiff. Hillsdale, NJ: Lawrence Erlbaum, 301–325.

Millar, S. 1994. *Understanding and Representing Space: Theory and Evidence from Studies with Blind and Sighted Children*. Oxford: Clarendon Press.

Millar, S. 1997. *Reading by Touch*. London: Routledge.

Millar, S., and Z. Al-Attar. 2005. What aspects of vision facilitate haptic processing? *Brain and Cognition* 59 (3):258–268.

Miller, A. I. 1984. *Imagery in Scientific Thought: Creating 20th-Century Physics*. Cambridge, MA: Harvard University Press.

Miller, E. K., C. A. Erickson, and R. Desimone. 1996. Neural mechanisms of visual working memory in prefrontal cortex of the macaque. *Journal of Neuroscience* 16 (16):5154–5167.

Mills, A. E. 1983. *Language Acquisition in the Blind Child: Normal and Deficient*. San Diego: College-Hill Press.

Milner, A. D., and M. A. Goodale. 1995. *The Visual Brain in Action*. Oxford: Oxford University Press.

Mintz-Hittner, H. A., and K. M. Fernandez. 2000. Successful amblyopia therapy initiated after age 7 years: Compliance cures. *Archives of Ophthalmology* 118 (11):1535–1541.

Mix, K. S. 1999. Preschoolers' recognition of numerical equivalence: sequential sets. *Journal of Experimental Child Psychology* 74 (4):309–332.

Mix, K. S., J. Huttenlocher, and S. C. Levine. 2002. Multiple cues for quantification in infancy: Is number one of them? *Psychological Bulletin* 128 (2):278–294.

Moidell, B., M. J. Steinbach, and H. Ono. 1988. Egocenter location in children enucleated at an early age. *Investigative Ophthalmology & Visual Science* 29 (8):1348–1351.

Monegato, M., Z. Cattaneo, A. Pece, and T. Vecchi. 2007. The effect of congenital and acquired visual impairments on visuo-spatial mental abilities. *Journal of Visual Impairment & Blindness* 101:278–295.

Montello, D. R., A. E. Richardson, M. Hegarty, and M. Provenza. 1999. A comparison of methods for estimating directions in egocentric space. *Perception* 28 (8):981–1000.

Morgan, M. 1999. Sensory perception: Supernormal hearing in the blind? *Current Biology* 9 (2):R53–R54.

Moro, V., G. Berlucchi, J. Lerch, F. Tomaiuolo, and S. M. Aglioti. 2008. Selective deficit of mental visual imagery with intact primary visual cortex and visual perception. *Cortex* 44 (2):109–118.

Morris, R. G., P. Garrud, J. N. Rowlins, and J. O'Keefe. 1982. Place navigation impaired in rats with hippocampal lesion. *Nature* 297:681–683.

Morrongiello, B. A. 1994. Effects of colocation on auditory-visual interactions and cross-modal perception in infants. In *The Development of Intersensory Perception: Comparative Perspectives*, ed. D. J. Lewkowicz and R. Lickliter. Hillsdale, NJ: Lawrence Erlbaum, 235–263.

Motter, B. C. 1994. Neural correlates of attentive selection for color or luminance in extrastriate area V4. *Journal of Neuroscience* 14 (4):2178–2189.

Mou, W., X. Li, and T. P. McNamara. 2008. Body- and environmental-stabilized processing of spatial knowledge. *Journal of Experimental Psychology: Learning, Memory, and Cognition* 34 (2):415–421.

Mou, W., T. P. McNamara, B. Rump, and C. Xiao. 2006. Roles of egocentric and allocentric spatial representations in locomotion and reorientation. *Journal of Experimental Psychology: Learning, Memory, and Cognition* 32 (6):1274–1290.

Moutoussis, K., and S. Zeki. 1997. A direct demonstration of perceptual asynchrony in vision. *Proceedings. Biological Sciences* 264 (1380):393–399.

Muchnik, C., M. Efrati, E. Nemeth, M. Malin, and M. Hildesheimer. 1991. Central auditory skills in blind and sighted subjects. *Scandinavian Audiology* 20 (1):19–23.

Murphy, C., and W. S. Cain. 1986. Odor identification: The blind are better. *Physiology & Behavior* 37 (1):177–180.

Nadel, L., and O. Hardt. 2004. The spatial brain. *Neuropsychology* 18 (3):473–476.

Naya, Y., M. Yoshida, and Y. Miyashita. 2001. Backward spreading of memory-retrieval signal in the primate temporal cortex. *Science* 291 (5504):661–664.

Neelon, M. F., D. S. Brungart, and B. D. Simpson. 2004. The isoazimuthal perception of sounds across distance: A preliminary investigation into the location of the audio egocenter. *Journal of Neuroscience* 24 (35):7640–7647.

Neville, H. J., and D. Bavelier. 2000. Cerebral organization of language and the effects of experience. In *Toward a Theory of Neural Plasticity*, ed. C. A. Shaw and J. C. McEachern. Philadelphia: Psychology Press, 261–274.

Neville, H., and D. Bavelier. 2002. Human brain plasticity: Evidence from sensory deprivation and altered language experience. *Progress in Brain Research* 138:177–188.

Neville, H. J., D. Bavelier, D. Corina, J. Rauschecker, A. Karni, A. Lalwani, A. Braun, V. Clark, P. Jezzard, and R. Turner. 1998. Cerebral organization for language in deaf and hearing subjects: Biological constraints and effects of experience. *Proceedings of the National Academy of Sciences of the United States of America* 95 (3):922–929.

Newcombe, N. S. 2002. The nativist-empiricist controversy in the context of recent research on spatial and quantitative development. *Psychological Science* 13:395–401.

Newell, F. N., M. O. Ernst, B. S. Tjan, and H. H. Bülthoff. 2001. Viewpoint dependence in visual and haptic object recognition. *Psychological Science* 12 (1):37–42.

Newell, F. N., A. T. Woods, M. Mernagh, and H. H. Bülthoff. 2005. Visual, haptic, and crossmodal recognition of scenes. *Experimental Brain Research* 161 (2):233–242.

Newstead, S. E., P. Pollard, and R. A. Griggs. 1986. Response bias in relational reasoning. *Bulletin of the Psychonomic Society* 24:95–98.

Nicholas, J. J., C. A. Heywood, and A. Cowey. 1996. Contrast sensitivity in one-eyed subjects. *Vision Research* 36 (1):175–180.

Niedermeyer, E. 1999. The normal EEG of the waking adult. In *Electroencephalography: Basic Principles, Clinical Applications, and Related Fields*, ed. E. Niedermeyer and F. Lopes Da Silva. Baltimore: Lippincott, Williams & Wilkins.

Niemeyer, W., and I. Starlinger. 1981. Do the blind hear better? Investigations on auditory processing in congenital or early acquired blindness. II. Central functions. *Audiology* 20 (6):510–515.

Nolan, C. Y., and C. J. Kederis. 1969. *Perceptual Factors in Braille Word Recognition.* New York: American Foundation for the Blind.

Noordzij, M. L., S. Zuidhoek, and A. Postma. 2006. The influence of visual experience on the ability to form spatial mental models based on route and survey descriptions. *Cognition* 100 (2):321–342.

Noppeney, U., K. J. Friston, J. Ashburner, R. Frackowiak, and C. J. Price. 2005. Early visual deprivation induces structural plasticity in gray and white matter. *Current Biology* 15 (13):R488–R490.

Noppeney, U., K. J. Friston, and C. J. Price. 2003. Effects of visual deprivation on the organization of the semantic system. *Brain* 126 (7):1620–1627.

Nunn, J. A., L. J. Gregory, M. Brammer, S. C. Williams, D. M. Parslow, M. J. Morgan, R. G. Morris, E. T. Bullmore, S. Baron-Cohen, and J. A. Gray. 2002. Functional magnetic resonance imaging of synesthesia: Activation of V4/V8 by spoken words. *Nature Neuroscience* 5 (4):371–375.

O'Craven, K., and N. Kanwisher. 2000. Mental imagery of faces and places activates corresponding stimulus-specific brain regions. *Journal of Cognitive Neuroscience* 12:1013–1023.

Obretenova, S., M. A. Halko, E. B. Plow, A. Pascual-Leone, and L. B. Merabet. 2010. Neuroplasticity associated with tactile language communication in a deaf-blind subject. *Frontiers in Human Neuroscience* 3 (60):1–14.

Occelli, V., C. Spence, and M. Zampini. 2008. Audiotactile temporal order judgments in sighted and blind individuals. *Neuropsychologia* 46 (11):2845–2850.

Ochaíta, E., and J. A. Huertas. 1993. Spatial representation by persons who are blind: A study of the effects of learning and development. *Journal of Visual Impairment & Blindness* 87:37–41.

Ogden, J. A., and K. Barker. 2001. Imagery used in autobiographical recall in early and late blind adults. *Journal of Mental Imagery* 25:135–152.

Ostrovsky, Y., A. Andalman, and P. Sinha. 2006. Vision following extended congenital blindness. *Psychological Science* 17 (12):1009–1014.

Ostrovsky, Y., E. Meyers, S. Ganesh, U. Mathur, and P. Sinha. 2009. Visual parsing after recovery from blindness. *Psychological Science* 20 (12):1484–1491.

Paillard, J. 1991. Motor and representational framing of space. In *Brain and Space*, ed. J. Paillard. Oxford: Oxford University Press, 163–182.

Paivio, A. 1971. *Imagery and Verbal Processes*. New York: Holt, Rinehart & Winston.

Paivio, A. 1986. *Mental Representations: A Dual Coding Approach*. Oxford: Oxford University Press.

Paivio, A. 1991. *Images in Mind: The Evolution of a Theory*. New York: Harvester Wheatsheaf.

Pantev, C., R. Oostenveld, A. Engelien, B. Ross, L. E. Roberts, and M. Hoke. 1998. Increased auditory cortical representation in musicians. *Nature* 392 (6678):811–814.

Pantev, C., B. Ross, T. Fujioka, L. J. Trainor, M. Schulte, and M. Schulz. 2003. Music and learning-induced cortical plasticity. *Annals of the New York Academy of Sciences* 999:438–450.

Park, H. J., J. D. Lee, E. Y. Kim, B. Park, M. K. Oh, S. Lee, and J. J. Kim. 2009. Morphological alterations in the congenital blind based on the analysis of cortical thickness and surface area. *NeuroImage* 47 (1):98–106.

Pascual-Leone, A., A. Amedi, F. Fregni, and L. B. Merabet. 2005. The plastic human brain cortex. *Annual Review of Neuroscience* 28:377–401.

Pascual-Leone, A., A. Cammarota, E. M. Wassermann, J. P. Brasil-Neto, L. G. Cohen, and M. Hallett. 1993. Modulation of motor cortical outputs to the reading hand of Braille readers. *Annals of Neurology* 34 (1):33–37.

Pascual-Leone, A., and R. Hamilton. 2001. The metamodal organization of the brain. *Progress in Brain Research* 134:427–445.

Pascual-Leone, A., H. Theoret, L. Merabet, T. Kauffmann, and G. Schlaug. 2006. The role of visual cortex in tactile processing: A metamodal brain. In *Touch and Blindness: Psychology and Neuroscience*, ed. M. A. Heller and S. Ballesteros. Mahwah, NJ: Lawrence Erlbaum, 171–195.

Pascual-Leone, A., and F. Torres. 1993. Plasticity of the sensorimotor cortex representation of the reading finger in Braille readers. *Brain* 116 (1):39–52.

Pasqualotto, A., C. M. Finucane, and F. N. Newell. 2005. Visual and haptic representations of scenes are updated with observer movement. *Experimental Brain Research* 166 (3–4):481–488.

Pasqualotto, A., and F. N. Newell. 2007. The role of visual experience on the representation and updating of novel haptic scenes. *Brain and Cognition* 65 (2):184–194.

Passini, R., G. Proulx, and C. Rainville. 1990. The spatio-cognitive abilities of the visually impaired population. *Environment and Behavior* 22 (1):91–118.

Paterson, M. 2006. "Seeing with the hands": Blindness, touch, and the Enlightenment spatial imaginary. *British Journal of Visual Impairment* 24 (2):52–59.

Paulesu, E., J. Harrison, S. Baron-Cohen, J. D. Watson, L. Goldstein, J. Heather, R. S. Frackowiak, and C. D. Frith. 1995. The physiology of coloured hearing: A PET activation study of colour-word synaesthesia. *Brain* 118 (3):661–676.

Pavani, F., C. Spence, and J. Driver. 2000. Visual capture of touch: Out-of-the-body experiences with rubber gloves. *Psychological Science* 11 (5):353–359.

Pazzaglia, F., and C. Cornoldi. 1999. The role of distinct components of visuo-spatial working memory in the processing of texts. *Memory* 7 (1):19–41.

Pearson, D. G., and R. H. Logie. 2003–2004. Effects of stimulus modality and working memory load on mental synthesis performance. *Imagination, Cognition, and Personality* 23 (2–3):183–191.

Pearson, D. G., R. H. Logie, and K. J. Gilhooly. 1999. Verbal representations and spatial manipulation during mental synthesis. *European Journal of Cognitive Psychology* 11 (3):259–314.

Pearson, J., and J. Brascamp. 2008. Sensory memory for ambiguous vision. *Trends in Cognitive Sciences* 12 (9):334–341.

Pearson, J., C. W. Clifford, and F. Tong. 2008. The functional impact of mental imagery on conscious perception. *Current Biology* 18 (13):982–986.

Perez-Pereira, M., and G. Conti-Ramsden. 1999. *Social Interaction and Language Development in Blind Children*. Hove: Psychology Press.

Perkel, D. J., J. Bullier, and H. Kennedy. 1986. Topography of the afferent connectivity of area 17 in the macaque monkey: A double-labelling study. *Journal of Comparative Neurology* 253 (3):374–402.

Perky, C. W. 1910. An experimental study of imagination. *American Journal of Psychology* 21 (3):422–452.

Phillips, J. R., R. S. Johansson, and K. O. Johnson. 1990. Representation of Braille characters in human nerve fibres. *Experimental Brain Research* 81 (3):589–592.

Piccolino, M. 2008. Visual images in Luigi Galvani's path to animal electricity. *Journal of the History of the Neurosciences* 17 (3):335–348.

Pick, A. D., H. L. Pick, Jr., and M. L. Thomas. 1966. Cross-modal transfer and improvement of form discrimination. *Journal of Experimental Child Psychology* 3 (3):279–288.

Pick, H. L., D. H. Warren, and J. C. Hay. 1969. Sensory conflict in judgments of spatial direction. *Perception & Psychophysics* 6:203–205.

Pietrini, P., M. L. Furey, E. Ricciardi, M. I. Gobbini, W.-H. C. Wu, L. Cohen, M. Guazzelli, and J. V. Haxby. 2004. Beyond sensory images: Object-based representation in the human ventral pathway. *Proceedings of the National Academy of Sciences of the United States of America* 101 (15):5658–5663.

Pietrini, P., M. Ptito, and R. Kupers. 2009. Blindness and consciousness: New light from the dark. In *The Neurology of Consciousness*, ed. G. Tononi and S. Laureys. Amsterdam: Elsevier, 360–374.

Pisella, L., M. Arzi, and Y. Rossetti. 1998. The timing of color and location processing in the motor context. *Experimental Brain Research* 121 (3):270–276.

Poirier, C., O. Collignon, A. G. De Volder, L. Renier, A. Vanlierde, D. Tranduy, and C. Scheiber. 2005. Specific activation of the V5 brain area by auditory motion processing: An fMRI study. *Brain Research. Cognitive Brain Research* 25 (3):650–658.

Poirier, C., O. Collignon, C. Scheiber, L. Renier, A. Vanlierde, D. Tranduy, C. Veraart, and A. G. De Volder. 2006. Auditory motion perception activates visual motion areas in early blind subjects. *NeuroImage* 31 (1):279–285.

Poirier, C., M.-A. Richard, D. T. Duy, and C. Veraart. 2006. Assessment of sensory substitution prosthesis potentialities in minimalist conditions of learning. *Applied Cognitive Psychology* 20:447–460.

Poirier, C., A. G. De Volder, and C. Scheiber. 2007. What neuroimaging tells us about sensory substitution. *Neuroscience and Biobehavioral Reviews* 31:1064–1070.

Pons, T. 1996. Novel sensations in the congenitally blind. *Nature* 380 (6574):479–480.

Porter, J., T. Anand, B. Johnson, R. M. Khan, and N. Sobel. 2005. Brain mechanisms for extracting spatial information from smell. *Neuron* 47 (4):581–592.

Posner, M. I. 2004. *Cognitive Neuroscience of Attention*. New York: Guilford.

Posner, M. I., M. J. Nissen, and R. M. Klein. 1976. Visual dominance: An information-processing account of its origins and significance. *Psychological Review* 83 (2):157–171.

Posner, M. I., M. J. Nissen, and W. C. Ogden. 1978. Attended and unattended processing modes: The role of set for spatial location. In *Modes of Perceiving and Processing Information*, ed. H. L. Pick and E. Saltzman. Hillsdale, NJ: Lawrence Erlbaum, 137–157.

Postma, A., S. Zuidhoek, M. L. Noordzij, and A. M. L. Kappers. 2007. Differences between early-blind, late-blind, and blindfolded-sighted people in haptic spatial-configuration learning and resulting memory traces. *Perception* 36 (8):1253–1265.

Postma, A., S. Zuidhoek, M. L. Noordzij, and A. M. L. Kappers. 2008. Haptic orientation perception benefits from visual experience: Evidence from early-blind, late-blind, and sighted people. *Perception & Psychophysics* 70 (7):1197–1206.

Power, R. P. 1981. The dominance of touch by vision: Occurs with familiar objects. *Perception* 10 (1):29–33.

Presmeg, N. C. 1986a. Visualization in high school mathematics. *For the Learning of Mathematics* 6 (3):42–48.

Presmeg, N. C. 1986b. Visualization and mathematical giftedness. *Educational Studies in Mathematics* 17:297–311.

Presmeg, N. C. 1992. Prototypes, metaphors, metonymies, and imaginative rationality in high school mathematics. *Educational Studies in Mathematics* 23:595–610.

Presmeg, N. C. 1997. Generalization using imagery in mathematics. In *Mathematical Reasoning: Analogies, Metaphors, and Images*, ed. L. D. English. Mahwah, NJ: Lawrence Erlbaum, 299–312.

Presmeg, N. C. 2006. Research on visualization in learning and teaching mathematics. In *Handbook of Research on Psychology of Mathematic Education: Past, Present, and Future*, ed. P. B. A. Gutierrez. Rotterdam: Sense Publishers, 205–235.

Presson, C. C., N. DeLange, and M. D. Hazelrigg. 1989. Orientation specificity in spatial memory: What makes a path different from a map of the path? *Journal of Experimental Psychology: Learning, Memory, and Cognition* 15 (5):887–897.

Price, D. J., J. M. Ferrer, C. Blakemore, and N. Kato. 1994. Functional organization of corticocortical projections from area 17 to area 18 in the cat's visual cortex. *Journal of Neuroscience* 14 (5):2732–2746.

Pring, E., and J. Rusted. 1985. Pictures for the blind: an investigation of the influence of pictures on the recall of texts by blind children. *British Journal of Developmental* Psychology 3:41–45.

Pring, L. 1988. The "reverse-generation" effect: A comparison of memory performance between blind and sighted children. *British Journal of Psychology* 79 (3):387–400.

Pring, L. 2005. *Autism and Blindness: Research and Reflections*. London: Wiley.

Pring, L., S. E. Freistone, and S. A. Katan. 1990. Recalling pictures and words: Reversing the generation effect. *Current Psychological Research & Reviews* 9 (1):35–45.

Pring, L., and L. Goddard. 2003. Autobiographical memory in individuals born totally blind. In *Touch and Blindness: Psychology and Neuroscience*, ed. M. A. Heller and S. Ballesteros. Hillsdale, NJ: Lawrence Erlbaum.

Pring, L., K. Woolf, and V. Tadic. 2008. Melody and pitch processing in five musical savants with congenital blindness. *Perception* 37 (2):290–307.

Prusky, G. T., N. M. Alam, and R. M. Douglas. 2006. Enhancement of vision by monocular deprivation in adult mice. *Journal of Neuroscience* 26 (45):11554–11561.

Ptito, M., A. Fumal, A. M. de Noordhout, J. Schoenen, A. Gjedde, and R. Kupers. 2008. TMS of the occipital cortex induces tactile sensations in the fingers of blind Braille readers. *Experimental Brain Research* 184 (2):193–200.

Ptito, M., J.-F. Giguère, D. Boire, D. O. Frost, and C. Casanova. 2001. When the auditory cortex turns visual. *Progress in Brain Research* 134:447–158.

Ptito, M., and R. Kupers. 2005. Cross-modal plasticity in early blindness. *Journal of Integrative Neuroscience* 4 (4):479–488.

Ptito, M., I. Matteau, A. Gjedde, and R. Kupers. 2009. Recruitment of the middle temporal area by tactile motion in congenital blindness. *Neuroreport* 20 (6):543–547.

Puche-Navarro, R., and R. Millan. 2007. Inferential functioning in visually impaired children. *Research in Developmental Disabilities* 28 (3):249–265.

Pujol, J., J. Roset-Llobet, D. Rosinés-Cubells, J. Deus, B. Narberhaus, J. Valls-Solé, A. Capdevila, and A. Pascual-Leone. 2000. Brain cortical activation during guitar-induced hand dystonia studied by functional MRI. *NeuroImage* 12 (3):257–267.

Putzar, L., I. Goerendt, K. Lange, F. Rösler, and B. Röder. 2007. Early visual deprivation impairs multisensory interactions in humans. *Nature Neuroscience* 10 (10):1243–1245.

Pylyshyn, Z. W. 1973. What the mind's eye tells the mind's brain: A critique of mental imagery. *Psychological Bulletin* 80:1–24.

Pylyshyn, Z. W. 1981. Psychological explanations and knowledge-dependent processes. *Cognition* 10 (1–3):267–274.

Pylyshyn, Z. W. 2003. Explaining mental imagery: Now you see it, now you don't. Reply to Kosslyn et al. *Trends in Cognitive Sciences* 7 (3):111–112.

Quinn, J. G. 2008. Movement and visual coding: The structure of visuo-spatial working memory. *Cognitive Processing* 9 (1):35–43.

Ragert, P., A. Schmidt, E. Altenmüller, and H. R. Dinse. 2004. Superior tactile performance and learning in professional pianists: Evidence for meta-plasticity in musicians. *European Journal of Neuroscience* 19 (2):473–478.

Ragni, M., M. Knauff, and B. Nebel. 2005. A computational model for spatial reasoning with mental models. In *Proceedings of the 27th Annual Cognitive Science Conference*, ed. B. G. Bara, L. Barsalou, and M. Bucciarelli. Mahwah, NJ: Lawrence Erlbaum.

Ramachandran, V. S., and E. M. Hubbard. 2001. Psychophysical investigations into the neural basis of synaesthesia. *Proceedings. Biological Sciences* 268 (1470):979–983.

Rao, A., A. C. Nobre, I. Alexander, and A. Cowey. 2007. Auditory evoked visual awareness following sudden ocular blindness: An EEG and TMS investigation. *Experimental Brain Research* 176 (2):288–298.

Rauschecker, J. P. 1999. Auditory cortical plasticity: A comparison with other sensory systems. *Trends in Neurosciences* 22 (2):74–80.

Rauschecker, J. P., and U. Kniepert. 1994. Auditory localization behaviour in visually deprived cats. *European Journal of Neuroscience* 6 (1):149–160.

Raz, N., A. Amedi, and E. Zohary. 2005. V1 activation in congenitally blind humans is associated with episodic retrieval. *Cerebral Cortex* 15 (9):1459–1468.

Raz, N., E. Striem, G. Pundak, T. Orlov, and E. Zohary. 2007. Superior serial memory in the blind: A case of cognitive compensatory adjustment. *Current Biology* 17 (13):1129–1133.

Reed, M. J., J. K. Steeves, and M. J. Steinbach. 1997. A comparison of contrast letter thresholds in unilateral eye enucleated subjects and binocular and monocular control subjects. *Vision Research* 37 (17):2465–2469.

Reed, M. J., J. K. Steeves, M. J. Steinbach, S. Kraft, and B. Gallie. 1996. Contrast letter thresholds in the non-affected eye of strabismic and unilateral eye enucleated subjects. *Vision Research* 36 (18):3011–3018.

Reed, M. J., M. J. Steinbach, S. M. Anstis, B. Gallie, D. Smith, and S. Kraft. 1991. The development of optokinetic nystagmus in strabismic and monocularly enucleated subjects. *Behavioural Brain Research* 46 (1):31–42.

Renier, L., and A. G. De Volder. 2010. Vision substitution and depth perception: Early blind subjects experience visual perspective through their ears. *Disability and Rehabilitation: Assistive Technology* 5 (3):175–183.

Resnikoff, S., D. Pascolini, D. Etya'ale, I. Kocur, R. Pararajasegaram, G. P. Pokharel, and S. P. Mariotti. 2004. Global data on visual impairment in the year 2002. *Bulletin of the World Health Organization* 82 (11):844–851.

Resnikoff, S., D. Pascolini, S. P. Mariotti, and G. P. Pokharel. 2008. Global magnitude of visual impairment caused by uncorrected refractive errors in 2004. *Bulletin of the World Health Organization* 86 (1):63–70.

Reynvoet, B., M. Brysbaert, and W. Fias. 2002. Semantic priming in number naming. *Quarterly Journal of Experimental Psychology A: Human Experimental Psychology* 55 (4):1127–1139.

Ricciardi, E., D. Bonino, C. Gentili, L. Sani, P. Pietrini, and T. Vecchi. 2006. Neural correlates of spatial working memory in humans: A functional magnetic resonance imaging study comparing visual and tactile processes. *Neuroscience* 139 (1):339–349.

Ricciardi, E., D. Bonino, L. Sani, T. Vecchi, M. Guazzelli, J. V. Haxby, L. Fadiga, and P. Pietrini. 2009. Do we really need vision? How blind people "see" the actions of others. *Journal of Neuroscience* 29 (31):9719–9724.

Ricciardi, E., N. Vanello, L. Sani, C. Gentili, E. P. Scilingo, L. Landini, M. Guazzelli, A. Bicchi, J. V. Haxby, and P. Pietrini. 2007. The effect of visual experience on the development of functional architecture in hMT+. *Cerebral Cortex* 17 (12):2933–2939.

Rice, C. E., S. H. Feinstein, and R. J. Schusterman. 1965. Echo-detection ability of the blind: Size and distance factors. *Journal of Experimental Psychology* 70:246–255.

Rieser, J. J., D. A. Guth, and E. W. Hill. 1986. Sensitivity to perspective structure while walking without vision. *Perception* 15 (2):173–188.

Rieser, J. J., E. W. Hill, C. R. Talor, A. Bradfield, and S. Rosen. 1992. Visual experience, visual field size, and the development of nonvisual sensitivity to the spatial structure of outdoor neighborhoods explored by walking. *Journal of Experimental Psychology: General* 121 (2):210–221.

Rieser, J. J., J. J. Lockman, H. L. Pick, Jr. 1980. The role of visual experience in knowledge of spatial layout. *Perception & Psychophysics* 28 (3):185–190.

Rinck, M., and M. Denis. 2004. The metrics of spatial distance traversed during mental imagery. *Journal of Experimental Psychology: Learning, Memory, and Cognition* 30 (6):1211–1218.

Rips, L. J. 1994. *The Psychology of Proof: Deductive Reasoning in Human Thinking*. Cambridge, MA: MIT Press.

Rizzolatti, G., L. Fadiga, V. Gallese, and L. Fogassi. 1996. Premotor cortex and the recognition of motor actions. *Brain Research: Cognitive Brain Research* 3 (2):131–141.

Rizzolatti, G., L. Fogassi, and V. Gallese. 2001. Neurophysiological mechanisms underlying the understanding and imitation of action. *Nature Reviews: Neuroscience* 2 (9):661–670.

Rizzolatti, G., L. Riggio, I. Dascola, and C. Umiltá. 1987. Reorienting attention across the horizontal and vertical meridians: Evidence in favor of a premotor theory of attention. *Neuropsychologia* 25 (1A):31–40.

Rock, I., and J. DiVita. 1987. A case of viewer-centered object perception. *Cognitive Psychology* 19 (2):280–293.

Rock, I., and J. Victor. 1964. Vision and touch: An experimentally created conflict between the two senses. *Science* 143:594–596.

Röder, B., L. Demuth, J. Streb, and F. Rösler. 2002. Semantic and syntactic priming in auditory word recognition in congenitally blind adults. *Language and Cognitive Processes* 18:1–20.

Röder, B., J. Föcker, K. Hötting, and C. Spence. 2008. Spatial coordinate systems for tactile spatial attention depend on developmental vision: Evidence from event-related potentials in sighted and congenitally blind adult humans. *European Journal of Neuroscience* 28 (3):475–483.

Röder, B., U. M. Krämer, and K. Lange. 2007. Congenitally blind humans use different stimulus selection strategies in hearing: An ERP study of spatial and temporal attention. *Restorative Neurology and Neuroscience* 25 (3–4):311–322.

Röder, B., A. Kusmierek, C. Spence, and T. Schicke. 2007. Developmental vision determines the reference frame for the multisensory control of action. *Proceedings of the National Academy of Sciences of the United States of America* 104 (11):4753–4758.

Röder, B., and H. Neville. 2003. Developmental functional plasticity. In *Handbook of Neuropsychology: Plasticity and Rehabilitation*, ed. J. Grafman and I. H. Robertson. Amsterdam: Elsevier Science, 231–270.

Röder, B., and F. Rösler. 1998. Visual input does not facilitate the scanning of spatial images. *Journal of Mental Imagery* 22:165–181.

Röder, B., and F. Rösler. 2003. Memory for environmental sounds in sighted, congenitally blind and late blind adults: Evidence for cross-modal compensation. *International Journal of Psychophysiology* 50 (1–2):27–39.

Röder, B., and F. Rösler. 2004. Compensatory plasticity as a consequence of sensory loss. In *The Handbook of Multisensory Processes*, ed. G. Calvert, C. Spence, and B. E. Stein. Cambridge, MA: MIT Press, 719–747.

Röder, B., and F. Rösler, M. Heil, and E. Hennighausen. 1993. [Haptic mental rotation in patients with congenital blindness, acquired blindness, and normal vision persons]. [Article in German.] *Zeitschrift für Experimentelle und Angewandte Psychologie* 40 (1):154–177.

Röder, B., F. Rösler, and E. Hennighausen. 1997. Different cortical activation patterns in blind and sighted humans during encoding and transformation of haptic images. *Psychophysiology* 34 (3):292–307.

Röder, B., F. Rösler, E. Hennighausen, and F. Näcker. 1996. Event-related potentials during auditory and somatosensory discrimination in sighted and blind human subjects. *Brain Research. Cognitive Brain Research* 4 (2):77–93.

Röder, B., F. Rösler, and H. J. Neville. 1999. Effects of interstimulus interval on auditory event-related potentials in congenitally blind and normally sighted humans. *Neuroscience Letters* 264 (1–3):53–56.

Röder, B., F. Rösler, and H. J. Neville. 2000. Event-related potentials during auditory language processing in congenitally blind and sighted people. *Neuropsychologia* 38 (11):1482–1502.

Röder, B., F. Rösler, and H. J. Neville. 2001. Auditory memory in congenitally blind adults: A behavioral-electrophysiological investigation. *Brain Research. Cognitive Brain Research* 11 (2):289–303.

Röder, B., F. Rösler, and C. Spence. 2004. Early vision impairs tactile perception in the blind. *Current Biology* 14 (2):121–124.

Röder, B., O. Stock, S. Bien, H. Neville, and F. Rösler. 2002. Speech processing activates visual cortex in congenitally blind humans. *European Journal of Neuroscience* 16 (5):930–936.

Röder, B., W. Teder-Salejarvi, A. Sterr, F. Rösler, S. A. Hillyard, and H. J. Neville. 1999. Improved auditory spatial tuning in blind humans. *Nature* 400 (6740):162–166.

Roeser, R., M. Valente, and H. Hosford-Dunn. 2000. *Audiology: Diagnosis*. New York: Thieme Medical Publishers.

Rokem, A., and M. Ahissar. 2009. Interactions of cognitive and auditory abilities in congenitally blind individuals. *Neuropsychologia* 47 (3):843–848.

Rorden, C., and J. Driver. 1999. Does auditory attention shift in the direction of an upcoming saccade? *Neuropsychologia* 37 (3):357–377.

Rosenbluth, R., E. S. Grossman, and M. Kaitz. 2000. Performance of early-blind and sighted children on olfactory tasks. *Perception* 29 (1):101–110.

Roskos-Ewoldsen, B., T. P. McNamara, A. L. Shelton, and W. Carr. 1998. Mental representations of large and small spatial layouts are orientation dependent. *Journal of Experimental Psychology: Learning, Memory, and Cognition* 24 (1):215–226.

Rösler, F., B. Röder, M. Heil, and E. Hennighausen. 1993. Topographic differences of slow event-related brain potentials in blind and sighted adult human subjects during haptic mental rotation. *Brain Research: Cognitive Brain Research* 1 (3):145–159.

Rossetti, Y. 1998. Implicit short-lived motor representations of space in brain damaged and healthy subjects. *Consciousness and Cognition* 7 (3):520–558.

Rossetti, Y., F. Gaunet, and C. Thinus-Blanc. 1996. Early visual experience affects memorization and spatial representation of proprioceptive targets. *Neuroreport* 7 (6):1219–1223.

Rossetti, Y., and L. Pisella. 2002. Several "vision for action" systems: A guide to dissociating and integrating dorsal and ventral functions. In *Attention and Performance XIX. Common Mechanisms in Perception and Action*, ed. W. Prinz and B. Hommel. Oxford: Oxford University Press, 62–119.

Rossetti, Y., and C. Régnier. 1995. Representations in action: pointing to a target with various representations. In *Studies in Perception and Action III*, ed. R. J. Bootsma, G. Bardy, and Y. Guiard. Mahwah, NJ: Lawrence Erlbaum, 233–236.

Rossi, P. 2000. *Logic and the Art of Memory*. Chicago: University of Chicago Press.

Rossi-Arnaud, C., L. Pieroni, and A. Baddeley. 2006. Symmetry and binding in visuo-spatial working memory. *Neuroscience* 139 (1):393–400.

Roth, H. L., A. N. Lora, and K. M. Heilman. 2002. Effects of monocular viewing and eye dominance on spatial attention. *Brain* 125 (9):2023–2035.

Rousselle, L., E. Palmers, and M. P. Noël. 2004. Magnitude comparison in preschoolers: What counts? Influence of perceptual variables. *Journal of Experimental Child Psychology* 87 (1):57–84.

Rudel, R. G., M. B. Denckla, and E. Spalten. 1974. The functional asymmetry of Braille letter learning in normal, sighted children. *Neurology* 24:733–738.

Ruff, C. C., F. Blankenburg, O. Bjoertomt, S. Bestmann, E. Freeman, J. D. Haynes, G. Rees, O. Josephs, R. Deichmann, and J. Driver. 2006. Concurrent TMS-fMRI and psychophysics reveal frontal influences on human retinotopic visual cortex. *Current Biology* 16 (15):1479–1488.

Ruff, C. C., A. Kristjánsson, and J. Driver. 2007. Readout from iconic memory and selective spatial attention involve similar neural processes. *Psychological Science* 18 (10):901–909.

Saariluoma, P., and V. Kalakoski. 1998. Apperception and imagery in blindfold chess. *Memory* 6 (1):67–90.

Sack, A. T., C. Jacobs, F. De Martino, N. Staeren, R. Goebel, and E. Formisano. 2008. Dynamic premotor-to-parietal interactions during spatial imagery. *Journal of Neuroscience* 28 (34):8417–8429.

Sacks, O. 1993. To see and not see—a neurologist's notebook. *New Yorker* (May 10): 59–73.

Sadato, N. 2005. How the blind "see" Braille: Lessons from functional magnetic resonance imaging. *Neuroscientist* 11 (6):577–582.

Sadato, N., and M. Hallett. 1999. fMRI occipital activation by tactile stimulation in a blind man. *Neurology* 52 (2):423.

Sadato, N., T. Okada, M. Honda, and Y. Yonekura. 2002. Critical period for cross-modal plasticity in blind humans: A functional MRI study. *NeuroImage* 16 (2):389–400.

Sadato, N., T. Okada, K. Kubota, and Y. Yonekura. 2004. Tactile discrimination activates the visual cortex of the recently blind naive to Braille: A functional magnetic resonance imaging study in humans. *Neuroscience Letters* 359 (1–2):49–52.

Sadato, N., A. Pascual-Leone, J. Grafman, M. P. Deiber, V. Ibañez, and M. Hallett. 1998. Neural networks for Braille reading by the blind. *Brain* 121 (7):1213–1229.

Sadato, N., A. Pascual-Leone, J. Grafman, V. Ibañez, M. P. Deiber, G. Dold, and M. Hallett. 1996. Activation of the primary visual cortex by Braille reading in blind subjects. *Nature* 380 (6574):526–528.

Sadoski, M., E. T. Goetz, and M. Rodriguez. 2000. Engaging texts: Effects of concreteness on comprehensibility, interest, and recall in four text types. *Journal of Educational Psychology* 92 (1):85–95.

Sadoski, M., and A. Paivio. 2001. Imagery and text: A dual coding theory of reading and writing. *Reading and Writing* 16 (3):259–262.

Sadoski, M., and A. Paivio. 2004. A dual coding theoretical model of reading. In *Theoretical Models and Processes of Reading,* 5th ed., ed. R. B. Ruddell and N. J. Unrau. Newark, DE: International Reading Association, 1329–1362.

Sadoski, M., A. Paivio, and E. T. Goetz. 1991. Commentary: A critique of schema theory in reading and a dual coding alternative. *Reading Research Quarterly* 26:463–484.

Sadoski, M., and Z. Quast. 1990. Reader recall and long term recall for journalistic text: The roles of imagery, affect, and importance. *Reading Research Quarterly* 25:256–272.

Saenz, M., L. B. Lewis, A. G. Huth, I. Fine, and C. Koch. 2008. Visual motion area MT+/V5 responds to auditory motion in human sight-recovery subjects. *Journal of Neuroscience* 28 (20):5141–5148.

Salillas, E., A. Grana, R. El-Yagoubi, and C. Semenza. 2009. Numbers in the blind's "eye." *PLoS ONE* 4 (7):6357.

Sampaio, E., S. Maris, and P. Bach-y-Rita. 2001. Brain plasticity: "Visual" acuity of blind persons via the tongue. *Brain Research* 908 (2):204–207.

Sandell, J. H., and P. H. Schiller. 1982. Effect of cooling area 18 on striate cortex cells in the squirrel monkey. *Journal of Neurophysiology* 48 (1):38–48.

Sanders, C. W., M. Sadoski, K. van Walsum, R. Bramson, R. Wiprud, and T. W. Fossum. 2008. Learning basic surgical skills with mental imagery: Using the simulation centre in the mind. *Medical Education* 42:607–612.

Sathian, K. 2005. Visual cortical activity during tactile perception in the sighted and the visually deprived. *Developmental Psychobiology* 46 (3):279–286.

Sathian, K., A. W. Goodwin, K. T. John, and I. Darian-Smith. 1989. Perceived roughness of a grating: Correlation with responses of mechanoreceptive afferents innervating the monkey's fingerpad. *Journal of Neuroscience* 9 (4):1273–1279.

Sathian, K., and R. Stilla. 2010. Cross-modal plasticity of tactile perception in blindness. *Restorative Neurology and Neuroscience* 28 (2):271–281.

Sathian, K., and A. Zangaladze. 2001. Feeling with the mind's eye: The role of visual imagery in tactile perception. *Optometry and Vision Science* 78 (5):276–281.

Sathian, K., A. Zangaladze, J. M. Hoffman, and S. T. Grafton. 1997. Feeling with the mind's eye. *Neuroreport* 8 (18):3877–3881.

Sato, M., and M. P. Stryker. 2008. Distinctive features of adult ocular dominance plasticity. *Journal of Neuroscience* 28 (41):10278–10286.

Schacter, D. L., and L. Nadel. 1991. *Varieties of Spatial Memory: A Problem for Cognitive Neuroscience*. New York: Oxford University Press.

Schendan, H. E., G. Ganis, and M. Kutas. 1998. Neurophysiological evidence for visual perceptual categorization of words and faces within 150 ms. *Psychophysiology* 35 (3):240–251.

Schendan, H. E., and M. Kutas. 2007. Neurophysiological evidence for the time course of activation of global shape, part, and local contour representations during visual object categorization and memory. *Journal of Cognitive Neuroscience* 19 (5):734–749.

Schlieder, C., and B. Berendt. 1998. Mental model construction in spatial reasoning: A comparison of two computational theories. In *Mind Modelling: A Cognitive Science Approach to Reasoning, Learning, and Discovery*, ed. U. Schmid, J. F. Krems, and F. Wysotzki. Lengerich: Pabst Science Publishers, 133–162.

Schneider, F., R. Kupers, and M. Ptito. 2006. MRI voxel-based morphometry reveals reduced visual pathways in early blind humans. *Society for Neuroscience Abstracts* 240:6.

Schwartz, D. L., and J. B. Black. 1996. Analog imagery in mental model reasoning: depictive models. *Cognitive Psychology* 30 (2):154–219.

Schwenn, O., I. Hundorf, B. Moll, S. Pitz, and J. W. Mann. 2002. [Do blind persons have a better sense of smell than normal sighted people?] [Article in German.] *Klinische Monatsblatter fur Augenheilkunde* 219 (9):649–654.

Seemungal, B. M., S. Glasauer, M. A. Gresty, and A. M. Bronstein. 2007. Vestibular perception and navigation in the congenitally blind. *Journal of Neurophysiology* 97 (6):4341–4356.

Semenza, C., M. Zoppello, O. Gidiuli, and F. Borgo. 1996. Dichaptic scanning of Braille letters by skilled blind readers: Lateralization effects. *Perceptual and Motor Skills* 82 (3):1071–1074.

Shapiro, K. L., W. J. Jacobs, and V. M. LoLordo. 1980. Stimulus-reinforcer interactions in Pavlovian conditioning of pigeons: Implications for selective associations. *Animal Learning and Behavior* 8:586–594.

Shao, Z., and A. Burkhalter. 1996. Different balance of excitation and inhibition in forward and feedback circuits of rat visual cortex. *Journal of Neuroscience* 16 (22):7353–7365.

Shaver, P. R., L. Pierson, and S. Lang. 1975. Converging evidence for the functional significance of imagery in problem solving. *Cognition* 3:359–375.

Shaw, C. A., and J. C. McEachern. 2001. *Towards a Theory of Neuroplasticity*. London: Psychology Press.

Shepard, R. N. 1978. Externalization of mental images and the act of creation. In *Visual Learning, Thinking and Communication*, ed. B. S. Randhawa and W. E. Coffman. San Diego: Academic Press.

Shepard, R. N., and L. Cooper. 1982. *Mental Images and Their Transformations*. Cambridge, MA: MIT Press.

Shepard, R. N., and J. Metzler. 1971. Mental rotation of three-dimensional objects. *Science* 171 (972):701–703.

Shimizu, Y., S. Saida, and H. Shimura. 1993. Tactile pattern recognition by graphic display: Importance of 3-D information for haptic perception of familiar objects. *Perception & Psychophysics* 53 (1):43–48.

Shimono, K., A. Higashiyama, and W. J. Tam. 2001. Location of the egocenter in kinesthetic space. *Journal of Experimental Psychology: Human Perception and Performance* 27 (4):848–861.

Shimony, J. S., H. Burton, A. A. Epstein, D. G. McLaren, S. W. Sun, and A. Z. Snyder. 2006. Diffusion tensor imaging reveals white matter reorganization in early blind humans. *Cerebral Cortex* 16 (11):1653–1661.

Shu, N., J. Li, K. Li, C. Yu, and T. Jiang. 2009. Abnormal diffusion of cerebral white matter in early blindness. *Human Brain Mapping* 30 (1):220–227.

Shu, N., Y. Liu, J. Li, Y. Li, C. Yu, and T. Jiang. 2009. Altered anatomical network in early blindness revealed by diffusion tensor tractography. *PLoS One* 4 (9):e7228.

Signoret, J. L., P. van Eeckhout, M. Poncet, and P. Castaigne. 1987. [Aphasia without amusia in a blind organist. Verbal alexia-agraphia without musical alexia-agraphia in Braille.] [Article in French.] *Revue Neurologique* 143 (3):172–181.

Silvanto, J., N. Lavie, and V. Walsh. 2006. Stimulation of the human frontal eye fields modulates sensitivity of extrastriate visual cortex. *Journal of Neurophysiology* 96 (2):941–945.

Silvanto, J., N. Muggleton, and V. Walsh. 2008. State-dependency in brain stimulation studies of perception and cognition. *Trends in Cognitive Sciences* 12 (12):447–454.

Silvanto, J., and A. Pascual-Leone. 2008. State-dependency of transcranial magnetic stimulation. *Brain Topography* 21 (1):1–10.

Simon, J. R., J. V. Hinrichs, and J. L. Craft. 1970. Auditory S-R compatibility: Reaction time as a function of ear-hand correspondence and ear-response-location correspondence. *Journal of Experimental Psychology* 86 (1):97–102.

Simon, T. J. 1997. Reconceptualizing the origins of number knowledge: A "non-numerical" account. *Cognitive Development* 12:349–372.

Simon, T. J. 1999. The foundations of numerical thinking in a brain without numbers. *Trends in Cognitive Sciences* 3 (10):363–365.

Simons, D. J., and R. F. Wang. 1998. Perceiving real-world viewpoint changes. *Psychological Science* 9:315–320.

Simons, D. J., R. F. Wang, and D. Roddenberry. 2002. Object recognition is mediated by extraretinal information. *Perception & Psychophysics* 64 (4):521–530.

Singer, G., and R. H. Day. 1969. Visual capture of haptically judged depth. *Perception & Psychophysics* 5 (5):315–316.

Slotnick, S. D. 2008. Imagery: Mental pictures disrupt perceptual rivalry. *Current Biology* 18 (14):R603–R605.

Slotnick, S. D., W. L. Thompson, and S. M. Kosslyn. 2005. Visual mental imagery induces retinotopically organized activation of early visual areas. *Cerebral Cortex* 15 (10):1570–1583.

Small, J. P. 1997. *Wax Tablets of the Mind*. London: Routledge.

Smirnakis, S. M., A. A. Brewer, M. C. Schmid, A. S. Tolias, A. Schüz, M. Augath, W. Inhoffen, B. A. Wandell, and N. K. Logothetis. 2005. Lack of long-term cortical reorganization after macaque retinal lesions. *Nature* 435 (7040):300–307.

Smith, D., and C. Wright. 2008. Imagery and sport performance. In *Topics in Applied Psychology: Sport and Exercise Psychology*, ed. A. Lane. London: Hodder Education, 139–150.

Smith, D. C., R. N. Holdefer, and T. M. Reeves. 1982. The visual field in monocularly deprived cats and its permanence. *Behavioural Brain Research* 5 (3):245–259.

Smith, E. E., and J. Jonides. 1999. Storage and executive processes in the frontal lobes. *Science* 283 (5408):1657–1661.

Smith, R. S., R. L. Doty, G. K. Burlingame, and D. A. McKeown. 1993. Smell and taste function in the visually impaired. *Perception & Psychophysics* 54 (5):649–655.

Spalek, T. M., and S. Hammad. 2005. The left-to-right bias in inhibition of return is due to the direction of reading. *Psychological Science* 16 (1):15–18.

Sparing, R., F. M. Mottaghy, G. Ganis, W. L. Thompson, R. Töpper, S. M. Kosslyn, and A. Pascual-Leone. 2002. Visual cortex excitability increases during visual mental imagery—a TMS study in healthy human subjects. *Brain Research* 938:92–97.

Spence, C. J., M. E. R. Nicholls, and J. Driver. 2001. The cost of expecting events in the wrong sensory modality. *Perception & Psychophysics* 63:330–336.

Spence, C. J., D. I. Shore, and R. M. Klein. 2001. Multisensory prior entry. *Journal of Experimental Psychology: General* 130 (4):799–832.

Sperling, G. 1960. The information available in brief visual presentations. *Psychological Monographs: General and Applied* 74 (11):1–29.

Starlinger, I., and W. Niemeyer. 1981. Do the blind hear better? Investigations on auditory processing in congenital or early acquired blindness. I. Peripheral functions. *Audiology* 20 (6):503–509.

Starr, F. 1893. Note on color-hearing. *American Journal of Psychology* 5:416–418.

Steeves, J. K., E. G. González, B. L. Gallie, and M. J. Steinbach. 2002. Early unilateral enucleation disrupts motion processing. *Vision Research* 42 (1):143–150.

Steeves, J. K., E. G. González, and M. J. Steinbach. 2008. Vision with one eye: A review of visual function following unilateral enucleation. *Spatial Vision* 21 (6):509–529.

Steeves, J. K., R. Gray, M. J. Steinbach, and D. Regan. 2000. Accuracy of estimating time to collision using only monocular information in unilaterally enucleated observers and monocularly viewing normal controls. *Vision Research* 40 (27):3783–3789.

Steeves, J. K., F. Wilkinson, E. G. González, H. R. Wilson, and M. J. Steinbach. 2004. Global shape discrimination at reduced contrast in enucleated observers. *Vision Research* 44 (9):943–949.

Stein, B. E., M. A. Meredith, and M. T. Wallace. 1993. The visually responsive neuron and beyond: Multisensory integration in cat and monkey. *Progress in Brain Research* 95:79–90.

Steinbach, M. J., I. P. Howard, and H. Ono. 1985. Monocular asymmetries in vision: We don't see eye-to-eye. *Canadian Journal of Psychology* 39 (3):476–478.

Sternberg, R. J. 1980. Representation and process in linear syllogistic reasoning. *Journal of Experimental Psychology. General* 109:119–159.

Sterr, A., L. Green, and T. Elbert. 2003. Blind Braille readers mislocate tactile stimuli. *Biological Psychology* 63 (2):117–127.

Sterr, A., M. Müller, T. Elbert, B. Rockstroh, and E. Taub. 1999. Development of cortical reorganization in the somatosensory cortex of adult Braille students. *Electroencephalography and Clinical Neurophysiology: Supplement* 49:292–298.

Sterr, A., M. M. Muller, T. Elbert, B. Rockstroh, C. Pantev, and E. Taub. 1998a. Perceptual correlates of changes in cortical representation of fingers in blind multifinger Braille readers. *Journal of Neu*roscience 18 (11):4417–4423.

Sterr, A., M. M. Müller, T. Elbert, B. Rockstroh, C. Pantev, and E. Taub. 1998b. Changed perceptions in Braille readers. *Nature* 391 (6663):134–135.

Steven, M. S., and C. Blakemore. 2004. Visual synaesthesia in the blind. *Perception* 33 (7):855–868.

Stevens, A. A., and K. Weaver. 2005. Auditory perceptual consolidation in early-onset blindness. *Neuropsychologia* 43 (13):1901–1910.

Stevens, A. A., and K. E. Weaver. 2009. Functional characteristics of auditory cortex in the blind. *Behavioural Brain Research* 196 (1):134–138.

Stevens, J. C., and K. K. Choo. 1996. Spatial acuity of the body surface over the life span. *Somatosensory & Motor Research* 13 (2):153–166.

Stevens, J. C., E. Foulke, and M. Q. Patterson. 1996. Tactile acuity, aging, and Braille reading in long-term blindness. *Journal of Experimental Psychology: Applied* 2 (2):91–106.

Stevenson, R. J., and T. I. Case. 2005. Olfactory imagery: A review. *Psychonomic Bulletin & Review* 12:244–264.

Stilla, R., G. Deshpande, S. LaConte, X. Hu, and K. Sathian. 2007. Posteromedial parietal cortical activity and inputs predict tactile spatial acuity. *Journal of Neuroscience* 27 (41):11091–11102.

Stilla, R., R. Hanna, X. Hu, E. Mariola, G. Deshpande, and K. Sathian. 2008. Neural processing underlying tactile microspatial discrimination in the blind: A functional magnetic resonance imaging study. *Journal of Vision* 8 (10):1–19.

Stoesz, M. R., M. Zhang, V. D. Weisser, S. C. Prather, H. Mao, and K. Sathian. 2003. Neural networks active during tactile form perception: Common and differential activity during macrospatial and microspatial tasks. *International Journal of Psychophysiology* 50 (1–2):41–49.

Strelow, E. R., and J. A. Brabyn. 1982. Locomotion of the blind controlled by natural sound cues. *Perception* 11 (6):635–640.

Struiksma, M. E., M. L. Noordzij, and A. Postma. 2009. What is the link between language and spatial images? Behavioral and neural findings in blind and sighted individuals. *Acta Psychologica* 132 (2):145–156.

Sukemiya, H., S. Nakamizo, and H. Ono. 2008. Location of the auditory egocentre in the blind and normally sighted. *Perception* 37 (10):1587–1595.

Sunness, J. S., T. Liu, and S. Yantis. 2004. Retinotopic mapping of the visual cortex using functional magnetic resonance imaging in a patient with central scotomas from atrophic macular degeneration. *Ophthalmology* 111 (8):1595–1598.

Sur, M., P. E. Garraghty, and A.W. Roe. 1988. Experimentally induced visual projections into auditory thalamus and cortex. *Science* 242:1437–1441.

Swindale, N. V. 2000. Brain development: Lightning is always seen, thunder always heard. *Current Biology* 10 (15):R569–R571.

Szucs, D., and V. Csepe. 2005. The effect of numerical distance and stimulus probability on ERP components elicited by numerical incongruencies in mental addition. *Brain Research: Cognitive Brain Research* 22 (2):289–300.

Taylor, P. C., A. C. Nobre, and M. F. Rushworth. 2007. FEF TMS affects visual cortical activity. *Cerebral Cortex* 17 (2):391–399.

Théoret, H., L. Merabet, and A. Pascual-Leone. 2004. Behavioral and neuroplastic changes in the blind: Evidence for functionally relevant cross-modal interactions. *Journal of Physiology Paris* 98 (1–3):221–233.

Thinus-Blanc, C., and F. Gaunet. 1997. Representation of space in blind persons: Vision as a spatial sense? *Psychological Bulletin* 121 (1):20–42.

Thompson, W. L., S. M. Kosslyn, M. S. Hoffman, and K. Van der Kooij. 2008. Inspecting visual mental images: Can people "see" implicit properties as easily in imagery and perception? *Memory & Cognition* 36 (5):1024–1032.

Thurrell, R. J., and T. S. Josephson. 1966. Retinoblastoma and intelligence. *Psychosomatics* 7 (6):368–370.

Tinti, C., M. Adenzato, M. Tamietto, and C. Cornoldi. 2006. Visual experience is not necessary for efficient survey spatial cognition: Evidence from blindness. *Quarterly Journal of Experimental Psychology* 59 (7):1306–1328.

Tinti, C., D. Galati, M. G. Vecchio, R. De Beni, and C. Cornoldi. 1999. Interactive auditory and visual images in totally blind persons. *Journal of Visual Impairment & Blindness* 93: 579–583.

Tlauka, M., and F. P. McKenna. 1998. Mental imagery yields stimulus-response compatibility. *Acta Psychologica* 98 (1):67–79.

Tomita, H., M. Ohbayashi, K. Nakahara, I. Hasegawa, and Y. Miyashita. 1999. Top-down signal from prefrontal cortex in executive control of memory retrieval. *Nature* 401 (6754):699–703.

Tootell, R. B., J. D. Mendola, N. K. Hadjikhani, A. K. Liu, and A. M. Dale. 1998. The representation of the ipsilateral visual field in human cerebral cortex. *Proceedings of the National Academy of Sciences of the United States of America* 95 (3):818–824.

Trachtenberg, J. T., and M. P. Stryker. 2001. Rapid anatomical plasticity of horizontal connections in the developing visual cortex. *Journal of Neuroscience* 21 (10):3476–3482.

Trainor, L. J., A. Shahin, and L. E. Roberts. 2003. Effects of musical training on the auditory cortex in children. *Annals of the New York Academy of Sciences* 999:506–513.

Trauzettel-Klosinski, S., M. MacKeben, J. Reinhard, A. Feucht, U. Dürrwächter, and G. Klosinski. 2002. Pictogram naming in dyslexic and normal children assessed by SLO. *Vision Research* 42 (6):789–799.

Trick, L. M., and Z. W. Pylyshyn. 1994. Why are small and large numbers enumerated differently? A limited-capacity preattentive stage in vision. *Psychological Review* 101 (1):80–102.

Trojano, L., D. Grossi, D. E. Linden, E. Formisano, R. Goebel, S. Cirillo, R. Elefante, and F. Di Salle. 2002. Coordinate and categorical judgements in spatial imagery: An fMRI study. *Neuropsychologia* 40 (10):1666–1674.

Trojano, L., D. Grossi, D. E. Linden, E. Formisano, H. Hacker, F. E. Zanella, R. Goebel, and F. Di Salle. 2000. Matching two imagined clocks: The functional anatomy of spatial analysis in the absence of visual stimulation. *Cerebral Cortex* 10 (5):473–481.

Tusa, R. J., M. J. Mustari, A. F. Burrows, and A. F. Fuchs. 2001. Gaze-stabilizing deficits and latent nystagmus in monkeys with brief, early-onset visual deprivation: Eye movement recordings. *Journal of Neurophysiology* 86 (2):651–661.

Tweney, R. D., M. E. Doherty, and C. R. Mynatt, eds. 1981. *On Scientific Thinking*. New York: Columbia University Press.

Tychsen, L., A. M. Wong, and A. Burkhalter. 2004. Paucity of horizontal connections for binocular vision in V1 of naturally strabismic macaques: Cytochrome oxidase compartment specificity. *Journal of Comparative Neurology* 474 (2):261–275.

Uetake, K., and Y. Kudo. 1994. Visual dominance over hearing in feed acquisition procedure of cattle. *Applied Animal Behaviour Science* 42:1–9.

Uhl, F., P. Franzen, G. Lindinger, W. Lang, and L. Deecke. 1991. On the functionality of the visually deprived occipital cortex in early blind persons. *Neuroscience Letters* 124 (2):256–259.

Uhl, F., P. Franzen, I. Podreka, M. Steiner, and L. Deecke. 1993. Increased regional cerebral blood flow in inferior occipital cortex and cerebellum of early blind humans. *Neuroscience Letters* 150 (2):162–164.

Uhl, F., I. Podreka, and L. Deecke. 1994. Anterior frontal cortex and the effect of proactive interference in word pair learning—results of Brain-SPECT. *Neuropsychologia* 32 (2):241–247.

Ungar, S. 2000. Cognitive mapping without visual experience. In *Cognitive Mapping: Past, Present, and Future*, ed. R. F. Kitchin. London: Routledge, 221.

Ungar, S., M. Blades, and C. Spencer. 1994. Can visually impaired children use tactile maps to estimate directions? *Journal of Visual Impairment & Blindness* 88:221–233.

Ungar, S., M. Blades, and C. Spencer. 1995a. Mental rotation of a tactile layout by young visually impaired children. *Perception* 24 (8):891–900.

Ungar, S., M. Blades, and C. Spencer. 1995b. Visually impaired children's strategies for memorising a map. *British Journal of Visual Impairment* 13:27–32.

Ungar, S., M. Blades, and C. Spencer. 1996. The ability of visually impaired children to locate themselves on a tactile map. *Journal of Visual Impairment & Blindness* 90:526–535.

Ungar, S., M. Blades, and C. Spencer. 1997a. Strategies for knowledge acquisition from cartographic maps by blind and visually impaired adults. *Cartographic Journal* 34:93–110.

Ungar, S., M. Blades, and C. Spencer. 1997b. Teaching visually impaired children to make distance judgements from a tactile map. *Journal of Visual Impairment & Blindness* 91:163–174.

Ungerleider, L. G., and M. Mishkin. 1982. Two cortical visual systems. In *Analysis of Visual Behavior*, ed. D. J. Ingle, M. A. Goodale, and R. J. W. Mansfield. Cambridge, MA: MIT Press.

Vallar, G. 2001. Extrapersonal visual unilateral spatial neglect and its neuroanatomy. *NeuroImage* 14 (1):S52–S58.

Valvo, A. 1971. *Sight Restoration after Long-term Blindness: The Problems and Behavior Patterns of Visual Rehabilitation*. New York: American Foundation for the Blind.

Van Boven, R. W., R. H. Hamilton, T. Kauffman, J. P. Keenan, and A. Pascual-Leone. 2000. Tactile spatial resolution in blind Braille readers. *Neurology* 54 (12):2230–2236.

Van der Lubbe, R. H., C. M. Van Mierlo, and A. Postma. 2009. The involvement of occipital cortex in the early blind in auditory and tactile duration discrimination tasks. *Journal of Cognitive Neuroscience* 7:1541–1556.

van Garderen, D. 2006. Spatial visualization, visual imagery, and mathematical problem solving of students with varying abilities. *Journal of Learning Disabilities* 39 (6):496–506.

Van Sluyters, R. C., and F. B. Levitt. 1980. Experimental strabismus in the kitten. *Journal of Neurophysiology* 43 (3):686–699.

Van Velzen, J., A. F. Eardley, B. Forster, and M. Eimer. 2006. Shifts of attention in the early blind: An erp study of attentional control processes in the absence of visual spatial information. *Neuropsychologia* 44 (12):2533–2546.

Vandierendonck, A., V. Dierckx, and G. De Vooght. 2004. Mental model construction in linear reasoning: Evidence for the construction of initial annotated models. *Quarterly Journal of Experimental Psychology. A, Human Experimental Psychology* 57 (8):1369–1391.

Vanlierde, A., A. G. De Volder, M. C. Wanet-Defalque, and C. Veraart. 2003. Occipito-parietal cortex activation during visuo-spatial imagery in early blind humans. *NeuroImage* 19 (3):698–709.

Vanlierde, A., and M. C. Wanet-Defalque. 2004. Abilities and strategies of blind and sighted subjects in visuo-spatial imagery. *Acta Psychologica* 116 (2):205–222.

Vanlierde, A., and M. C. Wanet-Defalque. 2005. The role of visual experience in mental imagery. *Journal of Visual Impairment and Blindness* 99:165–178.

Vecchi, T. 1998. Visuo-spatial imagery in congenitally totally blind people. *Memory* 6 (1):91–102.

Vecchi, T., Z. Cattaneo, M. Monegato, A. Pece, C. Cornoldi, and P. Pietrini. 2006. Why Cyclops could not compete with Ulysses: Monocular vision and mental images. *Neuroreport* 17 (7):723–726.

Vecchi, T., M. L. Monticellai, and C. Cornoldi. 1995. Visuo-spatial working memory: Structures and variables affecting a capacity measure. *Neuropsychologia* 33 (11):1549–1564.

Vecchi, T., C. Tinti, and C. Cornoldi. 2004. Spatial memory and integration processes in congenital blindness. *Neuroreport* 15 (18):2787–2790.

Veraart, C., A. G. De Volder, M. C. Wanet-Defalque, A. Bol, C. Michel, and A. M. Goffinet. 1990. Glucose utilization in human visual cortex is abnormally elevated in blindness of early onset but decreased in blindness of late onset. *Brain Research* 510 (1):115–121.

Vergauwe, E., P. Barrouillet, and V. Camos. 2009. Visual and spatial working memory are not that dissociated after all: A time-based resource-sharing account. *Journal of Experimental Psychology. Learning, Memory, and Cognition* 35 (4):1012–1028.

Verguts, T., and F. Van Opstal. 2005. Dissociation of the distance effect and size effect in one-digit numbers. *Psychonomic Bulletin & Review* 12 (5):925–930.

Volcic, R., and A. M. Kappers. 2008. Allocentric and egocentric reference frames in the processing of three-dimensional haptic space. *Experimental Brain Research* 188 (2):199–213.

Volcic, R., A. M. Kappers, and J. J. Koenderink. 2007. Haptic parallelity perception on the frontoparallel plane: The involvement of reference frames. *Perception & Psychophysics* 69 (2):276–286.

von Melchner, L., S. L. Pallas, and M. Sur. 2000. Visual behaviour mediated by retinal projections directed to the auditory pathway. *Nature* 404 (6780):871–876.

Von Senden, M. 1932. *Space and Sight: The Perception of Space and Shape in the Congentially Blind Before and After Operation.* Reprint, Glencoe, IL: Free Press, 1960.

Voss, P., F. Gougoux, M. Lassonde, R. J. Zatorre, and F. Lepore. 2006. A positron emission tomography study during auditory localization by late-onset blind individuals. *Neuroreport* 17 (4):383–388.

Voss, P., F. Gougoux, R. J. Zatorre, M. Lassonde, and F. Lepore. 2008. Differential occipital responses in early- and late-blind individuals during a sound-source discrimination task. *NeuroImage* 40 (2):746–758.

Voss, P., M. Lassonde, F. Gougoux, M. Fortin, J. P. Guillemot, and F. Lepore. 2004. Early- and late-onset blind individuals show supra-normal auditory abilities in far-space. *Current Biology* 14 (19):1734–1738.

Wade, A. R., A. A. Brewer, J. W. Rieger, and B. A. Wandell. 2002. Functional measurements of human ventral occipital cortex: Retinotopy and colour. *Philosophical Transactions of the Royal Society of London Series B: Biological Sciences* 357 (1424):963–973.

Wagemans, J. 1997. Characteristics and models of human symmetry detection. *Trends in Cognitive Sciences* 1 (9):346–352.

Wakefield, C. E., J. Homewood, and A. J. Taylor. 2004. Cognitive compensations for blindness in children: An investigation using odour naming. *Perception* 33 (4):429–442.

Walker, R., A. W. Young, and N. B. Lincoln. 1996. Eye patching and the rehabilitation of visual neglect. *Neuropsychological Rehabilitation* 6 (3):219–231.

Wallace, M. T., and B. E. Stein. 2000. Onset of cross-modal synthesis in the neonatal superior colliculus is gated by the development of cortical influences. *Journal of Neurophysiology* 83 (6):3578–3582.

Waller, D., and E. Hodgson. 2006. Transient and enduring spatial representations under disorientation and self-rotation. *Journal of Experimental Psychology: Learning, Memory, and Cognition* 32 (4):867–882.

Walsh, V., and A. Cowey. 2000. Transcranial magnetic stimulation and cognitive neuroscience. *Nature Reviews: Neuroscience* 1 (1):73–79.

Walsh, V., and A. Pascual-Leone. 2003. *Transcranial Magnetic Stimulation.* Cambridge, MA: MIT Press.

Wan, C. Y., A. G. Wood, D. C. Reutens, and S. J. Wilson. 2010a. Early but not late-blindness leads to enhanced auditory perception. *Neuropsychologia* 48 (1):344–348.

Wan, C. Y., A. G. Wood, D. C. Reutens, and S. J. Wilson. 2010b. Congenital blindness leads to enhanced vibrotactile perception. *Neuropsychologia* 48 (2):631–635.

Wanet-Defalque, M. C., C. Veraart, A. De Volder, R. Metz, C. Michel, G. Dooms, and A. Goffinet. 1988. High metabolic activity in the visual cortex of early blind human subjects. *Brain Research* 446 (2):369–373.

Warren, D. H., and B. B. Platt. 1974. The subject: A neglected factor in recombination research. *Perception* 3 (4):421–438.

Wason, P., and P. Johnson-Laird. 1972. *Psychology of Reasoning: Structure and Content.* Cambridge, MA: Harvard University Press.

Watson, J. D., R. Myers, R. S. Frackowiak, J. V. Hajnal, R. P. Woods, J. C. Mazziotta, S. Shipp, and S. Zeki. 1993. Area V5 of the human brain: Evidence from a combined study using positron emission tomography and magnetic resonance imaging. *Cerebral Cortex* 3 (2):79–94.

Weaver, K. E., and A. A. Stevens. 2006. Auditory gap detection in the early blind. *Hearing Research* 211 (1–2):1–6.

Weaver, K. E., and A. A. Stevens. 2007. Attention and sensory interactions within the occipital cortex in the early blind: An fMRI study. *Journal of Cognitive Neuroscience* 19 (2):315–330.

Weeks, R., B. Horwitz, A. Aziz-Sultan, B. Tian, C. M. Wessinger, L. G. Cohen, M. Hallett, and J. P. Rauschecker. 2000. A positron emission tomographic study of auditory localization in the congenitally blind. *Journal of Neuroscience* 20 (7):2664–2672.

Weisser, V., R. Stilla, S. Peltier, X. Hu, and K. Sathian. 2005. Short-term visual deprivation alters neural processing of tactile form. *Experimental Brain Research* 166 (3–4):572–582.

Weissman, B. M., A. O. DiScenna, and R. J. Leigh. 1989. Maturation of the vestibulo-ocular reflex in normal infants during the first 2 months of life. *Neurology* 39 (4):534–538.

Welch, R. B., L. D. DuttonHurt, and D. H. Warren. 1986. Contributions of audition and vision to temporal rate perception. *Perception & Psychophysics* 39 (4):294–300.

Welch, R. B., and D. H. Warren. 1980. Immediate perceptual response to intersensory discrepancy. *Psychological Bulletin* 88:638–667.

Wheatley, G. H. 1997. Reasoning with images in mathematical activity. In *Mathematical Reasoning: Analogies, Metaphors, and Images*, ed. L. D. English. Mahwah, NJ: Lawrence Erlbaum.

Wiesel, T. N., and D. H. Hubel. 1963. Single-cell responses in striate cortex of kittens deprived of vision in one eye. *Journal of Neurophysiology* 26:1003–1017.

Wiesel, T. N., and D. H. Hubel. 1965. Extent of recovery from the effects of visual deprivation in kittens. *Journal of Neurophysiology* 28 (6):1060–1072.

Wiggs, C. L., and A. Martin. 1998. Properties and mechanisms of perceptual priming. *Current Opinion in Neurobiology* 8 (2):227–233.

Williams, J. M., H. G. Healy, and N. C. Ellis. 1999. The effect of imageability and predicability of cues in autobiographical memory. *Quarterly Journal of Experimental Psychology A: Human Experimental Psychology* 52 (3):555–579.

Williams, M. 1968. Superior intelligence of children blinded from retinoblastoma. *Archives of Disease in Childhood* 43 (228):204–210.

Withington-Wray, D. J., K. E. Binns, and M. J. Keating. 1990. The developmental emergence of a map of auditory space in the superior colliculus of the guinea pig. *Brain Research: Developmental Brain Research* 51 (2):225–236.

Withington, D. J. 1992. The effect of binocular lid suture on auditory responses in the guinea-pig superior colliculus. *Neuroscience Letters* 136 (2):153–156.

Wittenberg, G. F., K. J. Werhahn, E. M. Wassermann, P. Herscovitch, and L. G. Cohen. 2004. Functional connectivity between somatosensory and visual cortex in early blind humans. *European Journal of Neuroscience* 20 (7):1923–1927.

Wolbers, T., P. Zahorik, and N. A. Giudice. 2010. Decoding the direction of auditory motion in blind humans. *Neuroimage*.

Wolffe, M. 1995. Role of peripheral vision in terms of critical perception—its relevance to the visually impaired. *Ophthalmic & Physiological Optics* 15 (5):471–474.

Woods, A. T., A. Moore, and F. N. Newell. 2008. Canonical views in haptic object perception. *Perception* 37 (12):1867–1878.

Yates, F. A. 1966. *The Art of Memory*. London: Routledge and Kegan Paul.

Yates, J. T., R. M. Johnson, and W. J. Starz. 1972. Loudness perception of the blind. *Audiology* 11 (5–6):368–376.

Yi, D. J., N. B. Turk-Browne, M. M. Chun, and M. K. Johnson. 2008. When a thought equals a look: Refreshing enhances perceptual memory. *Journal of Cognitive Neuroscience* 20 (8):1371–1380.

Yoo, S. S., D. K. Freeman, J. J. McCarthy III, and F. A. Jolesz. 2003. Neural substrates of tactile imagery: A functional MRI study. *Neuroreport* 14 (4):581–585.

Yoo, S. S., C. U. Lee, and B. G. Choi. 2001. Human brain mapping of auditory imagery: Event-related functional MRI study. *Neuroreport* 12 (14):3045–3049.

Young, M. P. 2000. The architecture of visual cortex and inferential processes in vision. *Spatial Vision* 13 (2–3):137–146.

Zacks, J. M. 2008. Neuroimaging studies of mental rotation: A meta-analysis and review. *Journal of Cognitive Neuroscience* 20 (1):1–19.

Zangaladze, A., C. M. Epstein, S. T. Grafton, and K. Sathian. 1999. Involvement of visual cortex in tactile discrimination of orientation. *Nature* 401 (6753):587–590.

Zatorre, R. J., P. Belin, and V. B. Penhune. 2002. Structure and function of auditory cortex: Music and speech. *Trends in Cognitive Sciences* 6 (1):37–46.

Zeki, S. 1993. *A Vision of the Brain*. Oxford: Blackwell.

Zeki, S. 2008. The disunity of consciousness. *Progress in Brain Research* 168:11–18.

Zeki, S., J. D. Watson, C. J. Lueck, K. J. Friston, C. Kennard, and R. S. Frackowiak. 1991. A direct demonstration of functional specialization in human visual cortex. *Journal of Neuroscience* 11 (3):641–649.

Zimler, J., and J. M. Keenan. 1983. Imagery in the congenitally blind: How visual are visual images? *Journal of Experimental Psychology: Learning, Memory, and Cognition* 9 (2):269–282.

Zimmer, H. D. 2008. Visual and spatial working memory: From boxes to networks. *Neuroscience and Biobehavioral Reviews* 32 (8):1373–1395.

Zimmer, U., J. Lewald, M. Erb, W. Grodd, and H. O. Karnath. 2004. Is there a role of visual cortex in spatial hearing? *European Journal of Neuroscience* 20 (11):3148–3156.

Zimmermann-Schlatter, A., C. Schuster, M. A. Puhan, E. Siekierka, and J. Steurer. 2008. Efficacy of motor imagery in post-stroke rehabilitation: A systematic review. *Journal of Neuroengineering and Rehabilitation* 5:8.

Zuidhoek, S., A. M. Kappers, R. H. van der Lubbe, and A. Postma. 2003. Delay improves performance on a haptic spatial matching task. *Experimental Brain Research* 149 (3):320–330.

Zuidhoek, S., A. Visser, M. E. Bredero, and A. Postma. 2004. Multisensory integration mechanisms in haptic space perception. *Experimental Brain Research* 157 (2):265–268.

Zwaan, R. A., and G. A. Radvansky. 1998. Situation models in language comprehension and memory. *Psychological Bulletin* 123 (2):162–185.

Zwiers, M. P., A. J. Van Opstal, and J. R. Cruysberg. 2001a. Two-dimensional sound-localization behavior of early-blind humans. *Experimental Brain Research* 140 (2):206–222.

Zwiers, M. P., A. J. Van Opstal, and J. R. Cruysberg. 2001b. A spatial hearing deficit in early-blind humans. *Journal of Neuroscience* 21 (9): RC142: 1–5.

Index

Allocentric, 7, 115–121, 127, 132
 and blindness onset, 167–168
Amblyopia, 9, 148, 150, 153
Amodal. *See* Supramodal
Auditory attention, 24–28
 and ERPs, 25
 and eye movements, 25
 selective and divided, 25–28
Auditory egocenter, 21–24
 and blindness onset, 163
Auditory memory, 26–27
Auditory sensory compensation, 15–29
 and blindness onset, 162
 ERPs, 17
 for intensity discrimination, 15–16
 for sound localization, 17–21
 for temporal resolution, 16–17
Autobiographical memory, 164–165

Braille, 33–43, 82, 108, 125
 and hemispheric asymmetry, 194
 and somatosensory cortex, 37, 174–176
 and synesthesia, 165
 and tactile acuity, 33–34, 38–39
 and visual cortex recruitment, 170–172, 177–179, 182–183, 192–193

Chess (blindfold), 57–58
Ciclopean eye. *See* Visual egocenter
Colavita effect, 4. *See also* Visual dominance
Color
 and blindness, 86
 color blindness, 9
 knowledge, 96, 111
 and synesthesia, 165
 V4, 65–66
 and visual imagery, 78
Contrast sensitivity, 9, 148–149, 152
Cortical plasticity, 173–200
 in auditory cortex, 174–175
 and blindness onset, 170–172
 and Braille reading, 175–176, 182–183
 critical period, 147–149, 155, 163
 crossmodal, 170–172, 173–174, 176–196
 intramodal, 36, 170–171, 173–176, 181, 194–196
 and language, 192–194
 in low vision, 140, 146–147
 maladaptive, 176
 and memory, 192–193
 modality-specific, 185–188
 in monocular vision, 152–153
 in multisensory areas, 182
 and musical training, 174, 176, 180
 in somatosensory cortex, 175–176
 structural changes, 196–198
 and synesthesia, 165
 task-dependent, 185–187
 and TMS, 177–179
 underlying mechanisms, 194–196

Dichotic listening, 17, 25, 28, 193
Dorsal stream, 55, 66, 106, 180, 183–184
Dreams, 79–80, 87, 165
Dual coding theory, 57, 79

Early blind. *See* Onset
Egocentric, 115–116, 120–121, 127, 132
Enucleation (monocular), 148–150
Extrapersonal space. *See* Locomotor space
Eye movements, 25

Far space. *See* Locomotor space

Grating orientation task, 33–34, 37, 41, 140–141, 163, 188

Haptic test battery, 31–33
Hearing, 12–15
Hippocampus, 198

Imagery, 49–73
 and creativity, 61
 definition, 49–50
 general and specific images, 64, 72–73
 imagery debate, 51–54, 75–76
 learning and memory, 56
 and long-term memory, 62–64
 mnemonics, 56–58,
 neural basis, 67–73
 and numerical cognition, 60–61
 parallelism with perception, 69–72
 and primary visual cortex, 63, 68–69, 188
 and reasoning, 58–60
 visual vs. spatial, 59, 72–73
 and working memory, 55–56
Imagery in the blind, 75–87
 and creativity, 93
 and drawing, 83, 86
 dreams, 79–80
 and memory, 77–79
 neural basis, 96–98
 perspective, 83–87
 picture recognition, 82–83
 and reasoning, 93–95
 vantage point, 84
 visual vs. spatial, 95–96
Individual differences, 131–134
 and blindness onset, 169

Language, 26–27, 57, 75, 110–111, 134
 lateralization, 193–194
 and occipital cortex, 178, 187, 192–193
 and spatial images, 104–105
Late blind. *See* Onset
Lateralization
 Braille, 194
 language, 193–194
 spatial processing, 194
Line bisection, 109–110, 151
Loci, method of, 56–57
Locomotor space, 47, 81, 126–131, 167
Long-term memory, 26, 31, 55–56, 61–64, 76, 118, 193
Low vision, 137–147
 sensory compensation, 138–141

Mathematics, 60–61
Matrix task, 88–91, 93, 95
 in low vision, 142, 145–146
 in monocular vision, 151–152
Mental images. *See* Imagery
Mental rotation, 52, 59, 76, 80–82, 87, 96, 131
 and blindness onset, 167
 haptic, 92, 125
 neural basis, 72
Mental scanning, 52, 63, 76, 80–82
 and blindness onset, 167
 in low vision, 144
Mirror neurons, 198–201
Molyneaux question, 98–102
Monocular vision, 147–153
Multimodal. *See* Supramodal

Multisensory interaction, 45–48, 114, 163
audiotactile spatial interaction, 48
auditory-tactile illusions, 46
and ERPs, 46
Myopia, 138–141

Navigation, 114–115, 126, 128–131, 133, 135
and blindness onset, 168–169
and echo processing, 17
and hearing, 129
mental navigation, 105
navigational devices, 134
vestibular, 129–131
Near space. *See* Peripersonal space
Nociceptive sensitivity, 42
Numerical cognition, 60–61, 106–110
Braille reading, 108
ERPs, 110

Occipital cortex. *See* Visual cortex
Olfactory, 43–45
Onset (of visual impairment or blindness), 133, 143–148, 155–172
Orientation and mobility (O&M), 133–135

Parallel setting task, 117–121, 132, 167
Path integration. *See* Navigation
Perceptual consolidation (auditory), 28–29
Peripersonal space, 46–47, 81, 116–125, 166
Perky's experiment, 50–51
Perspective, 83–84, 99–100, 102, 161
and blindness onset, 166
and drawing, 84, 86
perspective taking task, 85, 117, 121–125, 166
Phosphenes, 67, 97–98, 171, 189, 191
Picture recognition, 82–83
and blindness onset, 166
in low vision, 143
Pitch
absolute pitch, 13, 15, 181
discrimination, 13–16, 162, 181
and synesthesia, 134
Plasticity. *See* Cortical plasticity
Pointing task, 21–23, 84, 167
in near space, 117–120
Prakash project, 100
Primary visual cortex (V1), 63, 65–66, 68–69, 195
and blindness onset, 170
and Braille reading, 170, 172, 177–178
and memory, 192–193
in monocular vision, 147, 152–153
and phonological and semantic processing, 170–171, 192
and speech perception, 181
and verb generation, 182
Pseudoneglect, 109–110

Rehabilitation, 133–135
Restored vision, 98–102. *See also* Prakash project; Molyneaux question
Rotation. *See* Mental rotation
Route representation, 126–128, 130
and blindness onset, 168–169

Scanning. *See* Mental scanning
Self-positioning ability, 26, 163
Semantic knowledge, 110–112, 169
Sensory compensation, 11–48
and blindness onset, 162–164
in low vision, 138–141
Sensory substitution devices (SSD), 134–135, 189–192
SNARC effect, 61, 106, 108
Social cognition, 198–201
Sound
frequency, 12–13
intensity, 13, 15–16
sound processing and crossmodal plasticity, 180–181
spectrum, 13
temporal order, 14–15

Sound localization, 13, 17–21, 129
and blindness onset, 162–163
central vs. peripheral space, 20
echo, 14, 17, 27, 139, 163
and ERPs, 20
in low vision, 138–141
monaural and binaural cues, 14, 19–20, 171, 180–181
vertical vs. horizontal, 20–21
and visual cortex, 180–182, 188–189
Spatial cognition, 113–134
and blindness onset, 167–169
body-centred representations, 167
definition, 113–114
in low vision, 144
object memory/relocation, 121–124, 132, 168
reference frames, 46–47, 115–117, 126–127, 132
spatial inferences, 116, 142–143
spatial updating, 116, 122
Speech perception, 16–17
Strabismus, 147–150
Strategy (mental), 91–93, 125, 131
and blindness onset, 166–167
Supramodal, 102–106, 153, 183, 201
and occipital cortex, 187
Survey representation, 126–129
and blindness onset, 168–169
Symmetry, 33, 90–91
Synesthesia, 165

Tactile acuity, 30–31, 33
and blindness onset, 163–164
in low vision, 140–141
Tactile attention, 41–43
and ERPs, 42
selective and divided, 42
Tactile map, 80, 127, 146
Tactile pressure sensitivity, 31
Tactile sensory compensation, 31–43
passive vs. active, 39–40
for spatial discrimination, 33–38
for temporal perception, 32–33
Taste, 43–45
Texture, 29, 76, 100–101
texture discrimination task, 30, 33–34, 40–41, 163–164
Theory of mind, 198
Three-dimensionality (3D), 83–84, 88, 93, 117, 143, 166
Touch, 29–43
passive vs. active, 39–40
receptors, 29–30, 33–36
and visual cortex, 179

Ventral stream, 55, 66, 106, 183–185
Ventriloquist effect, 5, 14, 114. *See also* Visual dominance
Verbal memory, 26–27, 55, 94, 169, 192
Visual acuity, 8–9, 99–100, 133, 137, 139, 142, 145, 146, 187
in monocular vision, 148, 152
Visual buffer, 64, 69
Visual cortex, 65–67, 97–98, 141, 188. *See also* Primary visual cortex
and language, 192–193
and memory, 192–193
MT/V5, 66, 68, 100, 185, 188, 195
and tactile processing, 187
structural changes, 197
Visual deprivation (short-term), 179–180
Visual dominance, 4–5
Visual egocenter, 21–24, 163
in monocular vision, 150
Visual field, 8–9, 133, 144, 146, 149
peripheral vs. central, 19–20, 68, 137, 140
Visual impairment, 8–9
estimates, 8–10
forms of, 8–9, 137–138
Visual impedance effect, 94
Visual prostheses, 189–192
Visuo-spatial working memory (VSWM), 55–56, 64, 87–93
in low vision, 142
passive vs. active, 87, 131
simultaneous vs. sequential, 88–90, 96, 152–153

Vividness, 63–64, 67, 78
V1. *See* Primary visual cortex

Wayfinding. *See* Navigation
Weber's law, 108
What pathway. *See* Ventral stream
Where pathway. *See* Dorsal stream
Working memory (WM), 55–56, 77, 87, 132, 141

www.ingramcontent.com/pod-product-compliance
Lightning Source LLC
Chambersburg PA
CBHW041427270326
41932CB00027B/3408

* 9 7 8 0 2 6 2 5 4 9 8 8 2 *